Controversies in Critical Care

Jose Chacko • Swapnil Pawar • Ian Seppelt
Gagan Brar

Controversies in Critical Care

Springer

Jose Chacko
Department of Critical Care Medicine
Narayana Health
Bangalore, Karnataka, India

Swapnil Pawar
Intensive Care
St George Hospital
Sydney, NSW, Australia

Ian Seppelt
Intensive Care Medicine
Nepean Hospital
Sydney, NSW, Australia

Gagan Brar
Critical Care Medicine
Aster RV Hospital
Bangalore, Karnataka, India

ISBN 978-981-19-9939-0 ISBN 978-981-19-9940-6 (eBook)
https://doi.org/10.1007/978-981-19-9940-6

This Springer imprint is published by the registered company Springer Nature Singapore Pte Ltd.
The registered company address is: 152 Beach Road, #21-01/04 Gateway East, Singapore 189721, Singapore

Foreword

The authors of the first edition of *Controversies in Critical Care* are to be commended on an incredibly valuable contribution to the Australasian critical care literature. Intensive Care Medicine is a young specialty and has undergone significant development since the establishment of our specialty 70 years ago. The origin of the specialty can be traced to the tragic Copenhagen polio epidemic of 1952. This epidemic witnessed the initiation of positive pressure ventilation delivered by hand to hundreds of patients afflicted by respiratory and bulbar failure. It also generated the impetus to collocate critically ill patients, who could be cared for by a group of health professionals with the requisite interest, equipment, knowledge, and skill set. The subsequent seven decades have witnessed enormous progress: technological advances, new therapies for old diseases, old therapies for new diseases, and an enhanced understanding of the pathogenesis underlying a diverse range of conditions. In the last three years Intensive Care Medicine has received substantial public attention, predominantly related to potentially limited capacity and resources. It did, however, illustrate how rapidly critical care providers need to assimilate new knowledge.

The responsibility of providing clinical care to a heterogeneous population, unified only by the severity of their disease, is unique in medical practice. This incredible clinical diversity is precisely what attracts many to the specialty. However, it also provides an enormous challenge to the delivery of quality care. Quality research remains the key to resolving the controversies that may surround a particular aspect of care; however, the relatively small number of critical care patients and their heterogeneity can make studying this patient group difficult. Despite these obstacles, the volume of acute care literature generated on a weekly basis presents the practitioner with a daunting task of staying current. *Controversies in Critical Care* covers a wide range of contemporaneous and highly relevant critical care topics in an easy to access and digestible format. The topics covered range from the important basics of critical care including ventilation strategies and weaning, while also exploring more esoteric, yet important considerations, such as vitamin C use in the ICU. Every chapter provides a succinct review of the current literature, in a balanced and informative way.

The authors of this textbook have made a significant contribution to critical care, and I suspect this book will adorn many bookshelves, regardless of the individual's stage of career.

University of Queensland
Herston, QLD, Australia

Royal Brisbane & Women's Hospital
Brisbane, QLD, Australia

Australian and New Zealand Intensive Care Society
Melbourne, VIC, Australia

Anthony Holley

Preface

We are just about finding our feet after a global pandemic, often fraught with controversies. The specialty of critical care medicine played a pivotal role during the Covid-19 pandemic, with an unprecedented number of patients requiring respiratory support. The pandemic era has firmly entrenched critical care medicine as a crucial area of specialization during a crisis.

Although relatively young, our specialty has experienced its fair share of controversies. When Vivi Ebert, a 12-year-old girl, presented to the Blegdam Hospital, Copenhagen, in August 1952 with respiratory failure due to poliomyelitis, Bjorn Ibsen chose to perform a tracheostomy to apply positive pressure ventilation. Ibsen ushered in the era of modern intensive care; however, many of his colleagues did not see eye to eye with him. It is pertinent that we continue to face similar controversies with tracheostomy even today, particularly regarding the timing.

Medical science has evolved over the years; unlike in the past, we seek evidence before we embark upon any novel therapeutic intervention. Randomized controlled trials, although by no means perfect, are least prone to bias, and occupy the apex of the pyramid of evidence.

Several landmark papers have addressed ongoing controversies in critical care medicine. There have been practice-changing clinical trials, such as the ARDSNet trial that ushered in the epoch of lung-protective ventilation. On the contrary, other studies have failed to confirm the putative benefits of interventions that seemed to have a strong physiological rationale, like intensive glycemic control in critical illness. Besides, evidence keeps changing with time, given the dynamic nature of science. Many interventions remain steeped in controversy due to conflicting results from controlled clinical trials.

In this book, we have undertaken an evidence-based review of contentious topics in critical care medicine, highlighting landmark papers. Each topic addresses the putative mechanisms behind possible benefits of therapies, the relative advantages and disadvantages, and finally, how it fares when it boils down to real-world clinical practice. We have tried to include most of the controversies of contemporaneous interest, but this is by no means a comprehensive list. It has been an enlightening experience to work through the evidence. We hope our readers, including practitioners and trainees in critical care medicine, find it equally interesting and thought-provoking.

Bangalore, Karnataka, India — Jose Chacko
Sydney, NSW, Australia — Swapnil Pawar
Kingswood, NSW, Australia — Ian Seppelt
Bangalore, Karnataka, India — Gagan Brar

Contents

Part II Shock and Circulatory Support

Part VIII Organizational Challenges in the ICU

Part IX Coagulopathy and Transfusion

About the Authors

Jose Chacko MD, DA, DNB, EDIC, FICCM, MBA, graduated in medicine and completed postgraduation in anesthesia from Medical College, Trivandrum, India. He underwent advanced training in critical care medicine from leading hospitals in Australia and worked as a consultant in anesthesia and critical care with the National Health Services in the United Kingdom. He has completed the European Diploma in Intensive Care (EDIC) from the European Society of Intensive Care Medicine (ESICM) and currently works as a senior consultant in critical care medicine at Narayana Health, Bangalore, India. A renowned teacher and academician, he is a leading practitioner and teacher of critical care medicine in India. He has many publications in peer-reviewed journals and contributed to textbooks in critical care and emergency medicine. He contributes regularly to academic meetings in critical care medicine. Dr. Chacko runs a blog site (criticalcareblogspot.com) and cohosts podcasts (critcareedu.com.au) that address provocative topics in critical care medicine.

Swapnil Pawar MD, FCICM, EDIC, CHSE, completed his post-graduation in Anaesthesia in 2010 from the Post Graduate Institute of Medical Education and Research (PGIMER), Chandigarh, India. He is a fellow of the College of Intensive Care Medicine (FCICM), Australia and New Zealand, and has also completed his European Diploma in Intensive Care (EDIC) with the European Society of Intensive Care Medicine (ESICM).

He is a staff specialist in Intensive care medicine at St George Hospital and associate professor of Critical Care medicine at University of New South Wales (UNSW). He is the past chair of the of the Australia and New Zealand Intensive Care Society (ANZICS) education committee. He has a keen interest in simulation and medical education and is a certified simulation healthcare educator (CHSE) with the Society of Simulation in Healthcare (SSH). He is the recipient of prestigious Ramesh Nagappan Award 2023, given by ANZICS in recognition of contribution to the field of medical education in Intensive care. He is the host and producer of six educational podcast series and runs his educational website Critical Care Education (www.critcareedu.com.au). He is currently pursuing his Ph.D. in the field of cognitive load theory and has delivered numerous oral and poster presentations at international meetings. He is a trained Negotiator and enjoys grooming young talent as a captain of St George district cricket club metro team.

Ian Seppelt FANZCA, FCICM, graduated in medicine from the University of Sydney, Australia. He is a senior specialist in intensive care medicine at Nepean Hospital, University of Sydney, professor of anesthesia at Macquarie University, and professorial fellow at The George Institute for Global Health, Sydney. He has more than 100 peer-reviewed international publications and has delivered numerous invited presentations at international meetings. He is a past executive member of the ANZICS Clinical Trials Group and lead investigator for SuDDICU (Australia) for which he received a National Health and Medical Research Council Research Excellence Award in 2015. He is on the management committees for several clinical trials including SuDDICU, SPICE-IV, and REMAP-CAP. He chairs the Nepean Blue Mountains Local Health District Human Research Ethics Committee (HREC) and is a member of various data safety monitoring boards. He is a medical advisor to Equestrian Australia and assistant groom and transport technician for his wife and children when they are competing.

Gagan Brar MD, DNB, EDIC, IDCCM, graduated in medicine and completed postgraduation in anesthesia from Kasturba Medical College, Manipal, India. She underwent training in critical care medicine at Manipal Hospital and Fortis Hospital, Bangalore, India. She is a fellow of the National Board of Examinations in critical care medicine and has completed the European Diploma in Intensive Care (EDIC) with the European Society of Intensive Care Medicine (ESICM). She currently works as a consultant in critical care medicine, Aster RV Hospital, Bangalore. Dr. Brar has published several original papers in peer-reviewed journals and is an invited speaker for major academic meetings in critical care medicine.

Part I

Respiratory Support in the Critically Ill

Oxygenation Targets in the ICU: Conservative or Liberal?

1

1.1 Introduction

Our planet was born approximately 4.8 billion years ago. The earth's atmosphere contained no oxygen in the early stages of its origin. Cyanobacteria, among the earliest forms of life on earth, generated oxygen by photosynthesis leading to a rise in atmospheric oxygen, followed by the evolution of complex living beings, roughly a billion years after the birth of our planet [1]. Several billion years later, in 1774, Joseph Priestly identified oxygen as the gas that sustained life on earth [2]. More than a century later, in 1885, George Holtzapple reported on the administration of supplemental oxygen for the treatment of pneumonia [3]. Lorraine Smith first reported on the acute toxic effects of oxygen in experimental mice. He noted that the toxic effects of oxygen progressively increased at higher oxygen levels in the blood [4].

1.2 What Is Hyperoxia?

Hyperoxia implies exposure to higher than normal levels of partial pressure of oxygen at the cellular and tissue levels [5]. Conventionally, a liberal approach to oxygen therapy is often favored by many clinicians as a preventive measure against inadvertent hypoxemia [6]. Compounding the problem is the inability of continuous pulse oximetry to identify hyperoxia. In an observational cohort study from a mixed medical-surgical ICU, during the first week of mechanical ventilation, the mean time-weighted PaO_2 was 144 mmHg; besides, the PaO_2 was >80 mmHg during 80% of the total duration of mechanical ventilation [7]. Hyperoxia has been variably defined [8]; a PaO_2 of 100–125 mmHg is considered to represent mild hyperoxia, while levels higher than 200 mmHg represent severe hyperoxia [9].

J. Chacko et al., *Controversies in Critical Care*,
https://doi.org/10.1007/978-981-19-9940-6_1

1.3 What Are the Physiological Consequences of Hyperoxia?

Lorraine Smith first reported on the potential for harm from excessive oxygen administration and described acute lung changes related to hyperoxia in experimental mice [4]. The oxygen molecule possesses the unique property of being an "electron acceptor." The newly accepted electrons, however, remain unpaired and are called oxygen free radicals. The oxygen free radicals that are involved in biological reactions represent the reactive oxygen species (ROS) [10]. ROS play an important physiological role in the eradication of mutated or damaged cells. This process is called apoptosis and enables the generation of new cells that replace mutated or damaged cells. Hyperoxia may result in an increase in the ROS levels. Normally, antioxidants, including superoxide dismutase, catalase, and vitamins C and E scavenge excessive ROS. However, in the face of hyperoxia, the antioxidant mechanisms are rapidly overwhelmed, leading to the destruction of normal cells by excessive ROS, resulting in harmful effects in different organs [11] (Fig. 1.1). The clinical effects of hyperoxia are summarized in Table 1.1.

1.3.1 Lungs

Loss of ciliary activity, leading to tracheobronchitis is one of the early toxic manifestations of hyperoxia in the lung, characterized by substernal distress, cough, and

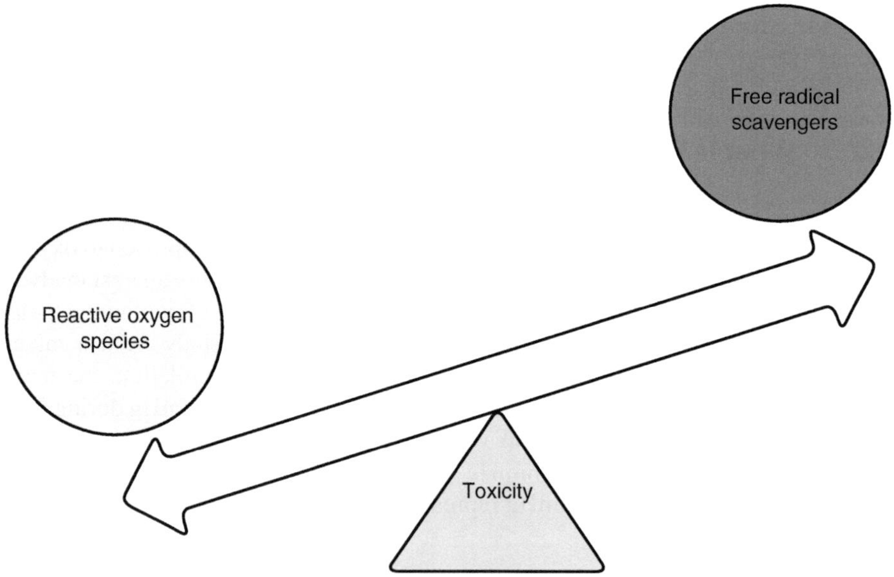

Fig. 1.1 ROS plays a physiological role in the eradication of mutated or damaged cells by apoptosis. Excess ROS is scavenged by antioxidants. In hyperoxia the ROS levels rise too high, and the antioxidant mechanisms are rapidly overwhelmed. Destruction of normal cells follows

Table 1.1 Clinical effects of excessive oxygen

Respiratory system	Blood flow	Control of breathing
• Loss of ciliary activity • Substernal distress, cough, and breathlessness • Tracheobronchitis • Absorption collapse • Prolonged high levels: ARDS-like changes	• Inhibits nitric oxide • Vasoconstriction and impaired blood flow to vital organs. Myocardial ischemia may occur	• Hypercapnia in patients with COPD • Oxygen administration leads to inhibition of the hypoxic vasoconstrictor response

breathlessness. Nitrogen, being less absorbable, exerts a "splinting" effect on the alveoli, keeping them open. As oxygen is absorbed much more rapidly than nitrogen from the alveoli, alveolar collapse occurs [12]. High FiO_2 levels lead to pathophysiological changes in the lung that are similar to the changes that occur in acute respiratory distress syndrome (ARDS). The findings on chest radiography and CT images are often indistinguishable from the radiological changes observed in ARDS (Table 1.1).

1.3.2 Vasoconstrictor Effect

Oxygen inhibits nitric oxide, a naturally occurring vasodilator. Nitric oxide inhibition leads to a vasoconstrictor effect at high levels of oxygen, leading to compromised blood flow to the vital organs [13]. Coronary vasoconstriction may ensue, leading to acute myocardial ischemia [14].

1.3.3 Control of Breathing

The administration of high FiO_2 often leads to the development of hypercapnia, particularly evident in patients with acute exacerbation of chronic obstructive pulmonary disease (COPD). Conventionally, the hypercapnic response has been attributed to the inhibition of hypoxia-induced respiratory drive [15]. High FiO_2 levels may lead to an initial decrease in minute ventilation and a rise in $PaCO_2$ levels. However, with continued oxygen therapy at the same FiO_2 level for longer than 15 min, the initial decrease in minute ventilation is attenuated to a large extent [16]. Oxygen-induced abolition of the hypoxic pulmonary vasoconstrictor mechanism is a more likely explanation for the development of hypercapnia. High FiO_2 levels lead to vasodilatation in the hypoxic regions of the lung, with the diversion of blood flow toward less ventilated regions, resulting in intrapulmonary shunting and hypercapnia [17, 18]. Besides, as FiO_2 levels rise, the oxygen saturation of hemoglobin increases. The rise in oxygen saturation leads to unloading of carbon dioxide from the hemoglobin in the lung by the reverse Haldane effect. However, if ventilation remains low, as may often occur in patients with COPD, carbon dioxide elimination is impaired, leading to hypercapnia.

1.4 What Does Clinical Evidence Suggest in Real-World Practice?

The clinical effects oxygen administration targeting different levels of PaO_2 or oxygen saturation have been the focus of several studies (Table 1.2).

1.4.1 Supplemental Oxygen in ST-Elevation Myocardial Infarction (STEMI): The AVOID Trial

Supplemental oxygen is administered to most patients with acute myocardial infarction. This therapeutic intervention is based on the premise that supplemental oxygen would improve oxygen delivery and reduce injury to the ischemic myocardium [19]. However, does supplemental oxygen in normoxic patients with ST-elevation myocardial infarction (STEMI) improve clinical outcomes?

The AVOID study was a multicentric, unblinded randomized controlled trial (RCT) conducted by the ambulance service in Melbourne, Australia [20]. The study included patients with STEMI and a baseline oxygen saturation of >94%. Supplemental oxygen at 8 L/min through a face mask was administered in the intervention group; the control group did not receive supplemental oxygen. Aspirin, 300 mg orally, was administered by paramedics to all patients. Continued antiplatelet therapy, the choice of anticoagulation, and percutaneous intervention were based on local protocols. Supplemental oxygen was not associated with beneficial effects in this study among patients with STEMI. In contrast, among patients who received supplemental oxygen, an increase in the infarct size was noted at 6 months on magnetic resonance imaging. Besides, a higher incidence of recurrent myocardial infarction and arrhythmias was also noted with oxygen administration.

1.4.2 The Oxygen-ICU Study

Several recently published RCTs have evaluated the effect of oxygen levels on mechanically ventilated patients in the ICU. The OXYGEN-ICU study, a single-center RCT, evaluated the impact of oxygen therapy in a medical-surgical ICU in Italy. The study included patients who were expected to have a duration of ICU stay of longer than 72 h. In the restrictive arm, the target PaO_2 level was set between 70 and 100 mmHg with saturation levels between 94 and 98%. In the liberal (conventional) arm, standard care was followed. In the latter group, maximum PaO_2 levels of up to 150 mmHg and saturation levels between 97 and 100% were allowed. There was a clear separation in the average, daily time-weighted PaO_2 levels between the liberal and conservative groups (102 mmHg, IQR: 88–116 vs. 87 mmHg, IQR: 79–97). This study revealed a significantly higher ICU mortality with liberal oxygen therapy (20.2% vs. 11.6%, $p = 0.01$). Furthermore, the incidence of new-onset shock, liver failure, and bacteremia was lower with conservative oxygen therapy [21].

Table 1.2 Main studies that have evaluated liberal vs. conservative oxygenation targets in critically ill patients

Study/year	Population	Liberal	Restrictive	Outcomes
AVOID (2012) [20]	Patients with STEMI and $SaO_2 > 94\%$	Oxygen 8 L/min by face mask	No supplemental oxygen	Supplemental oxygen associated with higher incidence of recurrent MI, arrhythmias, increase in infarct size at 6 months
Oxygen-ICU (2016) [21]	Medical-surgical ICU patients	PaO_2 up to 150 mmHg SaO_2: 94–100%	PaO_2: 70–100 mmHg SaO_2: 94–98%	Higher ICU mortality with liberal oxygen therapy. Less new-onset shock, liver failure, bacteremia with restrictive oxygen
ICU-ROX (2020) [22]	Mechanically ventilated patients	SaO_2: 91–100%	SaO_2: 91–96% FiO_2 reduced to 0.21 if SaO_2 maintained	No difference in ventilator-free days on day 28. No difference in the 90- and 180-day mortality. Possible harm in patients with HIE. Trend toward improved outcomes with liberal oxygen in patients with other types of brain injury
HYPER2S (2017) [24]	Patients in septic shock and mechanically ventilated	FiO_2 1.0 for the first 24 h of mechanical ventilation	SaO_2: 88–95%	Higher 28-day mortality, atelectasis, ICU-acquired weakness with liberal oxygen. Significantly higher adverse events with liberal oxygen
LOCO2 (2020) [25]	ARDS, mechanically ventilated patients	PaO_2: 90–105 mmHg SaO_2: 96% or higher	PaO_2: 55–70 mmHg SaO_2: 88–92%	28-day mortality not different 90-day mortality higher with restrictive oxygen Mesenteric ischemia noted in restrictive arm (5% vs. 0%)
HOT-ICU (2021) [27]	Acute hypoxic respiratory failure	PaO_2: 90 mmHg	PaO_2: 60 mmHg	90-day mortality not different No difference in days alive without life support No difference days alive after discharge
PILOT (2022) [28]	Mechanically ventilated patients in the emergency department and the ICU. Three-arm trial of low, intermediate, and high SaO_2 targets	Low SaO_2: 88–92%	Intermediate: 92–96%, and high: 96–100%	Duration of ventilator support, 28-d survival similar between groups
BOX (2022) [29]	Comatose survivors of out-of-hospital cardiac arrest	PaO_2: 68–75	PaO_2: 98–105 mm Hg	No difference in death or severe disability at 90 days

STEMI ST-segment elevation myocardial infarction, *MI* myocardial infarction, *HIE* hypoxic-ischemic encephalopathy, *ARDS* acute respiratory distress syndrome

1.4.3 The ICU-ROX Study

The Australian and New Zealand Intensive Care Society-Clinical Trials Group (ANZICS-CTG) conducted a multicentric study on mechanically ventilated patients expected to require ventilator support beyond the day of recruitment [22]. The ICU-ROX study randomized patients to a restrictive arm, with oxygen saturation maintained between 91 and 96%. If the oxygen saturation exceeded this range, the FiO_2 levels were turned down to the target level. The FiO_2 level was reduced to 0.21 if the target saturation level was met. In the liberal arm (usual care), no specific interventions were carried out to limit FiO_2 levels, with the maintenance of saturation levels between 91 and 100%. No significant difference was noted between the two groups in the number of ventilator-free days at day 28 (conservative vs. liberal: 21.3 days vs. 22.1 days). Besides, the 90- and 180-day mortality was also not significantly different between groups. On subgroup analysis, possible harmful effects were noted with liberal oxygen therapy in patients with hypoxic-ischemic encephalopathy (HIE). Patients with HIE who received liberal oxygen therapy had fewer ventilator-free days, higher 180-day mortality, and a higher incidence of adverse outcomes on the Glasgow Outcome Scale at 180 days. In patients with other types of brain injury, liberal oxygen therapy was found to be associated with improved outcomes on post hoc analysis. A post hoc analysis of septic patients revealed a trend toward improved 90-day survival with liberal oxygen therapy [23]. However, these findings are hypothesis-generating and need evaluation in future controlled studies.

1.4.4 The HYPERS2S Study

A multicentric French study compared two levels of oxygen therapy in patients with septic shock who underwent mechanical ventilation. In the liberal group, the FiO_2 was maintained at 1.0 for the initial 24 h of ventilation. In the restrictive group, the oxygen saturation was maintained between 88–95%. The study was stopped prematurely as concerns arose regarding the safety of the administration of 100% oxygen. At the time of cessation of the study, the 28-day mortality was higher in patients who received 100% oxygen. A significant increase in the overall incidence of serious adverse events was also noted with 100% oxygen administration. The incidence of ICU-acquired weakness was twice as high with liberal oxygen therapy; the incidence of atelectasis was also significantly higher [24].

1.4.5 The LOCO2 Trial

The LOCO2 trial was a multicentric RCT conducted across 13 ICUs in France [25]. The study included patients who were receiving mechanical ventilation for ARDS according to the Berlin criteria [26]. In the conservative group, the PaO_2 level was targeted between 55 and 70 mmHg with oxygen saturation maintained between 88 and 92%. In the liberal group, the set target was PaO_2 90–105 mmHg, with saturation levels of 96% or higher. No difference was observed in death from any cause at 28 days, the primary outcome. Among the secondary outcomes, the 90-day mortality was higher with conservative compared to liberal therapy. Importantly, a significantly higher incidence of mesenteric ischemia was noted in the conservative arm (5% vs. nil). Based on this adverse finding, the study was stopped after the enrolment of 205 patients due to safety concerns.

1.4.6 The HOT-ICU Trial

Critically ill patients with acute hypoxic respiratory failure from 35 ICUs were included in the HOT-ICU trial. Patients received supplemental oxygen at a minimum flow rate of 10 L/min through an open system or a minimum FiO_2 of 0.5 through a closed system (both invasive and noninvasive ventilation) and were expected to require supplemental oxygen for at least 24 h. In the conservative arm, the target PaO_2 was set at 60 mmHg compared to 90 mmHg in the liberal arm. The 90-day mortality, the primary outcome, was not significantly different between the conservative and the liberal groups (42.9% vs. 42.4%, $p = 0.64$). Among the secondary outcomes, there was no significant difference in the number of days alive without life support and days alive after hospital discharge. This study supported a lower PaO_2 target of 60 mmHg compared to 90 mmHg in patients with acute hypoxemic respiratory failure with no adverse clinical outcomes [27].

1.4.7 The PILOT Trial

The single-center PILOT cluster-randomized trial evaluated low (88–92%), intermediate (92–96%), and high (96–100%) oxygen saturation among mechanically ventilated patients in the emergency department and the ICU. This RCT enrolled 2987 patients; 2541 were included in the primary analysis. The number of ventilator-free days at day 28, the primary outcome, was similar in the three groups. The median number of ventilator-free days was 20 (IQR: 0–25), 21 (IQR: 0–25), and 21 (IQR: 0–26) in the low, intermediate, and high oxygen saturation groups respectively ($p = 0.81$). The 28-day mortality was also similar between the three groups. The PILOT trial suggested that aiming for a low oxygen saturation target of 90% or lower does not shorten the duration of ventilator support or improve survival compared to an intermediate or high target [28].

1.4.8 Oxygenation Targets in Hypoxic-Ischemic Encephalopathy

The BOX trial did not corroborate the subgroup analysis findings of the ICU-ROX study that suggested worse outcomes associated higher oxygenation targets in patients with hypoxic-ischemic encephalopathy. In this single center study, a restrictive oxygen target (PaO_2 68–75) was compared with a liberal target (PaO_2 98–105 mm Hg) among comatose survivors of out-of-hospital cardiac arrest. This RCT did not reveal a significant difference in death or severe disability at 90 days, the primary outcome, between a restrictive compared with a liberal oxygenation strategy [29]

Key Points

- There is robust clinical evidence that suggests adverse consequences associated with excessive oxygen use, including increased mortality.
- The safe limits of oxygen therapy remain unclear. The range of safety may vary depending on the underlying condition. Hypoxic-ischemic encephalopathy may exacerbate vulnerability to the adverse effects of excessive oxygen.
- Among mechanically ventilated patients, a target saturation level of 91–96% may be adequate under most clinical circumstances.
- The FiO_2 levels may be weaned down to target saturation levels, in contrast to setting an arbitrary lower limit of FiO_2.
- Oxygen must be considered as a drug and administered judiciously; adverse effects occur with unrestricted use.
- A target saturation level may be prescribed in critically ill patients, and the FiO_2 levels titrated accordingly.

References

1. Catling DC, Glein CR, Zahnle KJ, McKay CP. Why O2 is required by complex life on habitable planets and the concept of planetary oxygenation time. Astrobiology. 2005;5(3):415–38.
2. West JB. Joseph Priestley, oxygen, and the enlightenment. Am J Physiol Lung Cell Mol Physiol. 2014;306(2):L111–9.
3. Shultz SM, Hartmann PM. George E Holtzapple (1862-1946) and oxygen therapy for lobar pneumonia: the first reported case (1887) and a review of the contemporary literature to 1899. J Med Biogr. 2005;13(4):201–6.
4. Smith JL. The pathological effects due to increase of oxygen tension in the air breathed. J Physiol. 1899;24(1):19–35.
5. Mach WJ, Thimmesch AR, Pierce JT, Pierce JD. Consequences of Hyperoxia and the toxicity of oxygen in the lung. Nurs Res Pract. 2011;2011:260482.
6. Ferguson ND. Oxygen in the ICU: too much of a good thing? JAMA. 2016;316(15):1553–4.
7. Panwar R, Capellier G, Schmutz N, Davies A, Cooper DJ, Bailey M, et al. Current oxygenation practice in ventilated patients—an observational cohort study. Anaesth Intensive Care. 2013;41(4):505–14.
8. Ni YN, Wang YM, Liang BM, Liang ZA. The effect of hyperoxia on mortality in critically ill patients: a systematic review and meta analysis. BMC Pulm Med. 2019;19(1):53.
9. Durlinger EMJ, Spoelstra-de Man AME, Smit B, de Grooth HJ, Girbes ARJ, Oudemans-van Straaten HM, et al. Hyperoxia: at what level of SpO2 is a patient safe? A study in mechanically ventilated ICU patients. J Crit Care. 2017;39:199–204.

10. Lushchak VI. Free radicals, reactive oxygen species, oxidative stress and its classification. Chem Biol Interact. 2014;224:164–75.
11. Rahman I, Biswas SK, Kode A. Oxidant and antioxidant balance in the airways and airway diseases. Eur J Pharmacol. 2006;533(1–3):222–39.
12. Aboab J, Jonson B, Kouatchet A, Taille S, Niklason L, Brochard L. Effect of inspired oxygen fraction on alveolar derecruitment in acute respiratory distress syndrome. Intensive Care Med. 2006;32(12):1979–86.
13. Cornet AD, Kooter AJ, Peters MJ, Smulders YM. The potential harm of oxygen therapy in medical emergencies. Crit Care. 2013;17(2):313.
14. Büsing CM, Kreinsen U, Bühler F, Bleyl U. Light and electron microscopic examinations of experimentally produced heart muscle necroses following normobaric hyperoxia. Virchows Arch A Pathol Anat Histol. 1975;366(2):137–47.
15. Davies CE, Mackinnon J. Neurological effects of oxygen in chronic Cor pulmonale. Lancet. 1949;2(6585):883–5. illust.
16. Abdo WF, Heunks LM. Oxygen-induced hypercapnia in COPD: myths and facts. Crit Care. 2012;16(5):323.
17. Robinson TD, Freiberg DB, Regnis JA, Young IH. The role of hypoventilation and ventilation-perfusion redistribution in oxygen-induced hypercapnia during acute exacerbations of chronic obstructive pulmonary disease. Am J Respir Crit Care Med. 2000;161(5):1524–9.
18. Hanson CW, Marshall BE, Frasch HF, Marshall C. Causes of hypercarbia with oxygen therapy in patients with chronic obstructive pulmonary disease. Crit Care Med. 1996;24(1):23–8.
19. Madias JE, Madias NE, Hood WB. Precordial ST-segment mapping. 2. Effects of oxygen inhalation on ischemic injury in patients with acute myocardial infarction. Circulation. 1976;53(3):411–7.
20. Stub D, Smith K, Bernard S, Bray JE, Stephenson M, Cameron P, et al. A randomized controlled trial of oxygen therapy in acute myocardial infarction air verses oxygen in myocardial infarction study (AVOID study). Am Heart J. 2012;163(3):339–345.e1.
21. Girardis M, Busani S, Damiani E, Donati A, Rinaldi L, Marudi A, et al. Effect of conservative vs conventional oxygen therapy on mortality among patients in an intensive care unit: the oxygen-ICU randomized clinical trial. JAMA. 2016;316(15):1583–9.
22. ICU-ROX Investigators and the Australian and New Zealand Intensive Care Society Clinical Trials Group, Mackle D, Bellomo R, Bailey M, Beasley R, Deane A, et al. Conservative oxygen therapy during mechanical ventilation in the ICU. N Engl J Med. 2020;382(11):989–98.
23. Young P, Mackle D, Bellomo R, Bailey M, Beasley R, Deane A, et al. Conservative oxygen therapy for mechanically ventilated adults with sepsis: a post hoc analysis of data from the intensive care unit randomized trial comparing two approaches to oxygen therapy (ICU-ROX). Intensive Care Med. 2020;46(1):17–26.
24. Asfar P, Schortgen F, Boisramé-Helms J, Charpentier J, Guérot E, Megarbane B, et al. Hyperoxia and hypertonic saline in patients with septic shock (HYPERS2S): a two-by-two factorial, multicentre, randomised, clinical trial. Lancet Respir Med. 2017;5(3):180–90.
25. Barrot L, Asfar P, Mauny F, Winiszewski H, Montini F, Badie J, et al. Liberal or conservative oxygen therapy for acute respiratory distress syndrome. N Engl J Med. 2020;382(11):999–1008.
26. ARDS Definition Task Force, Ranieri VM, Rubenfeld GD, Thompson BT, Ferguson ND, Caldwell E, et al. Acute respiratory distress syndrome: the Berlin definition. JAMA. 2012;307(23):2526–33.
27. Schjørring OL, Klitgaard TL, Perner A, Wetterslev J, Lange T, Siegemund M, et al. Lower or higher oxygenation targets for acute hypoxemic respiratory failure. N Engl J Med. 2021;384(14):1301–11.
28. Semler MW, Casey JD, Lloyd BD, Hastings PG, Hays MA, Stollings JL, et al. Oxygen-Saturation Targets for Critically Ill Adults Receiving Mechanical Ventilation. N Engl J Med. 2022;387(19):1759–69.
29. Schmidt H, Kjaergaard J, Hassager C, Mølstrøm S, Grand J, Borregaard B, et al. Oxygen Targets in Comatose Survivors of Cardiac Arrest. N Engl J Med. 2022;387(16):1467–76.

2 The Hypoxic Drive, Supplemental Oxygen, and Hypercapnia

2.1 Introduction

Painstaking titration of oxygen flows with elaborate precision is often performed in carbon dioxide retainers with chronic obstructive pulmonary disease (COPD). The driving principle behind this line of thinking is the tradition-borne belief that supplemental oxygen may inhibit the hypoxic respiratory drive and lead to hypoventilation with a rise in the $PaCO_2$ levels. It has even been reasoned that hypoxia was a respiratory stimulant in these patients through the sino-aortic nerve activity [1]. How important is the contribution of the hypoxic drive in patients with respiratory failure, especially among those with hypercapnia? Does supplemental oxygen really suppress ventilation in spontaneously breathing patients with COPD and lead to a significant rise in CO_2 levels? Could other mechanisms including an increase in the dead space and the loss of hypoxic pulmonary vasoconstriction be more likely to induce hypercapnia?

2.2 Dead Space

2.2.1 Anatomical Dead Space

The anatomical dead space comprises the airways that allow passage of air to the respiratory bronchioles and alveoli. Gas exchange does not occur in this part of the respiratory system. The volume of the anatomical dead space is approximately 150 mL. Dead space volume/tidal volume (V_d/V_t) represents the proportion of dead space relative to the tidal volume. With low tidal volume breaths, the relative proportion of the dead space increases (high V_d/V_t) and may lead to hypercapnia if the minute ventilation does not increase.

J. Chacko et al., *Controversies in Critical Care*,
https://doi.org/10.1007/978-981-19-9940-6_2

2.2.2 Alveolar Dead Space

The alveolar dead space refers to a reduction in perfusion to ventilated alveoli (high *V*/*Q*) [2]. Thus, alveolar dead space representing areas of adequate ventilation, but impaired perfusion is in direct contrast to areas of the lung that are poorly ventilated, with normal perfusion (low *V*/*Q*, leading to shunting). In most parenchymal disease processes, the mechanism for hypercapnia is an increase in the alveolar dead space.

2.2.3 Physiological Dead Space

The combination of anatomical and alveolar dead spaces comprises the physiological dead space [2].

$$\text{Physiological dead space}\left(V_{\text{d phys}}\right) = \text{Anatomical dead space} + \text{alveolar dead space}.$$

2.3 Oxygen Administration and Respiratory Drive: The Evidence

Aubier et al. analyzed the breathing pattern of 20 patients with COPD during the acute phase of respiratory failure; in 12 patients, further analysis was carried out after recovery from the acute phase [3]. The results were compared with those of normal subjects in a similar age group. The minute ventilation was similar during the acute and chronic phases and was comparable to those of normal subjects. The respiratory drive, measured using mouth occlusion pressure, was fivefold higher during the acute phase compared to normal subjects. Following supplemental oxygen, the mouth occlusion pressure decreased by 40%, suggesting a significant reduction of the respiratory drive. Supplemental oxygen at 5 L/min for 30 min resulted in a 14% reduction in the minute ventilation, due to a reduced respiratory rate, indicating lower inspiratory flows. The $PaCO_2$ rose after oxygen administration, although the rise was not commensurate with the decrease in minute ventilation, suggesting other possible mechanisms for the hypercapnia. The authors proposed that an increase in dead space could explain hypercapnia that followed oxygen supplementation.

In a later study, Aubier et al. evaluated changes in ventilation and arterial blood gases on 22 patients with acute infective exacerbation of COPD, following switch over from room air to 100% oxygen [4]. Patients were hypoxic (mean PaO_2 38 ± 2 mmHg) and hypercapnic 65 ± 3 mmHg while breathing room air. Respiratory parameters were monitored throughout the 15-min period of breathing 100% oxygen. An initial decrease in minute ventilation was observed following administration of 100% oxygen; the lowest value was noted between 20 and 180 s of oxygen

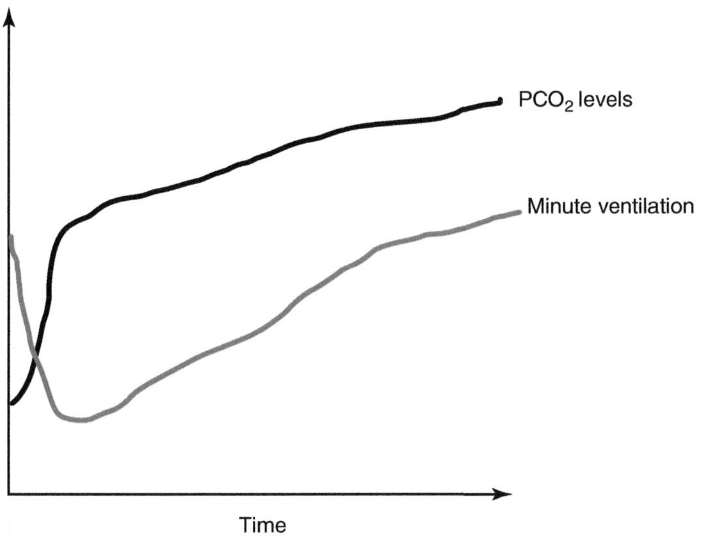

Fig. 2.1 Effect of switching from air to 100% oxygen in acute exacerbation of COPD. The minute ventilation decreased initially, and reached a plateau; however, the PaCO2 continued to rise, suggesting other mechanisms for hypercapnia

inhalation. Following the initial decrease, the minute ventilation gradually increased and plateaued off about 12 min after the commencement of 100% oxygen administration. The plateau level of minute ventilation at the end of the 15-min study period was 93 ± 6% of the baseline level. However, the $PaCO_2$ continued to rise during the entire study period and increased by a mean of 23 ± 5 mmHg (Fig. 2.1). The PaO_2 increased from a mean baseline level of 38 ± 2 mmHg to 225 ± 23 mmHg. No significant change was observed in the tidal volume or respiratory rate with inhalation of 100% oxygen. The rise in $PaCO_2$ was disproportionately high and could not be explained by the marginal decrease in minute ventilation. During acute exacerbation of COPD, a marked increase in the respiratory drive is commonly observed. The above studies suggest that although the respiratory drive may decrease marginally following oxygen supplementation, it still remains higher than normal. The decrease in respiratory drive alone does not explain the rise in $PaCO_2$ levels [3].

2.4 The Haldane Effect

Hemoglobin carries carbon dioxide as carbamino compounds. According to the Haldane effect, the carbon dioxide dissociation curve is shifted to the right as the oxyhemoglobin level rises [5]. Thus, oxygenated hemoglobin carries less carbon dioxide. In the normal lungs, as the hemoglobin gets oxygenated to oxyhemoglobin, the carbon dioxide is released and expired out. Consider the case of a patient with

COPD. Oxygen administration would lead to the release of carbon dioxide from the hemoglobin as expected. However, the expiration of carbon dioxide released from the hemoglobin remains inadequate as there is no proportional increase in ventilation in COPD patients. This leads to an increase in the $PaCO_2$ levels [6].

2.5 Loss of the Hypoxic Pulmonary Vasoconstrictor Effect

When the partial pressure of oxygen in the alveoli drops, the smooth muscle of the pulmonary circulation contracts, resulting in vasoconstriction [7]. This is a reflex mechanism to reduce intrapulmonary shunt in the presence of hypoxia. The vasoconstrictor response of the pulmonary vessels in response to hypoxia is in contrast to the hypoxia-induced vasodilator effect that occurs in the systemic circulation [8]. On administration of supplemental oxygen, the alveolar partial pressure of oxygen rises. The rise in oxygen level leads to inhibition of the hypoxic pulmonary vasoconstrictor response, leading to a redistribution of blood flow from better-ventilated to relatively less ventilated areas of the lung, with a regional reduction in the *V*/*Q* ratio. In contrast, in the better-ventilated areas of the lung (from which the blood was diverted away), the perfusion is reduced relative to ventilation leading to a higher *V*/*Q* ratio and an increase in the dead space ventilation. Aubier et al. also observed a significant increase in the dead space ventilation from 77 ± 2 to 82 ± 2 following 15 min of breathing 100% oxygen in their study [6]. Both the above mechanisms may contribute to a rise in $PaCO_2$ levels.

Robinson et al. evaluated the mechanism of oxygen-induced hypercapnia among 22 patients with acute exacerbation of COPD [9]. Patients were allowed to breathe air initially, followed by 100% oxygen through a nasal mask for at least 20 min. Ventilation, *V*/*Q* ratio, and cardiac output were measured while breathing air and 100% oxygen. Patients were classified as retainers if the $PaCO_2$ rose by more than 3 mmHg and non-retainers if the PCO_2 rise was less than 3 mmHg. Among 12 patients in the retainer group, the $PaCO_2$ level rose by 8.3 ± 5.6; in the non-retainer group, the $PaCO_2$ change was −1.3 ± 2.2 mmHg. The minute ventilation decreased from 9.0 ± 1.5 to 7.2 ± 1.2 L/min in the retainer group after 20 min of breathing 100% oxygen. However, the rise in CO_2 seemed disproportionate to the decrease in minute ventilation. The *V*/*Q* mismatch was of the same magnitude in both the groups, likely due to inhibition of the hypoxic pulmonary vasoconstrictor response. A significant increase in dead space ventilation was observed in the retainer group, which may have resulted in the rise in PCO_2.

Hanson et al. compared data derived from a simulated computer model of the pulmonary circulation with data from a series of patients with COPD [10]. The model with simulated oxygen therapy generated data comparable to COPD patients treated with supplemental oxygen. The authors observed that oxygen administration led to an increase in the physiological dead space resulting from inhibition of the hypoxic pulmonary vasoconstrictor response and through the Haldane effect. They concluded that the increase in physiological dead space alone was sufficient to explain the rise in $PaCO_2$ observed in patients who received supplemental oxygen. The plausible mechanisms of $PaCO_2$ rise with supplemental oxygen are depicted in Fig. 2.2.

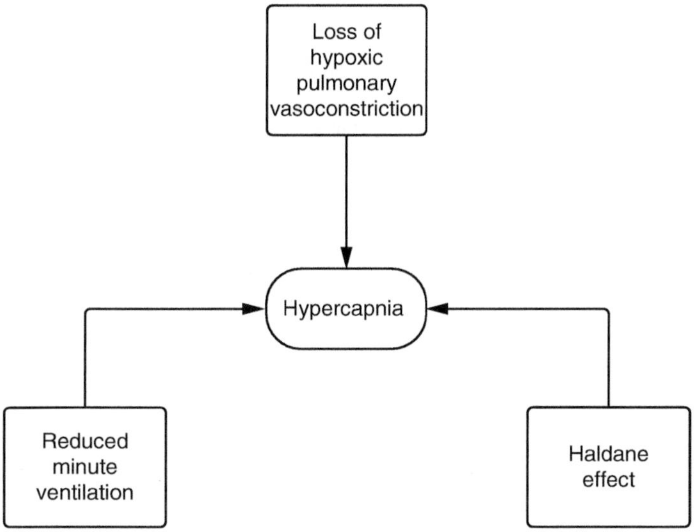

Fig. 2.2 The plausible mechanisms behind the hypercapnia observed with oxygen supplementation in acute exacerbation of COPD

Key Points

- There is a modest rise in $PaCO_2$ levels in patients with acute exacerbation of COPD who receive supplemental oxygen.
- There is a marginal decrease in minute ventilation associated with oxygen administration; however, the rise in $PaCO_2$ level cannot be explained solely on the basis of hypoventilation.
- Furthermore, the minute ventilation returns to baseline levels with minutes, although the $PaCO_2$ levels continue to remain high, suggesting an alternate mechanism for the hypercapnia.
- A more plausible mechanism for the rise in $PaCO_2$ levels is through inhibition of hypoxic pulmonary vasoconstriction resulting from a higher alveolar oxygen tension resulting from supplemental oxygen. Release of hypoxic pulmonary vasoconstriction results in redistribution of blood to less ventilated areas, with an increase in the dead space and hypercapnia.
- The Haldane effect results in reduced carbon dioxide carriage as the hemoglobin gets oxygenated in the lung. However, the carbon dioxide cannot be eliminated adequately as the ventilation remains low, contributing to the hypercapnia.
- It is important not to withhold oxygen in patients who are hypoxic based on an irrational fear of suppressing the "hypoxic drive."

References

1. Davies CE, Mackinnon J. Neurological effects of oxygen in chronic cor pulmonale. Lancet. 1949;2(6585):883–5. illust.
2. Intagliata S, Rizzo A, Gossman W. Physiology, lung dead space. In: StatPearls. Treasure Island, FL: StatPearls; 2021. http://www.ncbi.nlm.nih.gov/books/NBK482501/.
3. Aubier M, Murciano D, Fournier M, Milic-Emili J, Pariente R, Derenne JP. Central respiratory drive in acute respiratory failure of patients with chronic obstructive pulmonary disease. Am Rev Respir Dis. 1980;122(2):191–9.
4. Aubier M, Murciano D, Milic-Emili J, Touaty E, Daghfous J, Pariente R, et al. Effects of the administration of O2 on ventilation and blood gases in patients with chronic obstructive pulmonary disease during acute respiratory failure. Am Rev Respir Dis. 1980;122(5):747–54.
5. Teboul JL, Scheeren T. Understanding the Haldane effect. Intensive Care Med. 2017;43(1):91–3.
6. Abdo WF, Heunks LM. Oxygen-induced hypercapnia in COPD: myths and facts. Crit Care. 2012;16(5):323.
7. Lumb AB, Slinger P. Hypoxic pulmonary vasoconstriction: physiology and anesthetic implications. Anesthesiology. 2015;122(4):932–46.
8. Farhi LE, Sheehan DW. Pulmonary circulation and systemic circulation: similar problems, different solutions. Adv Exp Med Biol. 1990;277:579–86.
9. Robinson TD, Freiberg DB, Regnis JA, Young IH. The role of hypoventilation and ventilation-perfusion redistribution in oxygen-induced hypercapnia during acute exacerbations of chronic obstructive pulmonary disease. Am J Respir Crit Care Med. 2000;161(5):1524–9.
10. Hanson CW, Marshall BE, Frasch HF, Marshall C. Causes of hypercarbia with oxygen therapy in patients with chronic obstructive pulmonary disease. Crit Care Med. 1996;24(1):23–8.

Noninvasive Respiratory Support in Acute Hypoxemic Respiratory Failure

3

3.1 Introduction

Acute hypoxemic respiratory failure is usually characterized by tachypnea and PaO_2/FiO_2 ratios of less than 300 mmHg with supplemental oxygen therapy. Although in widespread use, the efficacy of noninvasive respiratory support in acute hypoxemic respiratory failure is not firmly established. The pathophysiology of hypoxemic respiratory failure is variable and may result from direct or indirect injury to the lung. It is characterized by interstitial and intra-alveolar edema with loss of aeration, arterial hypoxemia, and enhanced respiratory drive. Noninvasive modalities of respiratory support have evoked interest in the treatment of acute hypoxemic respiratory failure and carry the potential to reduce the requirement for invasive mechanical ventilation and the associated complications. Clinical practice guidelines do not offer evidence-based recommendations on the usefulness of noninvasive respiratory support in acute hypoxemic respiratory failure [1]. In the face of the COVID-19 pandemic, there has been renewed interest in the use of noninvasive modalities of respiratory support, especially considering the constraint on resources imposed by an overwhelming number of patients who develop respiratory failure.

3.2 Modalities and Potential Benefits of Noninvasive Respiratory Support

The use of noninvasive respiratory support potentially enables the reduction of complications related to invasive mechanical ventilation including ventilator-associated lung injury (VILI) [2], and ventilator-associated pneumonia (VAP) [3]. Noninvasive respiratory support allows a reduction in the use of sedative agents and avoidance of the use of neuromuscular blocking agents [4]. Preservation of spontaneous

J. Chacko et al., *Controversies in Critical Care*,
https://doi.org/10.1007/978-981-19-9940-6_3

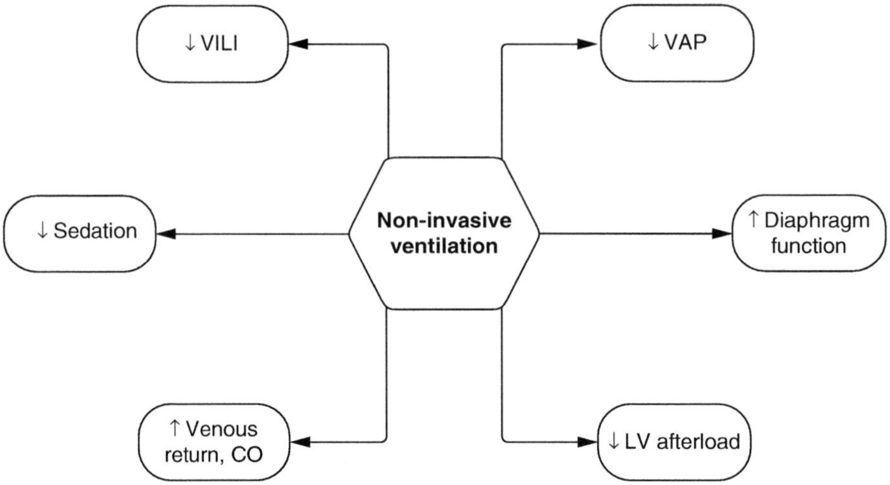

Fig. 3.1 The advantages of noninvasive respiratory support

respiratory efforts may also lessen the incidence of diaphragmatic atrophy and prolonged weaning often associated with invasive mechanical ventilation [5]. Besides, spontaneous respiratory efforts lead to improved venous return and cardiac output; the positive pleural pressure leads to a reduction in the transmural pressure of the left ventricle with a reduction in the afterload [6]. Figure 3.1 depicts the advantages of noninvasive respiratory support.

3.3 Potential Harm from Noninvasive Respiratory Support

3.3.1 Patients Self-Inflicted Lung Injury (P-SILI)

Although noninvasive respiratory support has the potential to reduce the incidence of complications commonly associated with invasive mechanical ventilation, harmful effects may occur. Unrelieved, vigorous spontaneous efforts may lead to injurious effects on the lung, termed patient self-inflicted lung injury (P-SILI) [7]. Vigorous inspiratory efforts lead to increasingly negative pleural pressures and an increase in the transpulmonary pressure (alveolar pressure-pleural pressure). Transpulmonary pressure is an important driver of lung injury. The pleural pressure is also distributed nonuniformly in the injured lung, with the dependent areas subjected to more negative pleural pressures. The nonuniform distribution of pleural pressure leads to the movement of gas from the nondependent to the dependent areas of the lung by the pendelluft effect [8]. Alveoli in the dependent areas, already prone to injury, are further subjected to the damaging effect of cyclical opening and closure due to the pendelluft effect. Besides, more negative pleural pressures lead to an increase in the transmural pressure across the already damaged pulmonary capillaries, leading to fluid leak and worsening of lung injury [9].

3.3.2 Diaphragmatic Dysfunction

Diaphragmatic injury may occur due to incorrectly applied ventilation strategies. Diaphragm atrophy may occur due to inappropriately high levels of inspiratory support. On the other hand, inadequate levels of support may injure the diaphragm through under-assistance, dyssynchrony, and excessive shortening at end-expiration due to high levels of PEEP.

3.4 Techniques of Noninvasive Respiratory Support

Three methods of noninvasive respiratory support are commonly employed, including (1) noninvasive ventilation (NIV) through a face mask (2), through a helmet interphase, and (3) use of a high-flow nasal cannula (HFNC). A face mask may be used to apply CPAP alone or with additional inspiratory pressure support.

The helmet is a relatively new interphase and employs a transparent hood that covers the head and sealed at the neck with a soft collar. Compared to the face mask, the helmet interphase seals better and offers an improved level of comfort, enabling the application of higher levels of PEEP for a longer duration. Both CPAP and pressure support modes may be employed through the helmet interphase [10, 11].

HFNC delivers gas flows of up to 60 L/min through wide-bored cannulae. Heated and humidified gas is delivered at a preset FiO_2. The high gas flow enables the washout of dead space gas from the upper airways, thereby reducing the arterial carbon dioxide level. The high gas flow employed matches the peak inspiratory flow of dyspneic patients more closely, thus alleviating distress. Furthermore, HFNC also generates a low level of PEEP leading to alveolar recruitment and improved gas exchange [12].

3.5 Predictors of Failure of Noninvasive Respiratory Support

The severity of hypoxemia may be an important predictor of outcomes with noninvasive respiratory support. A low PaO_2/FiO_2 ratio is closely associated with failure of NIV applied through a face mask. Several studies suggest that a PaO_2/FiO_2 ratio of less than 150 mmHg at baseline is a predictor of NIV failure [13, 14]. A greater severity of illness is also associated with an increased risk of poor outcomes with noninvasive respiratory support [13, 15]. High spontaneously generated tidal volumes during NIV are injurious. A tidal volume of higher than 9.5 mL/kg predicted NIV failure with a sensitivity of 82% and specificity of 87% [16]. The risk of NIV failure may be relatively higher in community-acquired pneumonia [13], especially if associated with worsening of infiltrates on the chest radiograph within 24 h of hospital admission [17]. There is robust evidence that delayed intubation in patients who receive NIV may lead to poor outcomes including mortality [17, 18].

3.6 What Does the Evidence Suggest?

The impact of noninvasive modalities of respiratory support on clinical outcomes has been addressed in recent studies (Table 3.1).

Duan et al. studied 449 patients with acute hypoxemic respiratory failure who received NIV, using a face mask as the first choice interphase [19]. They tested the validity of a scoring system including heart rate, acidosis, consciousness, oxygenation, and respiratory rate (the HACOR score, ranging from 0 to 25 points). In patients with a HACOR score of >5 after 1 h of initiation of NIV, they observed

Table 3.1 Recent studies on the impact of noninvasive respiratory support on clinical outcomes

Study/ year	Population	Noninvasive support group	Control	Outcomes
Duan et al. (2017) [19]	Acute hypoxemic respiratory failure	NIV applied through a full-face mask. PEEP 4–8 cmH_2O. Inspiratory pressure was initially set at 10 cmH_2O increased stepwise by 2 cmH_2O	None	A HACOR score of >5 points predicted NIV failure. Lower hospital mortality if invasive ventilation commenced within 12 h of NIV failure with a HACOR score of >5 at 1 h of NIV commencement
Frat et al. (2015) [20]	Acute hypoxemic respiratory failure, PaO_2/FiO_2 ratio <300, no hypercarbia	NIV through face mask or HFNC	Oxygen through face mask	28-day intubation rates similar in all three groups. Degree of discomfort and dyspnea better with HFNC. Invasive ventilation-free days at 28 days significantly more with HFNC. HR for mortality lower with HFNC
Patel et al. (2016) [10]	ARDS patients requiring mask for at least 8 h	Helmet NIV	Continued NIV through mask	Lower intubation rates with helmet NIV. More ventilation-free days with helmet NIV. 90-day mortality lower with helmet NIV
Franco et al. (2020) [21]	Acute respiratory failure due to COVID-19	Noninvasive support out-of-ICU with HFNC, NIV with CPAP alone, or NIPPV	None	Similar intubation rates and 30-day mortality with all three modalities. Study showed feasibility of noninvasive respiratory support outside the ICU

NIV noninvasive ventilation, *HACOR* heart rate, acidosis, consciousness oxygenation, respiratory rate, *HFNC* high-flow nasal cannula, *HR* hazard ratio, *NIPPV* noninvasive positive pressure ventilation

lower mortality among patients who received invasive ventilation within 12 h of commencement of NIV. Besides, a cutoff of 5 points on the HACOR scale predicted NIV failure in patient subgroups based on age, the severity of illness, and the presenting diagnosis.

In a multicenter randomized controlled trial (RCT), patients with acute hypoxemic respiratory failure with a PaO_2/FiO_2 ratio of $\leq$300 mmHg were assigned to receive conventional oxygen therapy, HFNC, or NIV through a face mask [20]. Intubation and invasive mechanical ventilation were performed based on prespecified criteria. Among 310 patients included in the final analysis, the intubation rates were not significantly different between the three groups (47% with conventional oxygen therapy, 38% with HFNC, and 50% with NIV). The degree of respiratory discomfort and the dyspnea score after 1 h of treatment were better with HFNC compared to the other modalities of support. Patients who received HFNC experienced significantly more ventilator-free days at day 28 (24 ± 8 days) compared to conventional oxygen therapy (22 ± 10 days) and NIV (19 ± 12 days) ($p = 0.02$). The hazard ratio for mortality at 90 days was also significantly lower with HFNC compared to conventional oxygen therapy ($p = 0.046$) and NIV ($p = 0.006$).

Considering the potential advantages of the helmet interphase allowing better tolerance and increased levels of PEEP with less air leak, Patel et al. compared it with NIV applied through a face mask [10]. Patients were initially commenced on face mask NIV; after 8 h, they were randomly assigned, if agreeable, in a 1:1 ratio to continue face mask NIV or switch to the helmet interphase. The study was terminated for efficacy after the enrolment of 83 patients. The helmet interphase resulted in significantly lower intubation rates compared to face mask NIV (18.2% vs. 61.5%, $p < 0.001$). Patients in the helmet group were ventilation-free for a longer duration compared to face mask NIV (28 vs. 12.5, $P < 0.001$). The 90-day mortality was also significantly lower with the use of helmet compared to face mask NIV (34.1% vs. 56.4%, $p = 0.02$). This study revealed significantly improved clinical outcomes with the use of the helmet compared to the face mask interphase for NIV therapy.

Noninvasive modalities of respiratory support have been extensively employed during the Covid-19 pandemic, particularly in resource-limited settings. A retrospective Italian study evaluated patients in acute respiratory failure due to COVID-19 infection [21]. Treatment was commenced in a non-ICU setting with respiratory support using HFNC, CPAP, or noninvasive positive pressure ventilation. The overall intubation rates were similar with different modalities of support: 29% with HFNC, 25% with CPAP, and 28% with noninvasive positive pressure ventilation. The 30-day mortality was also not different between groups after adjustment for potential confounders. This large observational cohort study suggests that the application of noninvasive respiratory support may be feasible outside the ICU in resource-constrained settings during a pandemic.

Ferreyro et al., in a network meta-analysis, compared the efficacy of different types of noninvasive oxygenation strategies in reducing mortality and intubation rates among patients with acute hypoxemic respiratory failure [22]. The meta-analysis included 25 RCTs, with 3804 patients. NIV administered through both face mask (RR, 0.83 [95% credible interval, 0.68–0.99]) and helmet (RR, 0.40 [95% credible interval, 0.24–0.63]) were associated with a significantly lower risk of mortality compared to standard oxygen administration. HFNC was not associated with a lower risk of mortality compared to standard oxygen administration. Helmet NIV was also associated with significantly lower mortality compared to HFNC and face mask NIV. The probability of reducing all-cause mortality was highest with helmet NIV, followed by face mask NIV, HFNC, and standard oxygen administration. The probability of endotracheal intubation also followed a similar pattern; it was lowest with helmet NIV, followed by face mask NIV, HFNC, and standard oxygen administration. The median duration of ICU and hospital stay was not significantly different between groups.

Key Points

- There is conflicting evidence regarding the efficacy of noninvasive respiratory support in acute hypoxemic respiratory failure with no firm recommendations in clinical practice guidelines.
- Judicious use of noninvasive respiratory support may improve clinical outcomes including intubation rates. However, persistence with noninvasive modalities in patients who do not respond may lead to delay in intubation and adverse outcomes.
- A continued high spontaneous respiratory drive may result in P-SILI and worsen outcomes.
- Increased severity of illness at baseline, low PaO_2/FiO_2 ratios, and high tidal volumes are associated with NIV failure.
- The helmet interphase may increase comfort and tolerance, reduce leak, and facilitate the application of higher levels of PEEP compared to face mask NIV.
- HFNC may be a viable option among selected patients in acute hypoxemic respiratory failure. Further studies are required to evaluate its efficacy in reducing intubation rates.
- Noninvasive modalities of respiratory support are a viable option in the face of resource constraints imposed by the COVID-19 pandemic.

References

1. Rochwerg B, Brochard L, Elliott MW, Hess D, Hill NS, Nava S, et al. Official ERS/ATS clinical practice guidelines: noninvasive ventilation for acute respiratory failure. Eur Respir J. 2017;50(2):1602426.
2. Slutsky AS, Ranieri VM. Ventilator-induced lung injury. N Engl J Med. 2013;369(22):2126–36.
3. Chanques G, Constantin JM, Devlin JW, Ely EW, Fraser GL, Gélinas C, et al. Analgesia and sedation in patients with ARDS. Intensive Care Med. 2020;46(12):2342–56.

4. Alhazzani W, Belley-Cote E, Møller MH, Angus DC, Papazian L, Arabi YM, et al. Neuromuscular blockade in patients with ARDS: a rapid practice guideline. Intensive Care Med. 2020;46(11):1977–86.
5. Goligher EC, Fan E, Herridge MS, Murray A, Vorona S, Brace D, et al. Evolution of diaphragm thickness during mechanical ventilation. Impact of inspiratory effort. Am J Respir Crit Care Med. 2015;192(9):1080–8.
6. MacIntyre NR. Physiologic effects of noninvasive ventilation. Respir Care. 2019;64(6):617–28.
7. Yoshida T, Grieco DL, Brochard L, Fujino Y. Patient self-inflicted lung injury and positive end-expiratory pressure for safe spontaneous breathing. Curr Opin Crit Care. 2020;26(1):59–65.
8. Yoshida T, Torsani V, Gomes S, De Santis RR, Beraldo MA, Costa ELV, et al. Spontaneous effort causes occult pendelluft during mechanical ventilation. Am J Respir Crit Care Med. 2013;188(12):1420–7.
9. Brochard L, Slutsky A, Pesenti A. Mechanical ventilation to minimize progression of lung injury in acute respiratory failure. Am J Respir Crit Care Med. 2017;195(4):438–42.
10. Patel BK, Wolfe KS, Pohlman AS, Hall JB, Kress JP. Effect of noninvasive ventilation delivered by helmet vs face mask on the rate of endotracheal intubation in patients with acute respiratory distress syndrome: a randomized clinical trial. JAMA. 2016;315(22):2435–41.
11. Antonelli M, Conti G, Pelosi P, Gregoretti C, Pennisi MA, Costa R, et al. New treatment of acute hypoxemic respiratory failure: noninvasive pressure support ventilation delivered by helmet—a pilot controlled trial. Crit Care Med. 2002;30(3):602–8.
12. Papazian L, Corley A, Hess D, Fraser JF, Frat JP, Guitton C, et al. Use of high-flow nasal cannula oxygenation in ICU adults: a narrative review. Intensive Care Med. 2016;42(9):1336–49.
13. Antonelli M, Conti G, Moro ML, Esquinas A, Gonzalez-Diaz G, Confalonieri M, et al. Predictors of failure of noninvasive positive pressure ventilation in patients with acute hypoxemic respiratory failure: a multi-center study. Intensive Care Med. 2001;27(11):1718–28.
14. Bellani G, Laffey JG, Pham T, Madotto F, Fan E, Brochard L, et al. Noninvasive ventilation of patients with acute respiratory distress syndrome. Insights from the LUNG SAFE study. Am J Respir Crit Care Med. 2017;195(1):67–77.
15. Frat JP, Ragot S, Coudroy R, Constantin JM, Girault C, Prat G, et al. Predictors of intubation in patients with acute hypoxemic respiratory failure treated with a noninvasive oxygenation strategy. Crit Care Med. 2018;46(2):208–15.
16. Carteaux G, Millán-Guilarte T, De Prost N, Razazi K, Abid S, Thille AW, et al. Failure of noninvasive ventilation for De novo acute hypoxemic respiratory failure: role of tidal volume. Crit Care Med. 2016;44(2):282–90.
17. Carrillo A, Gonzalez-Diaz G, Ferrer M, Martinez-Quintana ME, Lopez-Martinez A, Llamas N, et al. Non-invasive ventilation in community-acquired pneumonia and severe acute respiratory failure. Intensive Care Med. 2012;38(3):458–66.
18. Hraiech S, Alingrin J, Dizier S, Brunet J, Forel JM, La Scola B, et al. Time to intubation is associated with outcome in patients with community-acquired pneumonia. PLoS One. 2013;8(9):e74937.
19. Duan J, Han X, Bai L, Zhou L, Huang S. Assessment of heart rate, acidosis, consciousness, oxygenation, and respiratory rate to predict noninvasive ventilation failure in hypoxemic patients. Intensive Care Med. 2017;43(2):192–9.
20. Frat JP, Thille AW, Mercat A, Girault C, Ragot S, Perbet S, et al. High-flow oxygen through nasal cannula in acute hypoxemic respiratory failure. N Engl J Med. 2015;372(23):2185–96.
21. Franco C, Facciolongo N, Tonelli R, Dongilli R, Vianello A, Pisani L, et al. Feasibility and clinical impact of out-of-ICU noninvasive respiratory support in patients with COVID-19-related pneumonia. Eur Respir J. 2020;56(5):2002130.
22. Ferreyro BL, Angriman F, Munshi L, Del Sorbo L, Ferguson ND, Rochwerg B, et al. Association of noninvasive oxygenation strategies with all-cause mortality in adults with acute hypoxemic respiratory failure: a systematic review and meta-analysis. JAMA. 2020;324(1):57.

PEEP Titration by the Bedside: How Do We Set It Right?

4

The beneficial effects of mechanical ventilation are closely related to the prevention of ventilator-induced lung injury (VILI). The harmful effects of positive pressure ventilation may be mitigated by the judicious application of positive end-expiratory pressure (PEEP). In their seminal paper, Ashbaugh et al. observed the beneficial effect of PEEP on arterial oxygenation in patients with acute respiratory distress syndrome (ARDS) [1]. However, the potentially harmful effects of excessive PEEP, including hemodynamic compromise and barotrauma, were soon realized. How do we decide on what may be an appropriate level of PEEP among mechanically ventilated patients?

4.1 Physiological Effects of PEEP

The application of PEEP results in an increase in the end-expiratory lung volume, leading to improved lung compliance, thereby reducing the driving pressure (Pplat-PEEP). Improved compliance and lower driving pressures have been shown to improve survival [2]. If the airway and alveolar pressures remain low at end-expiration, unstable alveoli may repetitively open and collapse during tidal ventilation. The repetitive opening and closure perpetuates shear injury to the lung parenchyma and distal small airways. Besides, surfactant dysfunction occurs, leading to alveolar collapse [3]. Alveolar collapse in diseased areas of the lung leads to preferential ventilation and overdistension of alveoli in the relatively normal areas of the lung, causing strain. Thus, predilection to injury occurs in the better ventilated areas of the "baby" lung. The strain is selectively distributed along the margins of aerated and non-aerated alveoli [4]. The application of an appropriate level of PEEP attenuates tidal recruitment-derecruitment, thus reducing lung stress [2]. Furthermore, alleviation of lung stress mitigates the inflammatory response and the consequent biotrauma [5].

J. Chacko et al., *Controversies in Critical Care*,
https://doi.org/10.1007/978-981-19-9940-6_4

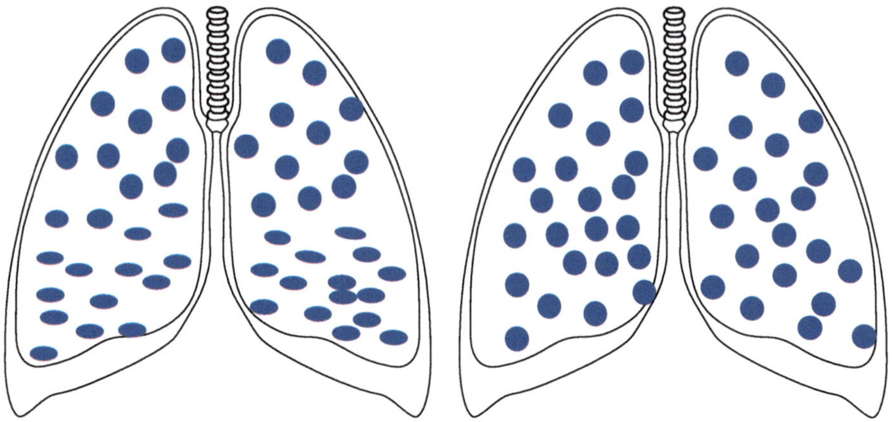

Fig. 4.1 Left: partially collapsed alveoli at the lung bases. Right: alveolar recruitment by increase in PEEP

The application of PEEP helps to maintain alveoli open during end-expiration, thus reducing the adverse impact of the tidal recruitment-derecruitment cycle [6]. As more alveoli remain open at end-expiration, there is less overinflation of the relatively normal lung (Fig. 4.1). Thus, the effect of stress at the margins of the aerated and collapsed lung is attenuated. Overall, optimal levels of PEEP offer more homogenous ventilation of the lung. Besides, by recruiting collapsed lung, PEEP results in reduction of the intrapulmonary shunt and improved oxygenation [7].

4.2 Adverse Effects of PEEP

The application of inappropriately high levels of PEEP may lead to increased inspiratory pressure, alveolar overdistension, and perpetuation of VILI. Besides, PEEP may not recruit collapsed alveoli as expected; instead, it may overinflate alveoli that are already aerated [8]. The extent of recruitment of collapsed alveoli compared to overinflation of already aerated alveoli may vary depending on the level of PEEP and the "recruitability" of the collapsed lung. Therefore, the application of PEEP may lead to recruitment, overinflation, or a combination of both.

Excessively high PEEP levels may also result in high intrathoracic pressures, impeding venous return, and thereby, reduce cardiac output [9]. Pulmonary capillaries may collapse as they are subjected to increased pressure, resulting in an increase in the pulmonary vascular resistance, thereby increasing the afterload to the right ventricle [10]. The alveolar pressure may rise above the pulmonary capillary pressure with excessive PEEP; this may result in collapse of pulmonary capillaries, thereby reducing the perfusion relative to ventilation, leading to an increase in the alveolar dead space [11]. High PEEP levels may also enhance the risk of barotrauma [12]. Table 4.1 depicts the potential advantages and possible adverse effects of increasing levels of PEEP.

Table 4.1 Increasing levels of PEEP: pros and cons

Advantages	Possible adverse effects
Maintains alveoli open at end-expiration	Increased inspiratory pressure, alveolar overdistension, and perpetuation of VILI
Attenuates adverse impacts of the tidal recruitment-derecruitment cycle	High intrathoracic pressures, reduced venous return and cardiac output
Less overinflation of the relatively normal lung; more homogenous ventilation	Increase in the pulmonary vascular resistance, increased RV afterload
Reduced stress at the margins of aerated and collapsed lung	Barotrauma
Alveolar recruitment with reduction of intrapulmonary shunt and improved oxygenation	PEEP may not recruit collapsed alveoli; instead, it may overinflate aerated alveoli. Increased alveolar dead space

4.3 How Do We Titrate PEEP?

4.3.1 PEEP Tables

The ARDS-net trial applied PEEP using a table based on the FiO_2 requirement [13]. Although simple to use, titration based on FiO_2 levels does not take into account lung recruitability, and improvement in oxygenation may not occur with incremental levels of PEEP. Indeed, there may be wide variability between patients in the individual response to PEEP [14].

4.3.2 Oxygenation Response

A commonly adopted approach is titration of PEEP based on the oxygenation response. If the lung is recruitable by PEEP, reduction of the intrapulmonary shunt should result in improved oxygenation. Although the correlation between alveolar recruitment and improved oxygenation may not be consistent, improvement in oxygenation in response to PEEP has been shown to improve survival [14]. An increase in the $PaCO_2$ levels in response to increasing levels of PEEP suggests alveolar overdistension.

4.3.3 Compliance

Improved compliance with PEEP application has been traditionally considered to suggest recruitment. In their landmark paper, Suter et al. demonstrated that maximal oxygen transport occurred when PEEP was titrated to obtain the highest level of static compliance [11]. Adjustment of PEEP levels targeting static compliance is associated with improved oxygenation and organ function [15]. However, an increase in the compliance may solely reflect cyclical opening and closure of alveoli, without resulting in recruitment.

4.3.4 Driving Pressure

Driving pressure is tidal volume/static compliance. Thus, for a constant tidal volume, a decrease in driving pressure with incremental PEEP suggests alveolar recruitment. However, a decrease in driving pressure occurs due to increased compliance. Hence, PEEP adjustment based on driving pressures may have the same limitations as adjustment based on static compliance. Amato et al. performed a multilevel mediation analysis of 3562 patients from nine randomized controlled trials. They demonstrated that driving pressure was most strongly associated with survival; higher driving pressures were associated with increased mortality. Changes in tidal volume and PEEP were associated with survival only through concomitant changes in driving pressure [16].

4.3.5 Esophageal Pressure

During mechanical ventilation, the airway pressure attempts to distend the lung, while the pleural pressure acts as a counterforce in the opposite direction. Thus the true distending pressure applied to the lung is the transpulmonary pressure.

$$\text{Transpulmonary pressure} = \text{airway pressure} - \text{pleural pressure}$$

Abnormalities of the chest wall and abdomen (chest trauma, pleural effusion, obesity, abdominal compartment syndrome, etc.) tend to increase the pleural pressure, thus, reducing the transpulmonary pressure. Any increase in the chest wall elastance (increased chest wall stiffness) offsets the transpulmonary pressure, thus opposing lung inflation. Setting the PEEP level at or above the pleural pressure at end-expiration may prevent alveolar collapse during expiration. The esophageal pressure is measured as a close approximation of the pleural pressure to set an appropriate level of PEEP.

Titration of PEEP guided by measurement of esophageal pressure was compared with empirically set PEEP, based on the FiO_2 requirement, in a randomized controlled trial. In the esophageal pressure-guided group, the PEEP level was set between 0 and 6 cmH_2O higher than the esophageal pressure, based on the FiO_2 requirement. There was no significant difference between groups in the primary composite outcome of death and mechanical ventilation-free days through day 28 [17].

4.3.6 Imaging-Guided PEEP Titration

CT imaging may enable analysis of compressive forces acting on the lung at different levels. However, the utility of CT imaging to guide PEEP levels has not been corroborated in clinical practice [18]. Considering the practical difficulty related to repeated CT imaging in critically ill patients, this approach does not hold promise in most settings. Bouhemad et al. employed lung ultrasonography to evaluate PEEP-induced lung recruitment. They observed a significant correlation between the ultrasonographic reaeration score and lung recruitment measured using pressure-volume curves [19]. Ultrasonography is easily performed by the bedside in the critically ill and, hence, more feasible compared to CT imaging. However, the use of ultrasonography is limited by the inability to identify alveolar overdistension.

4.4 Electrical Impedance Tomography (EIT) for PEEP Titration

EIT is a noninvasive tool that allows PEEP titration by the bedside. An alternating current is applied using one pair of electrodes applied to the chest wall, while the induced voltages are measured from other electrodes. The difference in conductivity is utilized to reconstruct a 2D image that depicts the distribution of ventilation and perfusion across different regions of the lung. Using EIT, changes in lung volume through recruitment may be assessed, allowing optimal titration of the PEEP level [20]. Early studies suggest that EIT may be a useful tool in the assessment of the potential for recruitment by the bedside and individualization of PEEP levels [21, 22].

4.5 High vs. Low Levels of PEEP

Several studies have compared high vs. low PEEP levels, using PEEP/FiO_2 tables [4, 23] or based on inspiratory plateau pressures [24], with no difference in clinical outcomes.

The PHARLAP study compared an open-lung strategy of ventilation, including recruitment maneuvers and titrated PEEP with a conventional lung-protective ventilation strategy among patients with moderate to severe ARDS [25]. In the open-lung strategy group, the PEEP level was increased to 20 cmH_2O, followed by stepwise increments to 30 and 40 cmH_2O for 2 min each. The PEEP level was then reduced to 25 cmH_2O and titrated downward in steps of 2.5 cmH_2O every 3 min until the saturation dropped by more than 2% or to a minimum PEEP level of 15 cmH_2O. In the control group, patients were ventilated with a tidal volume of 4–6 mL/kg predicted body weight at a plateau pressure of less than 30 cmH_2O, with PEEP levels based on the ARDS-net low PEEP table. No significant difference in the 28-day mortality, the primary outcome, was observed between the two groups. The secondary outcomes, including ICU mortality, hospital mortality, mortality at 90 days and 6 months, and the duration of ICU and hospital stay, were also not significantly different between groups. The open-lung strategy was associated with an increase in the incidence of adverse cardiovascular events; however, there was a lower requirement for rescue therapies for refractory hypoxemia.

In the multicenter ART trial, a lung recruitment maneuver combined with PEEP titration targeting best compliance was compared to a low PEEP strategy in patients with moderate to severe ARDS [26]. The original recruitment technique was to apply a PEEP of 25 cmH_2O for 1 min, 35 cmH_2O for 1 min, and 45 cmH_2O for 2 min, followed by application of PEEP levels based on the best lung compliance. The strategy was modified to lower levels of PEEP after three instances of cardiac arrests with the original technique. A significantly higher 28-day mortality was observed with the strategy of recruitment and PEEP titration compared with the low-PEEP strategy (55.3% vs. 49.3%; hazard ratio 1.20, 95% CI: 1.01 to 1.42; $P = 0.041$).

Kacmarek et al. compared an open-lung ventilation strategy with the ARDS Network low PEEP protocol-based strategy. The open-lung strategy included a recruitment maneuver followed by downward titration of PEEP levels. There was no significant difference in the 60-day mortality between the two groups; besides, the ICU mortality and ventilation-free days were also similar. In the open-lung strategy group, a significant improvement was noted in oxygenation, lung mechanics, and the driving pressures [27].

A beneficial impact of PEEP would occur only among patients with potential for lung recruitment. It is likely that an empirical strategy, without assessment of the potential for recruitment, may result in beneficial effects in patients with recruitable lung; in contrast, it may lead to overdistension-related harmful effects if the lung is non-recruitable. Any high PEEP-related benefit may thus be offset by harm among the subgroup of patients with no potential for alveolar recruitment. Patient heterogeneity may thus confound trials that use fixed levels of PEEP among patients with wide variability in the level of recruitability. Table 4.2 summarizes controlled studies that have compared different levels of PEEP.

Table 4.2 Studies that compare different levels of PEEP in ARDS

Study/year	Population	Lower PEEP	Higher PEEP (open-lung strategy)	Outcomes
Hodgson et al. (PHARLAP 2019) [25]	Moderate to severe ARDS	ARDS-net low PEEP strategy	PEEP increased to 20 cmH_2O, stepwise increments to 30 and 40 H_2O for 2 min each, followed by reduction to 25 H_2O. Titrated down in steps of 2.5 H_2O every 3 min, until drop in SaO_2 by >2% or to a minimum PEEP of 15 H_2O	Mortality at 28-day, in ICU, in hospital, at 90 day and 6 months similar. Duration of ICU and hospital stay similar. Higher incidence of adverse cardiovascular events with higher PEEP; lower requirement for rescue therapies

Table 4.2 (continued)

Study/year	Population	Lower PEEP	Higher PEEP (open-lung strategy)	Outcomes
Cavalcanti et al. (ART, 2017) [26]	Moderate to severe ARDS	Conventional low PEEP strategy	RM with stepwise increment of PEEP to 25 (1 min), 35 (1 min), and 45 cmH_2O (2 min), followed by PEEP application based on best compliance. Strategy modified after adverse events to RM using 25, 30, and then 35 cmH_2O for 1 min each	Significantly higher 28-day and 6-month mortality, less ventilator-free days, higher incidence of pneumothoraces in the higher PEEP group
Kacmarek et al. (2016) [27]	ARDS	ARDS-net low PEEP strategy	RM with PCV to Ppeak between 50–60 cmH_2O and PEEP 35–45 cmH_2O depending on patient's response. PEEP set using a decremental PEEP trial based on compliance	60-day and ICU mortality, ventilator-free days similar. Driving pressures lower, PaO_2/FiO_2 ratio higher at 24,48, and 72 h with the open-lung (higher PEEP) approach

ARDS acute respiratory distress syndrome, *PEEP* positive end-expiratory pressure, *RM* recruitment maneuver, *PCV* pressure-controlled ventilation

Key Points

- An appropriate level of PEEP must be individualized based on the potential for recruitment.
- Empirically applied high PEEP levels are unlikely to benefit.
- Oxygenation response to increasing levels of PEEP may be an appropriate physiological endpoint and has been shown to improve survival.
- Improved compliance and a reduction in the driving pressure may be clinically useful indicators of recruitability associated with increasing levels of PEEP.
- Although transpulmonary pressure-guided PEEP application has a strong physiological rationale, clinical outcomes have been disappointing.
- Future research should focus on improved methodology for the assessment of recruitability and more precise titration of PEEP.

References

1. Ashbaugh DG, Bigelow DB, Petty TL, Levine BE. Acute respiratory distress in adults. Lancet. 1967;2(7511):319–23.
2. Sahetya SK, Goligher EC, Brower RG. Fifty years of research in ARDS. Setting positive end-expiratory pressure in acute respiratory distress syndrome. Am J Respir Crit Care Med. 2017;195(11):1429–38.
3. Muscedere JG, Mullen JB, Gan K, Slutsky AS. Tidal ventilation at low airway pressures can augment lung injury. Am J Respir Crit Care Med. 1994;149(5):1327–34.
4. Mead J, Takishima T, Leith D. Stress distribution in lungs: a model of pulmonary elasticity. J Appl Physiol. 1970;28(5):596–608.
5. Schreiber T, Hueter L, Gaser E, Schmidt B, Schwarzkopf K, Rek H, et al. PEEP has beneficial effects on inflammation in the injured and no deleterious effects on the noninjured lung after unilateral lung acid instillation. Intensive Care Med. 2006;32(5):740–9.
6. Slutsky AS. Lung injury caused by mechanical ventilation. Chest. 1999;116(1 Suppl):9S–15S.
7. Karbing DS, Panigada M, Bottino N, Spinelli E, Protti A, Rees SE, et al. Changes in shunt, ventilation/perfusion mismatch, and lung aeration with PEEP in patients with ARDS: a prospective single-arm interventional study. Crit Care. 2020;24(1):111.
8. Chiumello D, Marino A, Brioni M, Cigada I, Menga F, Colombo A, et al. Lung recruitment assessed by respiratory mechanics and computed tomography in patients with acute respiratory distress syndrome. What is the relationship? Am J Respir Crit Care Med. 2016;193(11):1254–63.
9. Dorinsky PM, Whitcomb ME. The effect of PEEP on cardiac output. Chest. 1983;84(2):210–6.
10. Vieillard-Baron A, Schmitt JM, Augarde R, Fellahi JL, Prin S, Page B, et al. Acute cor pulmonale in acute respiratory distress syndrome submitted to protective ventilation: incidence, clinical implications, and prognosis. Crit Care Med. 2001;29(8):1551–5.
11. Suter PM, Fairley B, Isenberg MD. Optimum end-expiratory airway pressure in patients with acute pulmonary failure. N Engl J Med. 1975;292(6):284–9.
12. Eisner MD, Thompson BT, Schoenfeld D, Anzueto A, Matthay MA. Acute respiratory distress syndrome network. Airway pressures and early barotrauma in patients with acute lung injury and acute respiratory distress syndrome. Am J Respir Crit Care Med. 2002;165(7):978–82.
13. Acute Respiratory Distress Syndrome Network, Brower RG, Matthay MA, Morris A, Schoenfeld D, Thompson BT, et al. Ventilation with lower tidal volumes as compared with traditional tidal volumes for acute lung injury and the acute respiratory distress syndrome. N Engl J Med. 2000;342(18):1301–8.
14. Goligher EC, Kavanagh BP, Rubenfeld GD, Adhikari NKJ, Pinto R, Fan E, et al. Oxygenation response to positive end-expiratory pressure predicts mortality in acute respiratory distress syndrome. A secondary analysis of the LOVS and ExPress trials. Am J Respir Crit Care Med. 2014;190(1):70–6.
15. Pintado MC, de Pablo R, Trascasa M, Milicua JM, Rogero S, Daguerre M, et al. Individualized PEEP setting in subjects with ARDS: a randomized controlled pilot study. Respir Care. 2013;58(9):1416–23.
16. Amato MBP, Meade MO, Slutsky AS, Brochard L, Costa ELV, Schoenfeld DA, et al. Driving pressure and survival in the acute respiratory distress syndrome. N Engl J Med. 2015;372(8):747–55.
17. Beitler JR, Sarge T, Banner-Goodspeed VM, Gong MN, Cook D, Novack V, et al. Effect of titrating positive end-expiratory pressure (PEEP) with an esophageal pressure-guided strategy vs an empirical high PEEP-Fio2 strategy on death and days free from mechanical ventilation among patients with acute respiratory distress syndrome: a randomized clinical trial. JAMA. 2019;321(9):846–57.
18. Cressoni M, Chiumello D, Carlesso E, Chiurazzi C, Amini M, Brioni M, et al. Compressive forces and computed tomography-derived positive end-expiratory pressure in acute respiratory distress syndrome. Anesthesiology. 2014;121(3):572–81.

19. Bouhemad B, Brisson H, Le-Guen M, Arbelot C, Lu Q, Rouby JJ. Bedside ultrasound assessment of positive end-expiratory pressure-induced lung recruitment. Am J Respir Crit Care Med. 2011;183(3):341–7.
20. Sella N, Pettenuzzo T, Zarantonello F, Andreatta G, De Cassai A, Schiavolin C, et al. Electrical impedance tomography: a compass for the safe route to optimal PEEP. Respir Med. 2021;187:106555.
21. Perier F, Tuffet S, Maraffi T, Alcala G, Victor M, Haudebourg AF, et al. Electrical impedance tomography to titrate positive end-expiratory pressure in COVID-19 acute respiratory distress syndrome. Crit Care. 2020;24(1):678.
22. Sella N, Zarantonello F, Andreatta G, Gagliardi V, Boscolo A, Navalesi P. Positive end-expiratory pressure titration in COVID-19 acute respiratory failure: electrical impedance tomography vs. PEEP/FiO2 tables. Crit Care. 2020;24(1):540.
23. Brower RG, Lanken PN, MacIntyre N, Matthay MA, Morris A, Ancukiewicz M, et al. Higher versus lower positive end-expiratory pressures in patients with the acute respiratory distress syndrome. N Engl J Med. 2004;351(4):327–36.
24. Mercat A, Richard JCM, Vielle B, Jaber S, Osman D, Diehl JL, et al. Positive end-expiratory pressure setting in adults with acute lung injury and acute respiratory distress syndrome: a randomized controlled trial. JAMA. 2008;299(6):646–55.
25. Hodgson CL, Cooper DJ, Arabi Y, King V, Bersten A, Bihari S, et al. Maximal recruitment open lung ventilation in acute respiratory distress syndrome (PHARLAP). A phase II, multicenter randomized controlled clinical trial. Am J Respir Crit Care Med. 2019;200(11):1363–72.
26. Cavalcanti AB, Suzumura ÉA, Laranjeira LN, de Paisani DM, Damiani LP, Guimarães HP, et al. Effect of lung recruitment and titrated positive end-expiratory pressure (PEEP) vs low PEEP on mortality in patients with acute respiratory distress syndrome. JAMA. 2017;318(14):1335–45.
27. Kacmarek RM, Villar J, Sulemanji D, Montiel R, Ferrando C, Blanco J, et al. Open lung approach for the acute respiratory distress syndrome: a pilot, randomized controlled trial*. Crit Care Med. 2016;44(1):32–42.

Do Vigorous Spontaneous Respiratory Efforts Lead to Patient Self-Inflicted Lung Injury (P-SILI)?

5

5.1 Introduction

There is increasing concern that continued vigorous spontaneous respiratory efforts may be harmful in the presence of severe lung injury. The adverse outcomes associated with high tidal volumes during invasive mechanical ventilation are well established [1]. Transpulmonary pressure swings, representing lung stress, are comparable with spontaneous, controlled, or partially supported breaths when similar tidal volumes are delivered [2]. Thus, high tidal volumes may be equally injurious with spontaneous or assisted breaths compared to controlled breaths. Patients with de novo acute hypoxemic respiratory failure (AHRF) may have a strong respiratory drive, leading to the generation of large spontaneous tidal volumes. The intense respiratory efforts may exacerbate injury to the already damaged lung and has been termed patient self-inflicted lung injury (P-SILI) [3].

5.2 Mechanisms of P-SILI

Mascheroni et al., in a seminal study, evaluated the effect of metabolic acidosis-induced hyperventilation on adult sheep by injection of sodium salicylate into the cisternal magna [4]. They observed a drop in the PaO_2 levels, decrease in the lung compliance, and infiltrates on the chest radiograph. These changes did not occur in control animals who were mechanically ventilated with sedation and neuromuscular blockade. Vigorous spontaneous respiratory efforts lead to increased lung strain, with a similar risk for injury as with high tidal volume ventilation delivered during controlled mechanical ventilation, and may precipitate P-SILI. Recurrent, delayed-onset pulmonary edema has also been observed following hyperventilation due to diabetic ketoacidosis [5].

J. Chacko et al., *Controversies in Critical Care*,
https://doi.org/10.1007/978-981-19-9940-6_5

The force applied to the lung is the transpulmonary pressure and represents the stress experienced by the lung [6].

$$\text{Stress applied} = \text{transpulmonary pressure}$$

$$\text{Transpulmonary pressure} = \text{alveolar pressure} - \text{pleural pressure}$$

The resulting strain is the deformation that occurs in the lung and is represented by the ratio of the tidal volume (V_t) to the end-expiratory lung volume [6].

$$\text{Lung strain} = V_t / \text{end-expiratory lung volume.}$$

5.2.1 Nonuniform Distribution of Pleural Pressure

The delivery of V_t requires a transpulmonary pressure gradient. The transpulmonary pressure gradient may be achieved by either an increase in the alveolar pressure during controlled mechanical ventilation or a decrease in the pleural pressure during spontaneous breathing. The stress experienced by the lung, represented by the transpulmonary pressure, depends on the tidal volume delivered, regardless of whether the breaths are spontaneous or controlled [2]. The negative pleural pressure generated during a spontaneous respiratory effort is distributed uniformly throughout the normal lung. However, in the injured lung, during spontaneous breathing, the negative pleural pressure is selectively distributed to the dependent regions of the lung, which are in close proximity to the diaphragm. This leads to greater transpulmonary pressure swings leading to overdistension and increased lung stress localized to the dependent regions [7]. Furthermore, air may be drawn from the nondependent to the dependent regions of the lung, referred to as the "pendelluft" phenomenon [3] (Fig. 5.1). Pendelluft leads to cyclical inspiratory overdistension and expiratory collapse in the dependent areas, resulting in worsening of lung injury [8]. The nonuniform distribution of pleural and transpulmonary pressures during spontaneous breathing disappears with the abolition of spontaneous respiratory efforts with neuromuscular blockade [9].

5.2.2 Increase in the Transmural Pressure Within the Pulmonary Capillaries

During fully controlled ventilation, the alveolar pressure remains higher than the PEEP level during most of the respiratory cycle. However, with assisted modes of ventilation, during a spontaneous respiratory effort, the alveolar pressure often drops below the PEEP level [2]. The pleural pressure becomes more negative, leading to an increase in the transmural vascular pressure (pressure gradient across

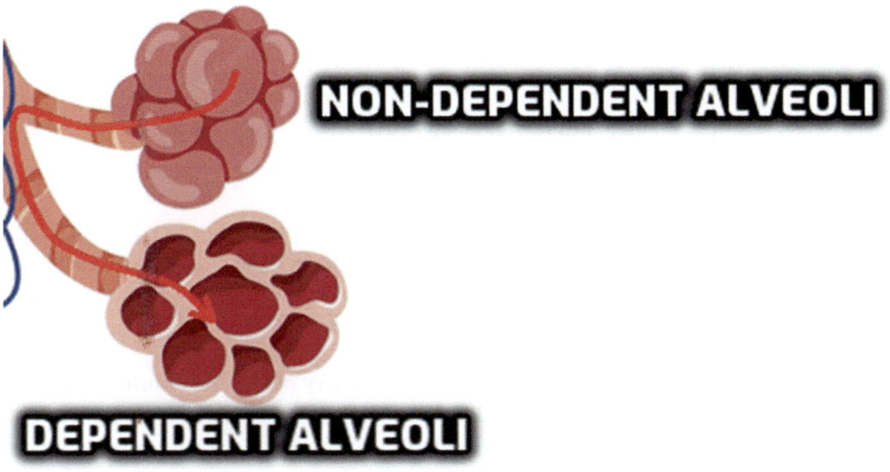

Fig. 5.1 The pendelluft phenomenon. In the injured lung, the pleural pressure is more negative in the dependent regions of the lung. Higher transpulmonary pressure swings lead to overdistension of the dependent alveoli. Air is drawn from the nondependent to the dependent regions of the lung

pulmonary vessels). In the injured lung with high pulmonary capillary permeability, the increase in the transmural vascular pressure leads to worsening of pulmonary edema [10]. An increase in the airway resistance may exacerbate this effect due to the development of more negative alveolar pressures during a spontaneous inspiratory effort [11].

5.3 Patient-Ventilator Dyssynchrony

5.3.1 Double Triggering

When the set inspiratory time on the ventilator is shorter than the inspiratory time of a spontaneous breath, the patient inspiratory effort continues into the expiratory phase of the ventilator-assisted breath. The continued patient inspiratory effort leads to triggering of a second assisted breath, resulting in the phenomenon of "double triggering" (Fig. 5.2), with delivery of twice the set tidal volume, and breath-stacking. Repeated delivery of high tidal volumes may lead to perpetuation of lung injury [12, 13].

5.3.2 Reverse Triggering

In the phenomenon of reverse triggering, a fully controlled mechanical breath is followed by reflex diaphragmatic contraction and triggering of another breath. The

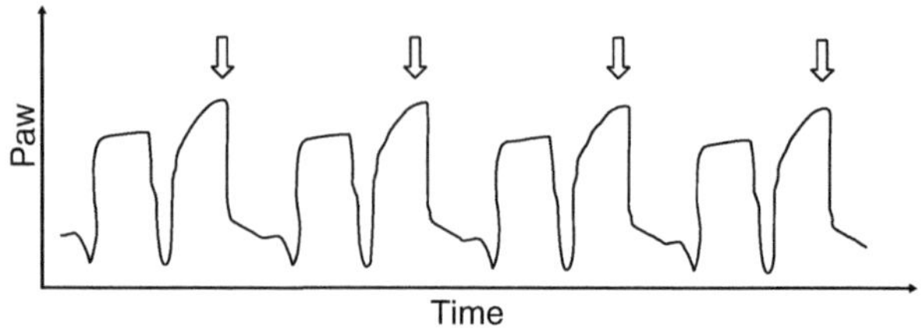

Fig. 5.2 Pressure-controlled ventilation with double triggering. The patient inspiratory effort continues into the expiratory phase of the ventilator-assisted breath, resulting in two ventilator breaths with a short expiratory time. Thus, a single inspiratory effort results in two breaths and leads to an increase in tidal volume that may trigger P-SILI

"reverse triggered" breath occurs during the inspiratory phase and continues into the expiratory phase of the fully controlled mechanical breath [14]. The phenomenon of reverse triggering may occur with deep sedation and when the sedative effect begins to wane [12]. Reverse triggering may also lead to breath-stacking, may increase in the transpulmonary pressure and tidal volume, and may initiate or perpetuate dependent lung injury through the pendelluft effect [15].

5.4 Evidence for P-SILI

Worsening of lung injury through uncontrolled spontaneous respiratory efforts may be difficult to establish, particularly considering the difficulty associated with monitoring of physiological variables in unintubated patients. Besides, worsening of lung injury may be attributed to the underlying disease process [3]. There is mainly indirect clinical evidence for the occurrence of P-SILI with exacerbation of lung injury. There are several reports of vigorous spontaneous respiratory efforts leading to worsening hypoxia, pulmonary edema, and barotrauma [16–18]. The abolition of vigorous spontaneous respiratory efforts using neuromuscular blockade has been demonstrated to improve clinical outcomes including survival [19, 20]. The available clinical data suggest that injury-provoking, vigorous, spontaneous respiratory effort is often difficult to control and may necessitate the use of neuromuscular blockade.

5.5 Monitoring of Respiratory Drive and Prevention of P-SILI

5.5.1 Clinical Monitoring

Clinical monitoring for the presence of a strong respiratory drive is the key to identifying the risk of P-SILI. During volume assist control ventilation, the presence of a spontaneous breath results in a decrease in the height of the airway pressure waveform, with the concavity directed upward. An intense inspiratory effort is usually

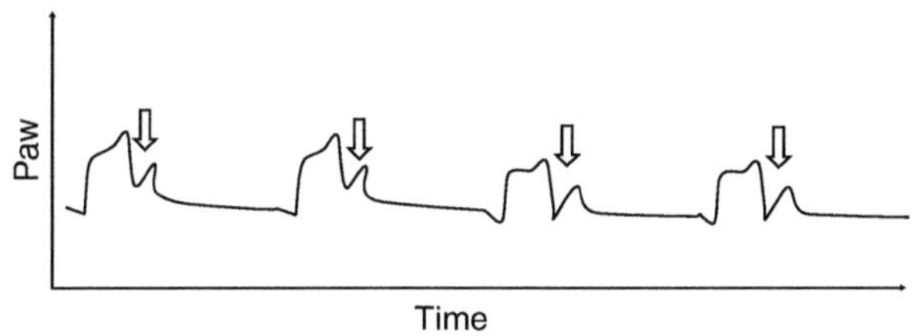

Fig. 5.3 Volume-controlled ventilation with the pressure waveform depicting vigorous spontaneous inspiratory efforts. A progressive increase in the inspiratory effort is seen as a deepening of the "cleft" (arrows)

easy to discern on the pressure waveform (Fig. 5.3). The presence of breath-stacking may also be evident on the airway pressure and flow waveforms [21]. The presence of double or reverse triggering should also be monitored. During pressure support ventilation, clinical signs of respiratory distress may be the only pointer toward injurious spontaneous respiratory efforts.

5.5.2 Objective Measures of Spontaneous Respiratory Efforts

The drop in esophageal pressure during inspiration can be directly monitored on some ventilators and enables detection of strong inspiratory efforts. Esophageal pressure may also be used to monitor the transpulmonary driving pressure [22]. The electrical activity of the diaphragm (EAdi) may be monitored with an eso-gastric electrode and a dedicated ventilator [23]. Other methods used to assess the intensity of spontaneous respiratory efforts include measurement of the airway occlusion pressure during the first 100 ms of the inspiratory phase ($P_{0.1}$) [24] and thickening fraction of the diaphragm by ultrasonography [25].

5.6 How Can P-SILI Be Prevented?

5.6.1 Noninvasive Ventilation (NIV) and High-Flow Nasal Oxygen (HFNO)

The application of PEEP may reduce the pendelluft effect and ameliorate atelectrauma to the dependent areas of the lung [26]. Experimental observations have revealed that following phrenic nerve stimulation, the pleural pressure change is reduced by increasing the PEEP level as the end-expiratory lung volume rises with the increase in PEEP. The more intense the spontaneous respiratory effort, the greater the pleural pressure change, and the higher the risk of lung injury [27]. The increase in the end-expiratory lung volume may also reduce muscular injury to the diaphragm by altering its curvature [28]. Besides, the application of an appropriate level of PEEP may improve gas exchange and reduce the respiratory drive. Patel et al. compared NIV applied through a helmet with conventional face mask NIV in a randomized controlled trial. The use of a helmet resulted in reduced respiratory drive accompanied by a lower respiratory rate, reduced requirement for intubation, more ventilator-free days, and improved survival. The improved outcomes associated with the use of the helmet NIV were attributed to more sustained PEEP levels compared to mask NIV [29].

HFNO enables elimination of carbon dioxide from the anatomical dead space, thereby reducing the requirement for ventilatory effort. However, the inability to monitor tidal volumes is a concern with HFNO use. In a prospective observational study, the ROX index, calculated by the ratio SpO_2/FiO_2 to respiratory rate, was used to identify patients at risk of failure with HFNO therapy. A ROX index of less than 2.85 at 2 h, 3.47 at 6 h, and 3.85 at 12 h after initiation of therapy predicted failure with HFNO [30].

5.6.2 Early Invasive Ventilation as a Part of a Lung-Protective Strategy

Identification of patients who may benefit from early invasive ventilation is crucial as part of the strategy to prevent possible harm from P-SILI due to enhanced respiratory drive. Abolition of spontaneous respiratory efforts with the use of neuromuscular blocking agents reduces the pro-inflammatory state in ARDS [28, 31]. The use of continuous neuromuscular blockade with cisatracurium in patients with early ARDS during the first 48 h of mechanical ventilation was evaluated in the ACURASYS study. The adjusted 90-day mortality, the primary outcome, was significantly lower with continuous neuromuscular blockade compared to the control group [19]. These studies reinforce the possibility of improved outcomes with a fully controlled ventilator strategy in severe ARDS.

The judicious use of PEEP may ameliorate the impact of P-SILI, as evidenced by the ROSE trial [32]. In contrast to the ACURASYS trial, the ROSE trial did not reveal a significant difference in the 90-day mortality with the use of cisatracurium infusion for 48 h after enrolment compared to a control group that received usual care. This was probably because of the relatively higher level of PEEP employed in the ROSE trial, with a possible protective effect against P-SILI in the control group.

The strategy of mechanical ventilation has undergone refinement in the past two decades with emphasis on lung-protective strategies, including the use of low tidal volumes, and increasing focus on optimizing transpulmonary and driving pressures (driving pressure = P_{plat} − PEEP). In this context, the important question arises whether persistence with NIV or other assisted modes of ventilation could lead to harm, compared with a strategy of early intubation, and controlled, lung-protective mechanical ventilation in patients with AHRF. Importantly, the crucial question regarding the appropriate timing of invasive ventilation needs to be investigated, considering the evidence of poor outcomes with NIV failure in AHRF [33].

Key Points

- A strong respiratory drive with vigorous spontaneous breathing efforts may exacerbate lung injury.
- In the injured lung, the negative pleural pressure generated through spontaneous respiratory efforts is prominently distributed to the dependent areas of the lung, which have a greater predilection to damage.
- Intense negative pleural pressures lead to an increase in the transmural vascular pressure across the pulmonary vasculature, leading to aggravation of capillary leak and pulmonary edema.
- Asynchrony with mechanically delivered breaths may result in double or reverse triggering, leading to worsening of lung injury.
- The intensity of the spontaneous respiratory drive must be closely monitored to recognize patients at risk of developing P-SILI. Clinical assessment combined with esophageal pressure monitoring may help to identify spontaneous respiratory efforts that may predispose to lung injury.
- NIV and HFNO therapy may attenuate the respiratory drive and reduce the risk of P-SILI.
- Optimizing PEEP levels may reduce injury by increasing the end-expiratory lung volume and inhibiting the adverse impact of pendelluft on the dependent areas of the lung.
- Timely intubation and judicious use of sedatives and neuromuscular blockade are important strategies in the prevention of P-SILI.

References

1. Acute Respiratory Distress Syndrome Network, Brower RG, Matthay MA, Morris A, Schoenfeld D, Thompson BT, et al. Ventilation with lower tidal volumes as compared with traditional tidal volumes for acute lung injury and the acute respiratory distress syndrome. N Engl J Med. 2000;342(18):1301–8.
2. Bellani G, Grasselli G, Teggia-Droghi M, Mauri T, Coppadoro A, Brochard L, et al. Do spontaneous and mechanical breathing have similar effects on average transpulmonary and alveolar pressure? A clinical crossover study. Crit Care. 2016;20(1):142.
3. Brochard L, Slutsky A, Pesenti A. Mechanical ventilation to minimize progression of lung injury in acute respiratory failure. Am J Respir Crit Care Med. 2017;195(4):438–42.
4. Mascheroni D, Kolobow T, Fumagalli R, Moretti MP, Chen V, Buckhold D. Acute respiratory failure following pharmacologically induced hyperventilation: an experimental animal study. Intensive Care Med. 1988;15(1):8–14.
5. Brun-Buisson CJ, Bonnet F, Bergeret S, Lemaire F, Rapin M. Recurrent high-permeability pulmonary edema associated with diabetic ketoacidosis. Crit Care Med. 1985;13(1):55–6.
6. Gattinoni L, Carlesso E, Caironi P. Stress and strain within the lung. Curr Opin Crit Care. 2012;18(1):42–7.
7. Yoshida T, Torsani V, Gomes S, De Santis RR, Beraldo MA, Costa ELV, et al. Spontaneous effort causes occult pendelluft during mechanical ventilation. Am J Respir Crit Care Med. 2013;188(12):1420–7.

8. Caironi P, Cressoni M, Chiumello D, Ranieri M, Quintel M, Russo SG, et al. Lung opening and closing during ventilation of acute respiratory distress syndrome. Am J Respir Crit Care Med. 2010;181(6):578–86.
9. Yoshida T, Nakahashi S, Nakamura MAM, Koyama Y, Roldan R, Torsani V, et al. Volume-controlled ventilation does not prevent injurious inflation during spontaneous effort. Am J Respir Crit Care Med. 2017;196(5):590–601.
10. Bhattacharya M, Kallet RH, Ware LB, Matthay MA. Negative-pressure pulmonary edema. Chest. 2016;150(4):927–33.
11. Loyd JE, Nolop KB, Parker RE, Roselli RJ, Brigham KL. Effects of inspiratory resistance loading on lung fluid balance in awake sheep. J Appl Physiol. 1985;60(1):198–203.
12. de Haro C, Ochagavia A, López-Aguilar J, Fernandez-Gonzalo S, Navarra-Ventura G, Magrans R, et al. Patient-ventilator asynchronies during mechanical ventilation: current knowledge and research priorities. Intensive Care Med Exp. 2019;7(Suppl 1):43.
13. Thille AW, Rodriguez P, Cabello B, Lellouche F, Brochard L. Patient-ventilator asynchrony during assisted mechanical ventilation. Intensive Care Med. 2006;32(10):1515–22.
14. Akoumianaki E, Lyazidi A, Rey N, Matamis D, Perez-Martinez N, Giraud R, et al. Mechanical ventilation-induced reverse-triggered breaths: a frequently unrecognized form of neuromechanical coupling. Chest. 2013;143(4):927–38.
15. Yoshida T, Nakamura MAM, Morais CCA, Amato MBP, Kavanagh BP. Reverse triggering causes an injurious inflation pattern during mechanical ventilation. Am J Respir Crit Care Med. 2018;198(8):1096–9.
16. Kallet RH, Alonso JA, Luce JM, Matthay MA. Exacerbation of acute pulmonary edema during assisted mechanical ventilation using a low-tidal volume, lung-protective ventilator strategy. Chest. 1999;116(6):1826–32.
17. Leray V, Bourdin G, Flandreau G, Bayle F, Wallet F, Richard JC, et al. A case of pneumomediastinum in a patient with acute respiratory distress syndrome on pressure support ventilation. Respir Care. 2010;55(6):770–3.
18. Sasidhar M, Chatburn RL. Tidal volume variability during airway pressure release ventilation: case summary and theoretical analysis. Respir Care. 2012;57(8):1325–33.
19. Papazian L, Forel JM, Gacouin A, Penot-Ragon C, Perrin G, Loundou A, et al. Neuromuscular blockers in early acute respiratory distress syndrome. N Engl J Med. 2010;363(12):1107–16.
20. Gainnier M, Roch A, Forel JM, Thirion X, Arnal JM, Donati S, et al. Effect of neuromuscular blocking agents on gas exchange in patients presenting with acute respiratory distress syndrome. Crit Care Med. 2004;32(1):113–9.
21. Carteaux G, Parfait M, Combet M, Haudebourg AF, Tuffet S, Mekontso DA. Patient-self inflicted lung injury: a practical review. J Clin Med. 2021;10(12):2738.
22. Goligher EC, Dres M, Patel BK, Sahetya SK, Beitler JR, Telias I, et al. Lung-and diaphragm-protective ventilation. Am J Respir Crit Care Med. 2020;202(7):950–61.
23. Beck J, Gottfried SB, Navalesi P, Skrobik Y, Comtois N, Rossini M, et al. Electrical activity of the diaphragm during pressure support ventilation in acute respiratory failure. Am J Respir Crit Care Med. 2001;164(3):419–24.
24. Vaporidi K, Akoumianaki E, Telias I, Goligher EC, Brochard L, Georgopoulos D. Respiratory drive in critically ill patients. Pathophysiology and clinical implications. Am J Respir Crit Care Med. 2020;201(1):20–32.
25. Tuinman PR, Jonkman AH, Dres M, Shi ZH, Goligher EC, Goffi A, et al. Respiratory muscle ultrasonography: methodology, basic and advanced principles and clinical applications in ICU and ED patients-a narrative review. Intensive Care Med. 2020;46(4):594–605.
26. Santini A, Mauri T, Dalla Corte F, Spinelli E, Pesenti A. Effects of inspiratory flow on lung stress, pendelluft, and ventilation heterogeneity in ARDS: a physiological study. Crit Care. 2019;23(1):369.
27. De Troyer A, Leduc D, Cappello M, Mine B, Gevenois PA, Wilson TA. Mechanisms of the inspiratory action of the diaphragm during isolated contraction. J Appl Physiol. 2009;107(6):1736–42.

28. Yoshida T, Grieco DL, Brochard L, Fujino Y. Patient self-inflicted lung injury and positive end-expiratory pressure for safe spontaneous breathing. Curr Opin Crit Care. 2020;26(1):59–65.
29. Patel BK, Wolfe KS, Pohlman AS, Hall JB, Kress JP. Effect of noninvasive ventilation delivered by helmet vs face mask on the rate of endotracheal intubation in patients with acute respiratory distress syndrome: a randomized clinical trial. JAMA. 2016;315(22):2435–41.
30. Roca O, Caralt B, Messika J, Samper M, Sztrymf B, Hernández G, et al. An index combining respiratory rate and oxygenation to predict outcome of nasal high-flow therapy. Am J Respir Crit Care Med. 2019;199(11):1368–76.
31. Forel JM, Roch A, Marin V, Michelet P, Demory D, Blache JL, et al. Neuromuscular blocking agents decrease inflammatory response in patients presenting with acute respiratory distress syndrome. Crit Care Med. 2006;34(11):2749–57.
32. National Heart, Lung, and Blood Institute PETAL Clinical Trials Network, Moss M, Huang DT, Brower RG, Ferguson ND, Ginde AA, et al. Early neuromuscular blockade in the acute respiratory distress syndrome. N Engl J Med. 2019;380(21):1997–2008.
33. Bellani G, Laffey JG, Pham T, Madotto F, Fan E, Brochard L, et al. Noninvasive ventilation of patients with acute respiratory distress syndrome. Insights from the LUNG SAFE study. Am J Respir Crit Care Med. 2017;195(1):67–77.

Prone Ventilation in Acute Respiratory Distress Syndrome

6

6.1 Introduction

Mechanical ventilation in the prone position has been employed for more than four decades to treat severe hypoxemia in acute respiratory failure. In a report from 1976, Piehl and Roberts described the use of prone ventilation in five patients using a special type of bed that could rotate the patient through 180° [1]. The authors reported a mean increase in PaO_2 of 47 ± 16 mmHg in the prone position with other ventilation parameters held constant. It was also observed that children with severe cystic fibrosis often positioned themselves on their hands and knees to ease breathing efforts [2]. Ventilation in the prone position became more widespread over the next two decades with the recognition of the nonhomogeneous nature of the diseased lung in acute respiratory distress syndrome (ARDS) and the concept of the "baby lung" [3]. What is the mechanism behind the beneficial effects of prone ventilation on the lung and chest wall mechanics and ventilation/perfusion matching?

6.2 How Does Prone Ventilation Result in More Homogenous Ventilation?

In ARDS, widespread edema occurs, leading to an increase in the weight of the lung. The dependent areas of the lung are compressed by the weight of the overlying, nondependent areas of the lung, due to gravitational effect. This results in collapse of the dependent areas of the lung as air is "squeezed out."

J. Chacko et al., *Controversies in Critical Care*,
https://doi.org/10.1007/978-981-19-9940-6_6

6.2.1 Difference in Lung Mass Between the Dorsal and Ventral Regions

The lung assumes the shape of a cone with the apex directed ventrally and the base directed dorsally. If a line is drawn halfway between the apex and the base of the cone, a relatively larger lung mass (75%) exists at the bottom, dorsal half of the cone compared to the ventral half (25%). In the supine position, gravity dictates that the relatively larger lung mass located in the dorsal areas undergo compression collapse. In contrast, in the prone position, the dorsal areas of the lung become nondependent and are relatively free from gravitational effect and compression by the overlying lung. This results in the larger, dorsal lung mass being released from the compression effect in the prone position. Thus, the distribution of ventilation becomes more uniform in the prone position [4] (Fig. 6.1).

6.2.2 Compression Effect Exerted by the Heart

Considering the conical shape of the lung, in the supine position, approximately 20% of the lung mass is located above the heart, compared to 50% below [5]. Thus, a larger lung mass is subjected to compression by the heart in the supine position. In contrast, on assuming the prone position, the larger part of the lung overlies the heart and is relieved from compression by the weight of the heart. This phenomenon also contributes to more homogenous ventilation in the prone position [6].

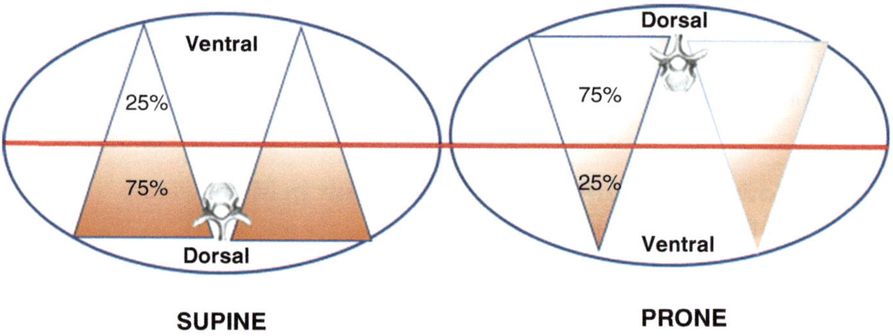

Fig. 6.1 The lung is shaped like a cone with the apex directed ventrally and the base directed dorsally. A relatively larger lung mass exists at the bottom, dorsal half of the cone compared to the ventral half. In the supine position, the force of gravity causes compression collapse of the dorsal lung regions. When prone, the dorsal areas, representing larger lung mass, become nondependent and freed from the gravitational effect and compression by the overlying lung. Thus, distribution of ventilation becomes more uniform in the prone position

6.2.3 Difference in Compliance Between the Ventral and Dorsal Chest Wall

In the supine position, the posterior wall of the chest is in contract with the surface; thus, it is relatively rigid with reduced movement. Compliance is determined by the anterior chest wall and the diaphragm. On turning prone, the posterior wall becomes nondependent and more mobile; however, the posterior wall is less compliant compared to the anterior wall. This leads to increased air movement and recruitment of the ventral areas of the lung, resulting in a more uniform distribution of ventilation [7].

6.2.4 The Shape of the Lung and the Chest Wall

In the supine position, the ventral regions of the lung, which constitute the apex of the lung cone, are relatively free to expand as it aligns with the more spherical shape of the anterior chest wall, allowing better ventilation of these areas. Gravitational forces also preferentially redistribute ventilation to the ventral regions. However, in the prone position, while the ventral areas of the lung remain free to expand and align with the chest wall, elimination of gravitational forces leads to better ventilation of the dorsal, nondependent lung. Thus the forces that dictate ventilation are more balanced in the prone position, allowing more uniform ventilation of different regions of the lung [4].

6.2.5 Effect of Intra-Abdominal Pressure

In the supine position, the intra-abdominal pressure exceeds the intrathoracic pressure; this phenomenon is exacerbated by obesity [8]. The compressive effect of intra-abdominal pressure is higher in the dorsal and inferior areas of the lung. The adverse impact of weight and pressure generated by the abdominal contents on the thoracic cavity is attenuated in the prone position, leading to better ventilation of the dorsal and inferior areas of the lung [9].

Overall, a more homogenous distribution of ventilation occurs in the prone position. More homogenous ventilation leads to a more uniform distribution of transpulmonary pressures, resulting in reduced lung stress [10].

6.3 Does the Prone Position Result in a More Homogenous Distribution of Lung Perfusion?

Gravitational effects may seem to favor increased blood flow to the ventral areas of the lung in the prone position. However, it has been clearly demonstrated in experimental [11] and human studies [12] that regardless of posture, perfusion is always higher in the dorsal regions of the lung. The perfusion bias to the dorsal lung regions, regardless of posture, is related to the unique vascular geometry of the lung. Thus, although the gravitational effect tends to redistribute perfusion ventrally, vascular geometry ensures preserved blood flow to the dorsal areas of the lung in the prone position [6]. The net result is a more homogenous distribution of perfusion in the prone compared to the supine position. The dorsal areas of the lung are better ventilated, while perfusion is maintained to these areas, thus, augmenting ventilation/perfusion matching.

6.4 What Is the Evidence?

Let us consider the major randomized controlled trials (RCT) that evaluated the physiological effects and clinical efficacy of the prone position in hypoxemic patients on mechanical ventilation (Table 6.1).

In one of the early RCTs on the efficacy of ventilation in the prone position, Gattinoni et al. studied 304 patients [13]. Patients were placed prone for 6 h or more daily, for 10 days. The PaO_2/FiO_2 ratio was significantly higher in the prone group; however, the relative risk of death was not different between groups at the end of the 10-day study period, at ICU discharge, and at 6 months. The low tidal volume strategy had not been established as practice during the study period; the mean baseline tidal volume was more than 650 mL in both groups. Besides, the study was stopped prematurely as recruitment slowed down over time. Although this study did not show improved mortality overall, on post hoc analysis, a significantly lower 10-day mortality was observed with prone ventilation in the quartile with the lowest PaO_2/FiO_2 ratios. This seminal study paved the way for further investigation of the possible clinical benefits of prone ventilation among severely hypoxemic patients.

Table 6.1 Major randomized controlled trials evaluating prone ventilation in patients with ARDS

Study/year	No of patients	Methodology	Outcomes	Comments
Gattinoni et al. (2001) [13]	304	Prone position for 6 h/day for 10 days	RR for death not different at ICU discharge and 6 months. P/F ratio higher in the prone position. Significantly lower mortality among patients with the lowest P/F ratios	Study was during the era before low Vt had become standard practice. The mean baseline V_t was around 650 mL in both groups
Guerin et al. (2004) [14]	791	P/F ratio <300 mmHg. Prone for 8 h/day	P/F ratios higher in the prone position. 28-day and 90-day mortality similar between groups. No difference in duration of ventilation and VAP	Adverse events more when prone

Table 6.1 (continued)

Study/year	No of patients	Methodology	Outcomes	Comments
Mancebo et al. (2006) [15]	136	Prone for 17 h/day for 10.1 day (mean)	Nonsignificant lower ICU mortality in the prone group. Improved P/F ratios with prone position	This study suggested that an extended duration of proning may improve survival
Taccone et al. (2009) [16]	342	Patients with moderate and severe hypoxemia. Prone for 18 h/day (mean)	Overall mortality similar at 28 day and 6 months. Trend toward lower mortality in patients with severe hypoxemia	This study suggested that patients with severe hypoxemia may benefit with prone ventilation
Guérin et al. (PROSEVA) (2013) [17]	466	Patients with severe hypoxemia, P/F ratio <150 mmHg. Prone for 17 h (mean). Mean of four sessions per patient	28- and 90-day mortality lower with prone position. Successful extubation at 90 day higher with prone; ventilator-free days at 28 and 90 day significantly more with prone ventilation	Lower requirement for rescue therapies (NO, ECMO) in the prone position. This landmark trial finally demonstrated improved survival with prone ventilation in ARDS

RR relative risk, *NO* nitric oxide, *ECMO* extracorporeal membrane oxygenation, *ARDS* acute respiratory distress syndrome

A French study conducted during the same period enrolled 791 patients with acute respiratory failure with a PaO_2/FiO_2 ratio of less than 300 mmHg [14]. Prone positioning was carried out for at least 8 h daily. The primary endpoint, the 28-day mortality, was similar between the prone and supine groups (32.4% vs. 31.5%, $p = 0.74$). There was no significant difference in the secondary endpoints, including the 90-day mortality, duration of mechanical ventilation, or the incidence of ventilator-associated pneumonia. Similar to the study by Gattinoni et al., the PaO_2/FiO_2 ratios were significantly higher with prone ventilation. Adverse events, including pressure sores, endobronchial intubation, and tube blocks were more common in the prone group. This study also demonstrated improvement in oxygenation with prone positioning, which did not translate to improved survival.

The Spanish study by Mancebo et al. represented a breakthrough, with the use of lower tidal volumes compared to the previous two studies and an extended duration of prone ventilation [15]. Plateau pressures employed were also lower in this study, with increasing awareness of the beneficial effects of a lung-protective ventilation strategy. Sixty patients with severe ARDS were randomized to supine and 76 to prone ventilation. Prone ventilation was carried out for an average of 17 h per day for a mean duration of 10.1 ± 10.3 days. Although not statistically significant, lower ICU mortality was observed among patients who underwent prone ventilation (43% vs. 58%, $p = 0.12$). On multivariate analysis, independent risk factors for mortality included randomization to the supine position, the simplified acute physiology score II (SAPS II) at baseline, and the time interval between the diagnosis of ARDS and study inclusion. Similar to previous studies, the authors observed a significantly higher PaO_2/FiO_2 ratio in patients who were prone ventilated. This study suggested that an extended duration of prone ventilation combined with a lung-protective strategy may improve survival in patients with severe ARDS.

Subsequently, Taccone et al. studied the clinical efficacy of prone ventilation among patients with moderate (PaO_2/FiO_2 100–200 mmHg) and severe (PaO_2/FiO_2 <100 mmHg) hypoxemia in the Prone-Supine II Study [16]. In the intervention arm, prone ventilation was carried out for 18 ± 4 h per day ($n = 174$), while in the control group, supine ventilation was carried out ($n = 168$). The overall mortality rate was similar between groups at 28 days and 6 months. Although not statistically significant, there was a trend toward lower mortality at 28 days and 6 months in the subgroup of patients with severe hypoxemia. This study set the background for further investigation of the clinical efficacy of prone ventilation among patients with severe hypoxemia.

The landmark PROSEVA trial unequivocally confirmed improved survival with prone ventilation among severely hypoxemic patients (PaO_2/FiO_2 ratio <150 mmHg, $FiO_2 \geq 0.6$, and PEEP ≥5 cmH_2O) [17]. This study included 466 patients who were from 26 ICUs in France and one in Spain. Prone ventilation was carried out in 237 patients, while 229 patients were ventilated in the supine position. The mean duration of prone ventilation was 17 ± 3 h per session; the average number of sessions was 4 ± 4 per patient. The unadjusted 28-day mortality, the primary endpoint, was significantly lower with prone ventilation [16% vs. 32.8%; hazard ratio: 0.39 (0.25–0.63); $p < 0.001$)]. The 90-day mortality was also significantly lower in the prone ventilated group. Improved survival was observed with prone ventilation after adjusting for baseline SOFA scores. Successful extubation at 90 days was significantly higher in patients who were prone ventilated; furthermore, ventilation-free days at 28 and 90 days were also significantly higher with prone ventilation. Besides, patients who were prone ventilated required less rescue therapy, including the use of extracorporeal membrane oxygenation and the administration of inhaled nitric oxide.

Several meta-analyses have evaluated the clinical efficacy of prone ventilation. In a meta-analysis of eight randomized trials, Munshi et al. reported a lower mortality with prone ventilation in severe ARDS, especially when the duration of prone ventilation was more than 12 h [18]. A network meta-analysis including 25 trials evaluated several ventilatory interventions among patients with moderate to severe ARDS who were ventilated with a lung-protective strategy. In this report, prone ventilation was associated with a significantly lower 28-day mortality (risk ratio: 0.69, 95% CI: 0.48–0.99) [19].

Key Points

- Prone positioning results in improved ventilation to the dorsal areas of the lung, which represent a larger tissue mass.
- In the prone position, perfusion to the dorsal areas of the lung is maintained by the unique vascular geometry of the lung that overrides gravitational effects.
- A more homogenous distribution of ventilation and perfusion results in more optimal ventilation/perfusion matching in the prone compared to the supine position.
- Early RCTs that evaluated the clinical efficacy of prone ventilation were carried out during the period when the lung-protective strategy was not in common practice; although these studies revealed improved oxygenation on assuming the prone position, no beneficial effect was observed in clinical outcomes.
- Later studies that carried out prone ventilation for extended periods, combined with low tidal volume ventilation and limitation of plateau pressures, revealed a trend toward improved survival.
- The PROSEVA trial conclusively demonstrated improved survival in patients who were severely hypoxic with a PaO_2/FiO_2 ratio <150 mmHg with extended use of prone ventilation combined with a lung-protective strategy.
- Most patients with severe ARDS should undergo a trial of prone ventilation prior to consideration of extracorporeal therapies.

References

1. Piehl MA, Brown RS. Use of extreme position changes in acute respiratory failure. Crit Care Med. 1976;4(1):13–4.
2. Mellins RB. Pulmonary physiotherapy in the pediatric age group. Am Rev Respir Dis. 1974;110(6P2):137–42.
3. Gattinoni L, Pesenti A, Avalli L, Rossi F, Bombino M. Pressure-volume curve of total respiratory system in acute respiratory failure. Computed tomographic scan study. Am Rev Respir Dis. 1987;136(3):730–6.
4. Gattinoni L, Busana M, Giosa L, Macrì M, Quintel M. Prone positioning in acute respiratory distress syndrome. Semin Respir Crit Care Med. 2019;40(01):094–100.
5. Gattinoni L, Pelosi P, Vitale G, Pesenti A, D'Andrea L, Mascheroni D. Body position changes redistribute lung computed-tomographic density in patients with acute respiratory failure. Anesthesiology. 1991;74(1):15–23.
6. Johnson NJ, Luks AM, Glenny RW. Gas exchange in the prone posture. Respir Care. 2017;62(8):1097–110.
7. Pelosi P, Tubiolo D, Mascheroni D, Vicardi P, Crotti S, Valenza F, et al. Effects of the prone position on respiratory mechanics and gas exchange during acute lung injury. Am J Respir Crit Care Med. 1998;157(2):387–93.

8. Chiumello D, Cressoni M, Racagni M, Landi L, Li Bassi G, Polli F, et al. Effects of thoraco-pelvic supports during prone position in patients with acute lung injury/acute respiratory distress syndrome: a physiological study. Crit Care. 2006;10(3):R87.
9. Mure M, Glenny RW, Domino KB, Hlastala MP. Pulmonary gas exchange improves in the prone position with abdominal distension. Am J Respir Crit Care Med. 1998;157(6 Pt 1):1785–90.
10. Protti A, Cressoni M, Santini A, Langer T, Mietto C, Febres D, et al. Lung stress and strain during mechanical ventilation: any safe threshold? Am J Respir Crit Care Med. 2011;183(10):1354–62.
11. Wiener CM, Kirk W, Albert RK. Prone position reverses gravitational distribution of perfusion in dog lungs with oleic acid-induced injury. J Appl Physiol. 1990;68(4):1386–92.
12. Nyrén S, Mure M, Jacobsson H, Larsson SA, Lindahl SG. Pulmonary perfusion is more uniform in the prone than in the supine position: scintigraphy in healthy humans. J Appl Physiol. 1999;86(4):1135–41.
13. Luciano G, Gianni T, Antonio P, Paolo T, Daniele M, Violeta L, et al. Effect of prone positioning on the survival of patients with acute respiratory failure. N Engl J Med. 2001;345:568–73.
14. Guerin C, Gaillard S, Lemasson S, Ayzac L, Girard R, Beuret P, et al. Effects of systematic prone positioning in hypoxemic acute respiratory failure: a randomized controlled trial. JAMA. 2004;292(19):2379.
15. Mancebo J, Fernández R, Blanch L, Rialp G, Gordo F, Ferrer M, et al. A multicenter trial of prolonged prone ventilation in severe acute respiratory distress syndrome. Am J Respir Crit Care Med. 2006;173(11):1233–9.
16. Taccone P, Pesenti A, Latini R, Polli F, Vagginelli F, Mietto C, et al. Prone positioning in patients with moderate and severe acute respiratory distress syndrome: a randomized controlled trial. JAMA. 2009;302(18):1977–84.
17. Guérin C, Reignier J, Richard JC, Beuret P, Gacouin A, Boulain T, et al. Prone positioning in severe acute respiratory distress syndrome. N Engl J Med. 2013;368(23):2159–68.
18. Munshi L, Del Sorbo L, Adhikari NKJ, Hodgson CL, Wunsch H, Meade MO, et al. Prone position for acute respiratory distress syndrome. A systematic review and meta-analysis. Ann Am Thorac Soc. 2017;14(Supplement_4):S280–8.
19. Aoyama H, Uchida K, Aoyama K, Pechlivanoglou P, Englesakis M, Yamada Y, et al. Assessment of therapeutic interventions and lung protective ventilation in patients with moderate to severe acute respiratory distress syndrome: a systematic review and network meta-analysis. JAMA Netw Open. 2019;2(7):e198116.

Neuromuscular Blocking Agents in Severe Acute Respiratory Distress Syndrome: Benefit or Harm?

7

7.1 Introduction

The acute respiratory distress syndrome (ARDS), characterized by hypoxemia and bilateral alveolar infiltrates, was described in 1967 by Ashbaugh et al. [1]. Ventilation strategies in ARDS have undergone considerable refinement over the years. A lung-protective ventilation strategy using low tidal volumes may be one of the key interventions to reduce ventilator-induced lung injury (VILI) [2].

7.2 Beneficial Effects of Neuromuscular Blocking Agents

The use of neuromuscular blocking agents (NMBs) may facilitate a lung-protective ventilation strategy. Vigorous spontaneous respiratory efforts may lead to worsening of lung injury through several mechanisms. Changes in transpulmonary pressure that predispose to lung injury are similar with spontaneously generated or ventilator-driven tidal volumes [3]. Changes in pleural pressure with respiration are transmitted uniformly in normal lungs. However, in the injured lung, transmission of pleural pressure is nonuniform. The dependent areas of the lung are in close physical contact with the diaphragm. As the diaphragm contracts forcefully during vigorous spontaneous efforts, the dependent areas of the lung experience a more pronounced negative pleural pressure. The nonuniform distribution of pleural pressure results in air movement from the nondependent to the dependent lung by the "pendelluft" phenomenon [4]. This intrapulmonary movement of air leads to injury to the dependent lung, one of the hallmarks of ARDS. Abolition of vigorous spontaneous efforts may thus prevent damage to the injured lung [3].

A spontaneous respiratory effort may be triggered at the end of the inspiratory phase of a mechanical breath in some patients, through a phenomenon called "reverse triggering," leading to patient-ventilator asynchrony [5]. These harmful

J. Chacko et al., *Controversies in Critical Care*,
https://doi.org/10.1007/978-981-19-9940-6_7

effects of spontaneous respiratory efforts in the injured lung are overcome with the use of NMBs. Besides, NMBs have been shown to improve oxygenation and reduce the release of inflammatory mediators [6, 7]. Abolition of spontaneous respiratory efforts may also reduce the oxygen consumption by decreasing the work of breathing and elimination of the resting muscle tone [8]. Furthermore, improved patient-ventilator synchrony may allow safer and more precise titration of tidal volumes and ventilation pressures [3].

7.3 Possible Harm from NMBs

ICU-acquired muscle weakness is of increasing concern in critically ill patients. Hence, the appropriate use of NMBs is of crucial importance. Studies in septic [9] and asthmatic patients [10] who were administered NMBs have revealed an increased incidence of skeletal muscle dysfunction-related morbidity. However, a direct cause and effect relationship attributable to NMBs and functional outcomes has not been demonstrated. Corticosteroids, often used in combination with NMBs have also been implicated in the causation of ICU-acquired muscle weakness [11]. Fan et al. conducted an epidemiological study on muscle weakness and health-related quality of life among survivors from acute lung injury. They observed that over the study period, skeletal muscle weakness was not associated with the cumulative dose of NMBs and corticosteroids [12]. ICU-acquired weakness is relatively more common with the use of the older NMBs, including vecuronium and atracurium, compared to cisatracurium [13]. Cisatracurium, unlike atracurium, does not lead to histamine release and hypotension [14]. Besides, it may decrease the release of pulmonary and systemic inflammatory cytokines with attenuation of lung injury [15].

Other complications related to prolonged immobility resulting from NMB include deep vein thrombosis and ocular complications, including dryness, scarring, and ulceration of the cornea. Awareness can be a significant problem if adequate sedation is not provided during NMB use. Continuous monitoring of awareness using bispectral index may enable early identification of awareness [16]. IgE-mediated anaphylaxis is a rare complication of NMB use with succinylcholine and rocuronium being the most implicated [17]. Figure 7.1 summarizes likely benefits and possible harm from the use of NMBs.

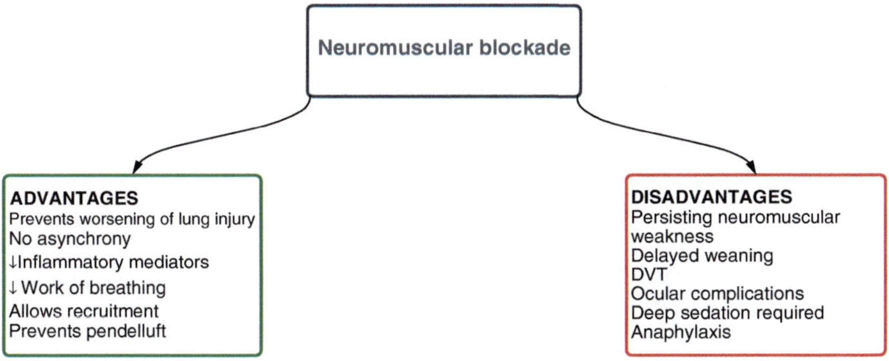

Fig. 7.1 Potential benefits and possible harm from the use of neuromuscular blocking agents

7.4 Evidence for NMB Use in ARDS

NMBs are commonly administered to ARDS patients who require invasive mechanical ventilation. In the international observational LUNG-SAFE study, NMBs were administered in 21.7% of invasively ventilated patients with ARDS, while 37.8% of patients with severe ARDS received NMBs [18]. The usefulness of neuromuscular blockade in ARDS has been addressed in several randomized controlled trials (RCTs) (Table 7.1).

In one of the early RCTs, 56 patients with ARDS with a PaO_2/FiO_2 ratio of less than 150 mmHg and a PEEP of ≥5 cmH_2O were studied. Patients were randomized to receive cisatracurium as a bolus followed by an infusion and compared with placebo. Gas exchange was followed up for a period of 120 h after randomization. There was a significant improvement in the PaO_2/FiO_2 ratio among patients who received cisatracurium at 48, 96, and 120 h after randomization. Besides, the use of cisatracurium resulted in a significant reduction of the PEEP level. This study demonstrated that the use of NMBs in early ARDS may result in improved gas exchange and enable reduction of PEEP levels [7].

Does the use of NMBs result in attenuation of the pulmonary and systemic inflammatory response in patients with ARDS? In a multicentric French study, 36 patients with ARDS and PaO_2/FiO_2 ratios of ≤200 on a positive end-expiratory pressure of ≥5 cmH_2O were studied. Patients were randomly assigned to receive cisatracurium as a loading dose followed by an infusion or an equivalent placebo within 48 h of disease onset. Lung-protective ventilation was carried out using tidal volumes of 4–8 mL/kg ideal body weight and a plateau pressure of ≤30 cmH_2O. Serum and bronchoalveolar fluid levels of tumor necrosis factor-alpha, IL-1, IL-6, and IL-8 were determined before randomization and after 48 h. Early cisatracurium administration during the initial 48-h period resulted in a significant reduction in the levels of pulmonary and systemic pro-inflammatory cytokines. Furthermore, a significantly greater improvement in the PaO_2/FiO_2 ratio was observed among patients who received cisatracurium [6].

Table 7.1 RCTs evaluating the efficacy of neuromuscular blockade in ARDS

Author/year	Population	Intervention	Control	Outcomes
Gainnier et al. (2004) [7]	56 ARDS patients with PaO_2/FiO_2 < 150 mmHg, PEEP ≥5 cmH_2O	Cisatracurium bolus followed by infusion	Placebo	Significant improvement in the PaO_2/FiO_2 ratio at 48, 96, and 120 h; significant reduction in PEEP with cisatracurium
Forel et al. (2006) [6]	36 ARDS patients with PaO_2/FiO_2 < 200 and PEEP ≥5 cmH_2O	Cisatracurium bolus followed by infusion	Placebo	Significant reduction in the level of pulmonary and systemic pro-inflammatory cytokines; improvement in the PaO_2/FiO_2 ratio with cisatracurium
Papazian et al. (2010) (ACURASYS) [19]	340 ARDS patients with PaO_2/FiO_2 < 150 mmHg, PEEP ≥5 cmH_2O	Cisatracurium bolus followed by infusion	Placebo	90-day in-hospital mortality similar. Significant reduction in 90-day mortality on adjusted analysis. More ventilator-free days at 28 and 90 day with cisatracurium. Similar incidence of ICU-acquired weakness
Moss et al. (ROSE) (2019) [20]	1006 ARDS patients with PaO_2/FiO_2 < 150 mmHg, PEEP ≥8 cmH_2O	Cisatracurium bolus followed by infusion, deep sedation, Ramsay score:6	Placebo. Sedation to Ramsay score 2–3	No significant difference in 90-day or 28-day all-cause mortality, ventilator, ICU-free days at day 28, ICU-acquired weakness

The ACURASYS trial was a multicenter RCT among patients with severe ARDS, characterized by a PaO_2/FiO_2 ratio of less than 150 mmHg while receiving a PEEP level of ≥5 cmH_2O [19]. Cisatracurium was administered as a bolus followed by a continuous infusion in 178 patients, while 162 patients received placebo. A lung-protective ventilation strategy was utilized, with tidal volumes of 6–8 mL/kg of predicted body weight. Cisatracurium was administered within 48 h of onset of ARDS and continued for 48 h. The overall in-hospital mortality at 90 days was not significantly different between patients who received cisatracurium compared to those who received placebo (31.6% vs. 40.7%, $p = 0.08$). On analysis after adjustment for the baseline PaO_2/FiO_2 ratio, plateau pressure, and the Simplified Acute Physiology II score (SAPS) score, the 90-day mortality was significantly lower in the cisatracurium group (hazard ratio, 0.68; 95% CI, 0.48–0.98; $p = 0.04$). The number of ventilator-free days at 28 and 90 days was also significantly more with cisatracurium administration. The incidence of ICU-acquired weakness was similar between groups.

The ROSE trial was conducted across multiple centers in the US by the National Heart, Lung, and Blood Institute PETAL Clinical Trials Network. Patients with severe ARDS and a PaO_2/FiO_2 ratio of <150 mmHg while receiving a PEEP >8 cmH_2O were included. Study enrolment was carried out within 1 week of disease onset. In the intervention group, cisatracurium was administered as a bolus followed by a continuous infusion after ensuring deep sedation (Ramsay sedation score: 6). In the control arm, light sedation was administered, titrated to a Ramsay sedation score of 2–3. A lung-protective ventilation strategy was followed in both groups. The study was stopped for futility at the second interim analysis after the enrolment of 1006 patients. There was no difference in the primary endpoint of 90-day all-cause hospital mortality between the cisatracurium and control groups (42.5% vs. 42.8%; $p = 0.93$). No significant difference was noted in the secondary endpoints, including 28-day mortality, ventilator- or ICU-free days at 28 days, and ICU-acquired weakness. The number of hospital-free days at day 28 and long-term quality of life also remained similar between groups [20].

The ROSE trial was ceased prematurely for futility although the stopping rules were not prespecified, leading to an underpowered study. Prone ventilation has been established to improve mortality in patients with severe ARDS [21]. In the ROSE trial, prone ventilation was carried out only in 16% of patients compared to 50% patients in the ACURASYS trial, which may have impacted outcomes. The use of a higher level of PEEP in the ROSE trial may have attenuated potentially injurious swings in the transpulmonary pressure [22], providing a lung-protective effect. Besides, 655 of 4848 patients who were screened were already on NMBs and hence excluded from the study. In contrast to the ACURASYS trial, the ROSE trial was unblinded, which may have resulted in bias.

Key Points

- The putative benefits of neuromuscular blockade in ARDS include elimination of patient-ventilator asynchrony, prevention of worsening of lung injury from vigorous spontaneous respiratory efforts, reduction in the pulmonary and systemic inflammatory response, and improvement in arterial oxygenation.
- These potential advantages may be offset by a higher incidence of neuromuscular weakness, complications related to prolonged immobility, and the need for deep sedation to prevent awareness.
- A consistent improvement in PaO_2/FiO_2 ratios has been demonstrated with the early administration of neuromuscular blocking drugs in ARDS.
- The impact of NMB usage on clinical outcomes, including mortality, remains inconclusive from the evidence available so far.
- However, there is a likely key role for the early administration of NMBs among patients with severe ARDS to enable lung-protective ventilation, reduce patient-ventilator asynchrony, allow prone ventilation, and mitigate arterial hypoxemia. Needless to say, a patient-centered approach is pivotal to guide the appropriate use of NMBs among mechanically ventilated patients with severe ARDS.

References

1. Ashbaugh DG, Bigelow DB, Petty TL, Levine BE. Acute respiratory distress in adults. Lancet. 1967;2(7511):319–23.
2. Acute Respiratory Distress Syndrome Network, Brower RG, Matthay MA, Morris A, Schoenfeld D, Thompson BT, et al. Ventilation with lower tidal volumes as compared with traditional tidal volumes for acute lung injury and the acute respiratory distress syndrome. N Engl J Med. 2000;342(18):1301–8.
3. Brochard L, Slutsky A, Pesenti A. Mechanical ventilation to minimize progression of lung injury in acute respiratory failure. Am J Respir Crit Care Med. 2017;195(4):438–42.
4. Yoshida T, Torsani V, Gomes S, De Santis RR, Beraldo MA, Costa ELV, et al. Spontaneous effort causes occult Pendelluft during mechanical ventilation. Am J Respir Crit Care Med. 2013;188(12):1420–7.
5. Akoumianaki E, Lyazidi A, Rey N, Matamis D, Perez-Martinez N, Giraud R, et al. Mechanical ventilation-induced reverse-triggered breaths. Chest. 2013;143(4):927–38.
6. Forel JM, Roch A, Marin V, Michelet P, Demory D, Blache JL, et al. Neuromuscular blocking agents decrease inflammatory response in patients presenting with acute respiratory distress syndrome*. Crit Care Med. 2006;34(11):2749–57.
7. Gainnier M, Roch A, Forel JM, Thirion X, Arnal JM, Donati S, et al. Effect of neuromuscular blocking agents on gas exchange in patients presenting with acute respiratory distress syndrome*. Crit Care Med. 2004;32(1):113–9.
8. deBacker J, Hart N, Fan E. Neuromuscular blockade in the 21st century management of the critically ill patient. Chest. 2017;151(3):697–706.
9. Garnacho-Montero J, Madrazo-Osuna J, García-Garmendia JL, Ortiz-Leyba C, Jiménez-Jiménez FJ, Barrero-Almodóvar A, et al. Critical illness polyneuropathy: risk factors and clinical consequences. A cohort study in septic patients. Intensive Care Med. 2001;27(8):1288–96.
10. Adnet F, Dhissi G, Borron SW, Galinski M, Rayeh F, Cupa M, et al. Complication profiles of adult asthmatics requiring paralysis during mechanical ventilation. Intensive Care Med. 2001;27(11):1729–36.
11. Schakman O, Gilson H, Thissen JP. Mechanisms of glucocorticoid-induced myopathy. J Endocrinol. 2008;197(1):1–10.
12. Fan E, Dowdy DW, Colantuoni E, Mendez-Tellez PA, Sevransky JE, Shanholtz C, et al. Physical complications in acute lung injury survivors: a two-year longitudinal prospective study. Crit Care Med. 2014;42(4):849–59.
13. Hansen-Flaschen J, Cowen J, Raps EC. Neuromuscular blockade in the intensive care unit. More than we bargained for. Am Rev Respir Dis. 1993;147(1):234–6.
14. Savarese JJ, Wastila WB. The future of the benzylisoquinolinium relaxants. Acta Anaesthesiol Scand Suppl. 1995;106:91–3.
15. Qadir N, Chang SY. Pharmacologic treatments for acute respiratory distress syndrome. Crit Care Clin. 2021;37(4):877–93.
16. Wang ZH, Chen H, Yang YL, Shi ZH, Guo QH, Li YW, et al. Bispectral index can reliably detect deep sedation in mechanically ventilated patients: a prospective multicenter validation study. Anesth Analg. 2017;125(1):176–83.
17. Mertes PM, Laxenaire MC, GERAP. Anaphylactic and anaphylactoid reactions occurring during anaesthesia in France. Seventh epidemiologic survey (January 2001-December 2002). Ann Fr Anesth Reanim. 2004;23(12):1133–43.
18. Bellani G, Laffey JG, Pham T, Fan E, Brochard L, Esteban A, et al. Epidemiology, patterns of care, and mortality for patients with acute respiratory distress syndrome in intensive care units in 50 countries. JAMA. 2016;315(8):788–800.
19. Papazian L, Forel JM, Gacouin A, Penot-Ragon C, Perrin G, Loundou A, et al. Neuromuscular blockers in early acute respiratory distress syndrome. N Engl J Med. 2010;363(12):1107–16.

20. The National Heart, Lung, and Blood Institute PETAL Clinical Trials Network. Early neuromuscular blockade in the acute respiratory distress syndrome. N Engl J Med. 2019;380(21):1997–2008.
21. Guérin C, Reignier J, Richard JC, Beuret P, Gacouin A, Boulain T, et al. Prone positioning in severe acute respiratory distress syndrome. N Engl J Med. 2013;368(23):2159–68.
22. Borges JB, Morais CCA, Costa ELV. High PEEP may have reduced injurious transpulmonary pressure swings in the ROSE trial. Crit Care. 2019;23(1):404.

Ventilator-Associated Pneumonia: Newer Definitions, Controversies, and Perspectives

8

8.1 Introduction

Ventilator-associated pneumonia (VAP) is among the most common hospital-acquired infections. A multinational study including 56 centers across 11 countries revealed a VAP incidence of 15.6%. VAP may lead to adverse clinical outcomes including prolongation of ICU and hospital stay, increased antibiotic use, and add substantially to the cost of care [1, 2]. VAP is considered to be an important measure of the quality of ICU care. However, changing definitions, lack of timely and reliable diagnostic techniques, and heterogeneity of clinical studies have besieged this topic.

8.2 Definitions: Diagnosis

In 2013, The National Healthcare Safety Network (NHSN) of the Center for Disease Control and Prevention (CDC) in the USA introduced new surveillance definitions to evaluate ventilator-associated events (VAE). There are three tiers of VAEs, including ventilator-associated complications (VAC), infection-related ventilator-associated complications (IVAC), and possible or probable VAP. According to the new criteria, possible or probable VAP meets the following criteria.

1. An increase in daily minimum PEEP $\geq$3 cmH_2O or $FiO_2 \geq 0.20$ sustained for at least 2 calendar days following a baseline period (2 calendar days) of stability or improvement (VAC).
2. Altered leukocyte count ($\geq$12,000 cells/mm^3 or $\leq$4000 cells/mm^3) and/or temperature (>38 °C or <36 °C); a new antimicrobial prescription has been started and sustained for at least 4 calendar days (IVAC).
3. Microbiological confirmation of a lower respiratory tract infection (possible or probable VAP).

J. Chacko et al., *Controversies in Critical Care*,
https://doi.org/10.1007/978-981-19-9940-6_8

Compared to previous definitions, the new definition does not include radiological infiltrates as a prerequisite for the diagnosis of VAP. An increase in the FiO_2 level and PEEP is considered to imply deterioration. The new design was meant primarily to identify deterioration of the respiratory status; it further aimed to reduce the subjectivity associated with previous definitions of VAP, including the development of new or progressive radiographic infiltrates and the volume and character of tracheal secretions. However, microbiological confirmation is required to diagnose possible or probable VAP. Considering the lack of certainty regarding the timing of microbiological testing, the sensitivity of these criteria may be less than optimal. Besides, several clinical conditions unrelated to pneumonia may fulfil the definition of VAE, leading to a lack of specificity. While 20–40% of all VAEs may be due to pneumonia, 30–40% of VAEs may occur from fluid overload, and 10–20% each due to collapse or acute respiratory distress syndrome (ARDS) [3]. Thus, the positive predictive value of VAE as a screening tool for VAP is low, because, by definition, it includes several other conditions that result in a deterioration of the respiratory status. In a study by Klompas et al., among 597 mechanically ventilated patients, 9.3% had VAP by conventional definition compared to 23% who had VAC [4].

Conversely, other studies have revealed poor sensitivity of the VAE criteria as a screening tool. In a prospective cohort study of 8408 mechanically ventilated patients, the VAE-VAC criteria identified less than one-third of VAPs diagnosed according to traditional criteria, using chest radiographs as the primary screening tool [5]. However, VAP may often be overdiagnosed by clinicians leading to excessive antibiotic prescription [6]. In an autopsy study, the accuracy of three common conventional definitions of VAP was found to be poor [7].

Overall, the utility of VAE as a surveillance tool for VAP appears to be less than optimal and of questionable value as an ICU quality indicator, considering its poor sensitivity and low positive predictive value.

8.3 VAP and Clinical Outcomes

Does VAP lead to attributable mortality in mechanically ventilated patients or could it be that sicker patients, likely to require a longer duration of ventilation, are more prone to develop VAP? Considering such confounders, the true attributable mortality due to VAP may be difficult to estimate. Fagon et al., in an early study, reported a high mortality rate of 71.4% with VAP caused by *Pseudomonas* or *Acinetobacter* species, with an attributable mortality of 42.8% [8]. In contrast, Papazian et al., in a study of VAP with matched controls, revealed no excess mortality when confounding factors were eliminated [9]. Bekaert et al. evaluated the attributable mortality of VAP from a multicenter database from France, including patients who underwent mechanical ventilation within 48 h of ICU admission and remained in the ICU for a minimum period of 2 days. The study included 4479 patients; 685 (15.3%) developed pneumonia within 30 days of ICU admission. The authors used statistical modeling techniques to eliminate possible confounders. In contrast to previous reports, the study estimated a relatively low attributable mortality due to VAP—about 1% at 30 days and 1.5% at 60 days [10]. An epidemiological analysis evaluated the mortality of patients with ARDS who developed VAP. This epidemiological study involved the analysis of data from the ACURASYS trial that evaluated the use of cisatracurium in ARDS [11]. The authors observed an increase in crude ICU mortality in patients who developed VAP compared to those who did not; however, the difference was nonsignificant on adjusted analysis [12].

Steen et al. analyzed data of 2720 adult patients who received mechanical ventilation within 48 h of admission to medical and surgical ICUs. Among these patients, 210 (7.7%) developed VAP. According to this study, the hypothetical eradication of VAP would lead to a relative reduction of ICU mortality reduction by only 1.7% (95% confidence interval, −1.3–4.6) by day 10 and 3.6% (95% confidence interval, 0.7–6.5) by day 60. The authors concluded that the attributable mortality of VAP is low, in light of the current preventive measures commonly employed [13]. In patients with cancer, VAP was not associated with adverse outcomes in a retrospective study [14]. Similarly, the development of VAP was not associated with mortality in patients with traumatic brain injury [15]. However, VAP may be associated with an increased duration of mechanical ventilation, ICU, and hospital stay and add to the overall cost of care [2].

8.4 Ventilator-Associated Tracheobronchitis Vs. VAP

Lower respiratory infection among mechanically ventilated patients without new or progressive radiological infiltrates is often referred to as ventilator-associated tracheobronchitis (VAT) [16]. According to this definition, positive endotracheal aspirate cultures without corroborative radiological findings could be interpreted as either colonization or VAT. Although new-onset systemic symptoms would point toward infection, it may be difficult to distinguish pulmonary from an extrapulmonary source of infection among critically ill patients. It is debatable whether VAT requires antibiotic treatment. However, untreated VAT has the potential for progression to VAP and an increase in the duration of mechanical ventilation or ICU stay [17, 18]. Martin-Loeches et al. conducted a multicenter, prospective observational study including 114 ICUs, aiming to evaluate the incidence and impact of VAT. They observed that appropriate antibiotic therapy of patients with VAT led to a significantly lower progression to VAP compared to those who were provided with inappropriate treatment [19]. Similar findings were observed in an earlier RCT that found a lower rate of progression to VAP, more ventilator-free days, and lower mortality in patients with VAT who were treated with antibiotics compared to those who were not [20].

The universal treatment of all cases suspected of VAT may lead to excessive antibiotic usage, adding to the burden of resistant strains, especially considering the uncertainty regarding diagnosis. Hence, the decision to administer antibiotics is not always straightforward and needs to be individualized weighing the risks of treatment compared to possible benefit [21]. As an alternative to intravenous administration, inhalational antibiotics have been proposed for the treatment of VAT; however, the efficacy of this modality of treatment remains unclear [22].

8.5 Efficacy of VAP Prevention Bundles

8.5.1 Semi-Recumbent Position, Sedation Hold, and Spontaneous Breathing Trials

The efficacy of several measures has been evaluated in the prevention of VAP, providing a bundled approach toward the care of mechanically ventilated patients. The individual elements of the bundle that may be effective in the prevention of VAP are depicted in Fig. 8.1. As VAP occurs due to the microaspiration of orogastric organisms, measures directed toward reducing the duration of mechanical ventilation are likely to be effective. These include daily interruption of sedation [23] and regular assessment for weaning and extubation with spontaneous breathing trials [24]. A semi-recumbent position, with ≥30° head up, may reduce the incidence of VAP compared to a 0–10° position [25]. A network meta-analysis of RCTs compared different body positions including lateral, prone, and semi-recumbent, among mechanically ventilated patients. In this study, the semi-recumbent and prone positions were associated with a significantly lower risk of VAP and mortality, compared to the supine position [26]. However, optimal positioning of mechanically ventilated patients remains contentious, with a relative lack of high-quality evidence.

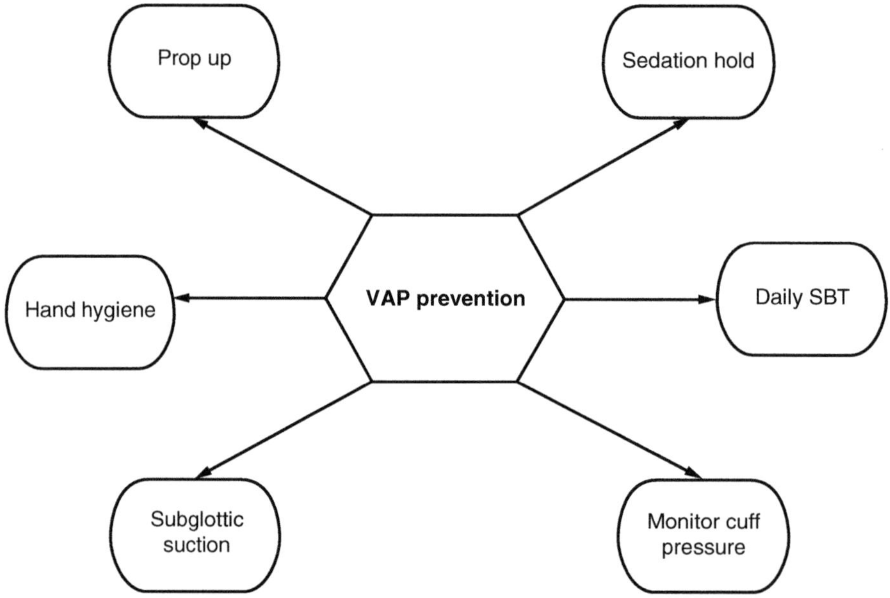

Fig. 8.1 Elements of preventive bundles that may reduce the incidence of VAP

8.5.2 Subglottic Secretion Drainage

Endotracheal tubes with the provision for subglottic drainage of accumulated secretions above the cuff are one of the commonly employed preventive interventions. A meta-analysis of 17 RCTs including 3369 patients revealed a significantly reduced incidence of VAP (risk ratio, 0.58; 95% CI, 0.51–0.67; $I^2 = 0\%$). However, this study did not reveal any beneficial effect on clinical outcomes including the duration of stay in the ICU and in hospital, duration of mechanical ventilation, VAEs, or mortality [27].

8.5.3 Maintenance of Cuff Pressure

Inadequate cuff inflation may constitute an important risk factor for microaspiration and VAP in mechanically ventilated patients. There are several devices that continuously monitor and maintain cuff pressures at preset threshold levels [28]. Nseir et al. performed a meta-analysis of three prospective, controlled trials that assessed the efficacy of continuous control of cuff pressure on the incidence of VAP. Continuous control was compared with usual care with measurement and adjustment of cuff pressure using a conventional manometer. Continuous cuff pressure control resulted in a significantly lower incidence of VAP compared to usual care (13.6% vs. 25.7%, HR: 0.47, 95% CI 0.31–0.71, $p < 0.001$). This study did not find a significant difference in the duration of mechanical ventilation, ICU stay, or mortality [29].

8.5.4 Modified Tube Surface and Coated Endotracheal Tubes

Coating the endotracheal tube surface with different types of material, including silver, to prevent the development of biofilms has been studied; however, there is no firm evidence to support this practice [30]. Another approach has been the creation of grooves or roughening of the inner surface of endotracheal tubes, thereby, reducing bacterial adhesion [31].

8.5.5 Hand Hygiene and Oral Care

Hand hygiene of healthcare workers is an important facet of the VAP prevention bundle. However, questions remain regarding the optimal hand hygiene technique, dose and strength of alcohol-based hand rubs, and their dry times for optimal efficacy [32]. Chlorhexidine-based oral care has been in widespread practice as a VAP prevention technique. However, most studies have included postoperative cardiac surgical patients who generally undergo less than a day of mechanical ventilation. It is unclear if these findings are extrapolatable to general critically ill patients. Besides, the use of chlorhexidine, an antiseptic, might result in negative cultures from endotracheal aspirates; however, the incidence of pneumonia may remain unchanged. Furthermore, a meta-analysis suggested a possible increase in mortality among noncardiac surgical patients with chlorhexidine-based oral care [33]. Adverse outcomes may be related to respiratory complications arising from the microaspiration of chlorhexidine [34].

8.5.6 Selective Digestive Decontamination

Selective digestive decontamination (SDD) uses a combination of nonabsorbable enteral antibiotics and parenteral antibiotics as a technique to prevent the growth of pathogenic organisms in the oropharynx and intestines. Although the efficacy of this technique has been demonstrated in the prevention of VAP, the ICUs involved had a low incidence of resistant organisms [35]. Excessive use of antibiotics with SDD regimes may also potentially lead to increased antibiotic resistance with the modification of ICU flora. Table 8.1 summarizes clinical trials and meta-analyses on the efficacy of interventions in the prevention VAP.

Table 8.1 Clinical trials and meta-analyses on interventions to prevent VAP

Study/year	Design	Intervention	Control	Outcomes
Kress et al. (2000) [23]	RCT; patients on mechanical ventilation in a medical ICU	Sedative agents interrupted daily until patients were awake	Sedation ceased at clinician discretion	Decreased duration of mechanical ventilation and ICU LOS with daily interruption of sedation
Wang et al. (2016) [25]	Meta-analysis of RCTs; patients on mechanical ventilation	Semi-recumbent position	Supine position	A semi-recumbent position (≥30°) reduced the incidence of VAP. Studies with high risk of bias
Pozuelo-Carrascosa et al. (2022) [26]	Network meta-analysis of RCTs; patients on mechanical ventilation	Lateral, prone, semi-recumbent, or other position	Supine position	Semi-recumbent associated with the lowest incidence of VAP. Prone position did not reduce the incidence of VAP
Caroff et al. (2016) [27]	Meta-analysis of RCTs; patients on mechanical ventilation	Subglottic secretion drainage	No subglottic secretion drainage	Lower incidence of VAP with subglottic secretion drainage. No decrease in the duration of ventilation, ICU LOS, VAEs, mortality, and antibiotic usage

Table 8.1 (continued)

Study/year	Design	Intervention	Control	Outcomes
Nseir et al. (2014) [29]	Pooled analysis of two RCTs and one quasi-randomized controlled trial; mechanically ventilated patients	Continuous monitoring and maintenance of cuff pressure using a dedicated device	Intermittent monitoring and maintenance of cuff pressure	Lower incidence of VAP with continuous cuff pressure monitoring
Klompas et al. (2014) [33]	Meta-analysis of RCTs; separate analysis of post-cardiac surgical and noncardiac surgical patients	Oral care with chlorhexidine	Any inert comparator for oral care	Lower incidence of respiratory infection with chlorhexidine oral care in cardiac surgical patients. No difference in VAP incidence in noncardiac surgical patients. Trend toward increased mortality with chlorhexidine use in noncardiac surgical patients

RCT randomized controlled trial, *LOS* length of stay, *VAP* ventilator-associated pneumonia, *VAE* ventilator-associated event

8.6 Duration of Therapy

The diagnosis of VAP may often be presumptive, and antibiotics may be commenced early based on signs of clinical worsening. Deterioration of respiratory function may not always be due to VAP; hence, in some patients, continued antibiotic treatment may not be required once the noninfective origin is apparent [6]. Clearly, a shorter duration of antibiotic treatment would have favorable effects on the bacterial ecology and reduce the emergence of resistant strains [36]. If antibiotics are commenced initially on clinical suspicion of VAP, it may be appropriate to cease therapy if the probability of an infective etiology appears low on later evaluation. This was demonstrated in a retrospective study, with an ultrashort antibiotic course of 1–3 days compared with >3 days of treatment in patients with suspected VAP [37]. On sensitivity analyses using propensity scores to match patients in both cohorts, the hospital mortality, duration of mechanical ventilation, and hospital length of stay were not significantly different between the two groups of patients. This study underlines the importance of early cessation of antibiotics in patients who are initially suspected to have VAP, but may have an alternate, noninfective etiology for the deterioration of respiratory status.

In a landmark RCT, Chastre et al. compared 8 days vs. 15 days of antibiotic treatment in patients with VAP [38]. The 28-day mortality, incidence of recurrent infection, mechanical ventilation-free days, organ failure-free days, and duration of ICU stay were similar between the two groups. A French study compared an 8-day compared to a 15-day antibiotic therapy in early-onset VAP [39]. The rate of clinical cure was similar between the two groups; the 21-day mortality was also not significantly different between both patient cohorts. Robust evidence supports a shorter duration of antibiotic therapy in VAP.

Key Points

- VAP is the most common nosocomial infection in critically ill, mechanically ventilated patients.
- The attributable mortality of VAP has been low in recent studies, probably related to the implementation of preventive bundles. However, it may lead to prolonged duration of mechanical ventilation, ICU stay, and increase of overall cost of care.
- Newer definitions were introduced as a surveillance technique for VAP. Although the new definitions improve objectivity, they have poor positive predictive value and sensitivity for the diagnosis of VAP.
- VAT may often be the harbinger of VAP and may require antibiotic treatment. However, treatment should be individualized; universal treatment of suspected VAT leads to excessive antibiotic usage and the emergence of resistant strains.
- Preventive bundles have been introduced to reduce the incidence of VAP. The interventions that may be useful include meticulous hand hygiene of healthcare personnel, daily interruption of sedation combined with spontaneous breathing trials, adoption of a semi-recumbent position of >30°, subglottic secretion drainage, and maintenance of tracheal cuff pressures to prevent microaspiration.
- Oropharyngeal decontamination with chlorhexidine and SDD are unlikely to be effective in the prevention of VAP.
- A shorter duration of antibiotic therapy of 7 days is as effective compared with longer durations of therapy in VAP. Longer duration of antibiotic usage results in an increase in the resistance burden. Ultrashort duration of antibiotic administration for 1–3 days may be appropriate when empirical treatment is commenced based on clinical suspicion alone and later turns out to be noninfective deterioration of the respiratory status.

References

1. Restrepo MI, Anzueto A, Arroliga AC, Afessa B, Atkinson MJ, Ho NJ, et al. Economic burden of ventilator-associated pneumonia based on total resource utilization. Infect Control Hosp Epidemiol. 2010;31(5):509–15.
2. Kollef MH, Hamilton CW, Ernst FR. Economic impact of ventilator-associated pneumonia in a large matched cohort. Infect Control Hosp Epidemiol. 2012;33(3):250–6.
3. Klompas M, Berra L. Should ventilator-associated events become a quality indicator for ICUs? Respir Care. 2016;61(6):723–36.
4. Klompas M, Khan Y, Kleinman K, Evans RS, Lloyd JF, Stevenson K, et al. Multicenter evaluation of a novel surveillance paradigm for complications of mechanical ventilation. PLoS One. 2011;6(3):e18062.
5. Lilly CM, Landry KE, Sood RN, Dunnington CH, Ellison RT, Bagley PH, et al. Prevalence and test characteristics of national health safety network ventilator-associated events. Crit Care Med. 2014;42(9):2019–28.
6. Nussenblatt V, Avdic E, Berenholtz S, Daugherty E, Hadhazy E, Lipsett PA, et al. Ventilator-associated pneumonia: overdiagnosis and treatment are common in medical and surgical intensive care units. Infect Control Hosp Epidemiol. 2014;35(3):278–84.
7. Tejerina E, Esteban A, Fernández-Segoviano P, Frutos-Vivar F, Aramburu J, Ballesteros D, et al. Accuracy of clinical definitions of ventilator-associated pneumonia: comparison with autopsy findings. J Crit Care. 2010;25(1):62–8.
8. Fagon JY, Chastre J, Hance AJ, Montravers P, Novara A, Gibert C. Nosocomial pneumonia in ventilated patients: a cohort study evaluating attributable mortality and hospital stay. Am J Med. 1993;94(3):281–8.
9. Papazian L, Bregeon F, Thirion X, Gregoire R, Saux P, Denis JP, et al. Effect of ventilator-associated pneumonia on mortality and morbidity. Am J Respir Crit Care Med. 1996;154(1):91–7.
10. Bekaert M, Timsit JF, Vansteelandt S, Depuydt P, Vésin A, Garrouste-Orgeas M, et al. Attributable mortality of ventilator-associated pneumonia: a reappraisal using causal analysis. Am J Respir Crit Care Med. 2011;184(10):1133–9.
11. Papazian L, Forel JM, Gacouin A, Penot-Ragon C, Perrin G, Loundou A, et al. Neuromuscular blockers in early acute respiratory distress syndrome. N Engl J Med. 2010;363(12):1107–16.
12. Forel JM, Voillet F, Pulina D, Gacouin A, Perrin G, Barrau K, et al. Ventilator-associated pneumonia and ICU mortality in severe ARDS patients ventilated according to a lung-protective strategy. Crit Care. 2012;16(2):R65.
13. Steen J, Vansteelandt S, De Bus L, Depuydt P, Gadeyne B, Benoit DD, et al. Attributable mortality of ventilator-associated pneumonia. Replicating findings, revisiting methods. Ann Am Thorac Soc. 2021;18(5):830–7.
14. Stoclin A, Rotolo F, Hicheri Y, Mons M, Chachaty E, Gachot B, et al. Ventilator-associated pneumonia and bloodstream infections in intensive care unit cancer patients: a retrospective 12-year study on 3388 prospectively monitored patients. Support Care Cancer. 2020;28(1):193–200.
15. Li Y, Liu C, Xiao W, Song T, Wang S. Incidence, risk factors, and outcomes of ventilator-associated pneumonia in traumatic brain injury: a meta-analysis. Neurocrit Care. 2020;32(1):272–85.
16. Niederman MS. Hospital-acquired pneumonia, health care-associated pneumonia, ventilator-associated pneumonia, and ventilator-associated tracheobronchitis: definitions and challenges in trial design. Clin Infect Dis. 2010;51(Suppl 1):S12–7.
17. Dallas J, Skrupky L, Abebe N, Boyle WA, Kollef MH. Ventilator-associated tracheobronchitis in a mixed surgical and medical ICU population. Chest. 2011;139(3):513–8.

18. Karvouniaris M, Makris D, Manoulakas E, Zygoulis P, Mantzarlis K, Triantaris A, et al. Ventilator-associated tracheobronchitis increases the length of intensive care unit stay. Infect Control Hosp Epidemiol. 2013;34(8):800–8.
19. Martin-Loeches I, Povoa P, Rodríguez A, Curcio D, Suarez D, Mira JP, et al. Incidence and prognosis of ventilator-associated tracheobronchitis (TAVeM): a multicentre, prospective, observational study. Lancet Respir Med. 2015;3(11):859–68.
20. Nseir S, Favory R, Jozefowicz E, Decamps F, Dewavrin F, Brunin G, et al. Antimicrobial treatment for ventilator-associated tracheobronchitis: a randomized, controlled, multicenter study. Crit Care. 2008;12(3):R62.
21. Kalil AC, Metersky ML, Klompas M, Muscedere J, Sweeney DA, Palmer LB, et al. Management of adults with hospital-acquired and ventilator-associated pneumonia: 2016 clinical practice guidelines by the Infectious Diseases Society of America and the American Thoracic Society. Clin Infect Dis. 2016;63(5):e61–111.
22. Solé-Lleonart C, Rouby JJ, Blot S, Poulakou G, Chastre J, Palmer LB, et al. Nebulization of antiinfective agents in invasively mechanically ventilated adults: a systematic review and meta-analysis. Anesthesiology. 2017;126(5):890–908.
23. Kress JP, Pohlman AS, O'Connor MF, Hall JB. Daily interruption of sedative infusions in critically ill patients undergoing mechanical ventilation. N Engl J Med. 2000;342(20):1471–7.
24. Girard TD, Kress JP, Fuchs BD, Thomason JWW, Schweickert WD, Pun BT, et al. Efficacy and safety of a paired sedation and ventilator weaning protocol for mechanically ventilated patients in intensive care (awakening and breathing controlled trial): a randomised controlled trial. Lancet. 2008;371(9607):126–34.
25. Wang L, Li X, Yang Z, Tang X, Yuan Q, Deng L, et al. Semi-recumbent position versus supine position for the prevention of ventilator-associated pneumonia in adults requiring mechanical ventilation. Cochrane Database Syst Rev. 2016;2016(1):CD009946.
26. Pozuelo-Carrascosa DP, Cobo-Cuenca AI, Carmona-Torres JM, Laredo-Aguilera JA, Santacruz-Salas E, Fernandez-Rodriguez R. Body position for preventing ventilator-associated pneumonia for critically ill patients: a systematic review and network meta-analysis. J Intensive Care. 2022;10(1):9.
27. Caroff DA, Li L, Muscedere J, Klompas M. Subglottic secretion drainage and objective outcomes: a systematic review and meta-analysis. Crit Care Med. 2016;44(4):830–40.
28. Babic SA, Chatburn RL. Laboratory evaluation of cuff pressure control methods. Respir Care. 2020;65(1):62–7.
29. Nseir S, Lorente L, Ferrer M, Rouzé A, Gonzalez O, Bassi GL, et al. Continuous control of tracheal cuff pressure for VAP prevention: a collaborative meta-analysis of individual participant data. Ann Intensive Care. 2015;5(1):43.
30. Tokmaji G, Vermeulen H, Müller MCA, Kwakman PHS, Schultz MJ, Zaat SAJ. Silver-coated endotracheal tubes for prevention of ventilator-associated pneumonia in critically ill patients. Cochrane Database Syst Rev. 2015;2015(8):CD009201.
31. Mann EE, Magin CM, Mettetal MR, May RM, Henry MM, DeLoid H, et al. Micropatterned endotracheal tubes reduce secretion-related lumen occlusion. Ann Biomed Eng. 2016;44(12):3645–54.
32. Boyce JM. Current issues in hand hygiene. Am J Infect Control. 2019;47S:A46–52.
33. Klompas M, Speck K, Howell MD, Greene LR, Berenholtz SM. Reappraisal of routine oral care with chlorhexidine gluconate for patients receiving mechanical ventilation: systematic review and meta-analysis. JAMA Intern Med. 2014;174(5):751–61.
34. Colombo SM, Palomeque AC, Li BG. The zero-VAP sophistry and controversies surrounding prevention of ventilator-associated pneumonia. Intensive Care Med. 2020;46(2):368–71.
35. Liberati A, D'Amico R, Pifferi S, Torri V, Brazzi L, Parmelli E. Antibiotic prophylaxis to reduce respiratory tract infections and mortality in adults receiving intensive care. Cochrane Database Syst Rev. 2009;(4):CD000022.
36. Bottery MJ, Pitchford JW, Friman VP. Ecology and evolution of antimicrobial resistance in bacterial communities. ISME J. 2021;15(4):939–48.

37. Klompas M, Li L, Menchaca JT, Gruber S, For the CDC Prevention Epicenters Program. Ultra short course antibiotics for patients with suspected ventilator-associated pneumonia but minimal and stable ventilator settings. Clin Infect Dis. 2016;64:ciw870.
38. Chastre J, Wolff M, Fagon JY, Chevret S, Thomas F, Wermert D, et al. Comparison of 8 vs 15 days of antibiotic therapy for ventilator-associated pneumonia in adults: a randomized trial. JAMA. 2003;290(19):2588–98.
39. Capellier G, Mockly H, Charpentier C, Annane D, Blasco G, Desmettre T, et al. Early-onset ventilator-associated pneumonia in adults randomized clinical trial: comparison of 8 versus 15 days of antibiotic treatment. PLoS One. 2012;7(8):e41290.

Lung-Protective Ventilation and Hypercapnia: How Much Is Permissible?

9

9.1 Introduction

The harmful effects of mechanical ventilation with the triggering of ventilator-induced lung injury (VILI) have been clearly established. The use of low tidal volumes with limitation of plateau pressure (P_{plat}) was shown to improve clinical outcomes, including survival, in the ARDS network randomized controlled trial (RCT) [1]. Lung-protective ventilation using low tidal volumes often leads to hypercapnic acidosis [2]. Permissive hypercapnia is the concept of tolerance to high carbon dioxide levels with the use of a lung-protective ventilation strategy [3]. There is conflicting evidence regarding the physiological impact of high carbon dioxide levels and their association with clinical outcomes. Some studies have suggested a beneficial effect [4] while others have reported possible harm [5].

9.2 The Physiologic Effects of Hypercapnia

9.2.1 Effects on the Lung

Hypercapnia seems to exert a net anti-inflammatory effect in the lung. In an animal model, hypercapnic acidosis attenuated VILI through a nuclear factor-κB-related mechanism [6]. Nuclear factor-κB inhibition also leads to downregulation of intercellular adhesion molecule-1 and interleukin-8. This results in the suppression of neutrophil adherence to the endothelial cells in the lung [7]. This beneficial effect may be offset by impaired repair of injury resulting from pulmonary epithelial damage related to VILI [8]. Hypercapnia may also lead to impairment of alveolar epithelial cell function, resulting in reduced fluid absorption from the alveoli [9].

J. Chacko et al., *Controversies in Critical Care*,
https://doi.org/10.1007/978-981-19-9940-6_9

9.2.2 Effects on the Pulmonary and Systemic Circulation

Hypercapnia augments the hypoxic pulmonary vasoconstrictor response and decreases the intrapulmonary shunt, leading to an improvement in gas exchange [10]. Hypercapnia and the associated acidosis cause a rightward shift of the hemoglobin-oxygen dissociation curve with improved oxygen delivery to the tissues. Hypercapnia also increases the cardiac output through an increase in the preload, afterload, and contractility and an increase in the heart rate, through an enhanced sympathetic response [11].

Hypercapnia may lead to pulmonary vasoconstriction with an increase in pulmonary vascular resistance (PVR). The rise in PVR may impair right ventricular function due an increase in the afterload, leading to hemodynamic instability [12]. Worsening pulmonary hypertension and right ventricular dysfunction may predispose to adverse clinical outcomes with the use of permissive hypercapnia in ARDS [5].

9.2.3 Neurological Effects

Hypercapnia results in cerebral vasodilatation and increased cerebral blood flow; this leads to an increase in the cerebral blood volume with a commensurate rise in the intracranial pressure. The effect is generally transient and wears off after 48 h of continued hypercapnia [13]. Acute hypercapnia may result in agitation or a decreased level of consciousness [14]. Hypercapnia may also lower the seizure threshold [15]. However, it is unknown whether the predisposition to seizures occurs only in those with a known seizure disorder.

9.2.4 Effect on the Diaphragm

Hypercapnia of less than 80 mmHg augments the myogenic tone of the diaphragm. Above this level, inhibition of myogenic tone may occur, with a more pronounced effect above 100 mmHg [16]. Skeletal muscle atrophy may occur due to prolonged hypercapnia [17] and may lead to a prolongation of the recovery phase in patients with ARDS, especially in the presence coexisting chronic lung disease. In spontaneously breathing patients, hypercapnic acidosis may impair diaphragmatic function by inhibition of afferent transmission through the vagus nerve [18].

9.2.5 Miscellaneous Effects

Hypercapnia may cause intracellular acidosis [4], leading to inhibition of actin-myosin linkage and impairment of muscle contractility [19]. The effect of hypercapnia on the host response to bacterial infection may be variable, with attenuation of lung injury due to acute bacterial pneumonia in an animal model [20]. Overall, it

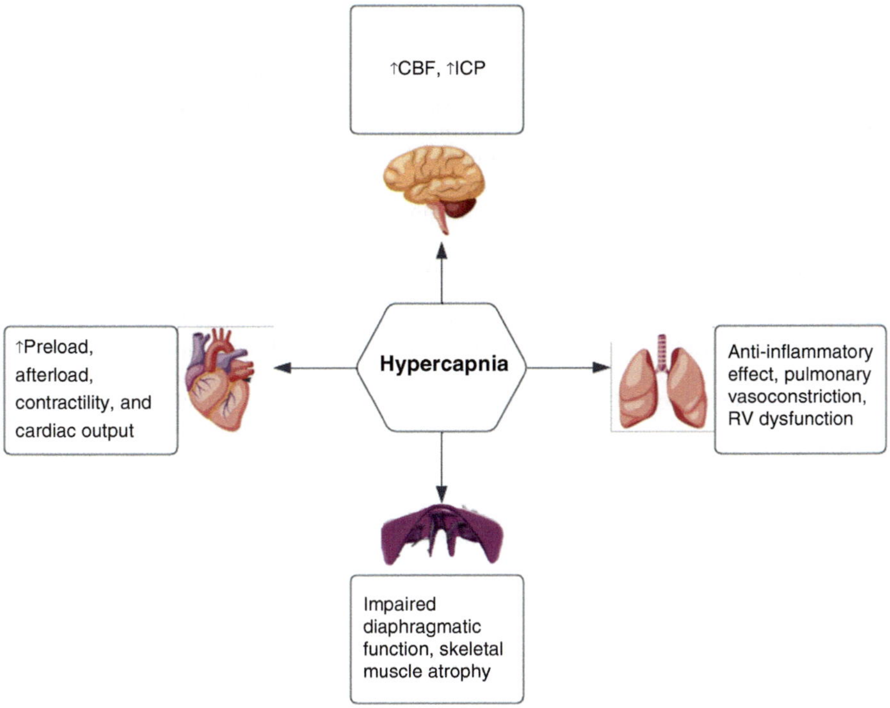

Fig. 9.1 The systemic effects of hypercapnia

is unclear if there is an increased risk of infection due to hypercapnia. The systemic effects of hypercapnia are depicted in Fig. 9.1.

9.3 What Does Clinical Evidence Suggest (Table 9.1)?

Tiruvoipati et al. analyzed the impact of hypercapnia across 171 ICUs from the Australian and New Zealand Intensive Care Society database during a 14-year period. The study included 252,812 patients with normocapnia, compensated hypercapnia, or hypercapnia with acidosis. On multivariable logistic regression analysis, the odds ratio (OR) for hospital mortality was highest among patients with hypercapnic acidosis, followed by those with compensated hypercapnia, and lowest for patients with normocapnia. The increased mortality with hypercapnia was observed regardless of the PaO_2/FiO_2 ratios. In patients with hypercapnic acidosis, the mortality rose to a $PaCO_2$ level of 65 mmHg and plateaued off thereafter. This retrospective observational study revealed a strong association between increasing levels of hypercapnia and mortality [21].

Kregenow et al. performed a secondary analysis of data from the landmark ARDS Network randomized controlled trial (RCT) that established improved survival with a lung-protective ventilation strategy in acute respiratory distress

Table 9.1 Main studies that have evaluated the effect of hypercapnia on outcomes in critically ill patients

Study/year	Design	Patient characteristics	Findings
Tiruvoipati et al. (2017) [21]	Retrospective observational database study	Patients were analyzed based on normocapnia, compensated hypercapnia, or hypercapnia with acidosis	Mortality highest among patients with hypercapnic acidosis, followed by those with compensated hypercapnia, and lowest in patients with normocapnia
Kregenow et al. (2006) [22]	Secondary analysis from the ARDS Network randomized controlled trial	Patients with hypercapnic acidosis on day 1, defined as a pH less than 7.35 and $PaCO_2 > 45$ mmHg compared to normocapnic patients	In the 12 mL/kg V_t group, OR for 28-days mortality significantly lower in patients with hypercapnic acidosis. In contrast, in the 6 mL/kg V_t group, mortality significantly higher with hypercapnic acidosis. Hypercapnia may mitigate the adverse effect of ventilation with high V_t
Tiruvoipati et al. (2021) [23]	Retrospective observational study	Critically ill, septic patients	Hypercapnia not an independent predictor of hospital mortality in ventilated or non-ventilated patients. In mechanically ventilated patients, both prolonged hypercapnia and acidemia were associated with higher mortality. Highest mortality with >120 h of hypercapnia and acidemia
Nin et al. (2017) [24]	Secondary analysis of 3 cohort studies	ARDS patients ventilated for more than 12 h	Mortality significantly higher in patients with a $PCO_2 \geq 50$ mmHg in the first 48 h of mechanical ventilation on both univariate and multivariate analysis. Incidence of complications higher with hypercapnia

V_t tidal volume, *ARDS* acute respiratory distress syndrome

syndrome (ARDS) [22]. The authors evaluated the 28-days mortality in patients with hypercapnic acidosis on day 1, defined as a pH less than 7.35 and $PaCO_2 > 45$ mmHg. The OR for 28-days mortality was significantly lower in patients with hypercapnic acidosis compared to those with normocapnia in the high tidal volume (12 mL/kg predicted body weight) group. However, in the low tidal volume (6 mL/kg predicted body weight) arm, the mortality was significantly higher among patients with hypercapnic acidosis. This study suggests that hypercapnia may mitigate the harm resulting from injurious ventilation strategies including the use of high tidal volumes. In patients who are ventilated with a lung-protective strategy using low tidal volumes, the protective effect of hypercapnia is not discernible; indeed a deleterious effect may occur.

The impact of hypercapnia in septic patients was evaluated in a retrospective study from three ICUs in Victoria, Australia [23]. The study included critically ill patients admitted with a diagnosis of sepsis over an 8-year period. The authors analyzed $PaCO_2$ values from more than 3000 patients. Adjustment for likely confounders was carried out through logistic regression modeling. Hypercapnia was not independently associated with hospital mortality in ventilated or non-ventilated patients. Furthermore, no association between hypercapnia and mortality was observed in patients with sepsis of pulmonary compared with non-pulmonary origin. However, among mechanically ventilated patients, both hypercapnia and acidemia of prolonged duration were associated with higher mortality. The highest mortality rate was observed with 120 h or more of exposure to hypercapnia and acidemia. An increased risk of mortality was also observed in mechanically ventilated patients with non-pulmonary sepsis with hypercapnic academia between 48 and 120 h of exposure.

Nin et al. carried out a secondary analysis of three cohort studies including 1899 patients with ARDS who were ventilated for more than 12 h. On univariate analysis, mortality was significantly higher in patients with a $PCO_2 \geq 50$ mmHg in the first 48 h of mechanical ventilation. Based on this finding, a multivariable regression analysis was performed including the PaO_2/FiO_2 ratio, PEEP level, respiratory rate, presence of acidosis, the use of a pressure-limited strategy during the first 48 h after commencing mechanical ventilation, and the period of study. Severe hypercapnia of $\geq$50 mmHg remained independently associated with ICU mortality (OR 1.93, 95% CI 1.32–2.81; $p = 0.001$). The incidence of complications including barotrauma and renal and cardiovascular dysfunction was also higher in patients with severe hypercapnia [24]. Table 9.1 summarizes the main studies that have evaluated the effect of hypercapnia on outcomes in critically ill patients.

9.4 Interventions to Reduce Carbon Dioxide Levels

9.4.1 Increasing Minute Ventilation

An increase in the minute ventilation may offset a rise in carbon dioxide levels. While using a low tidal volume, lung-protective strategy, the respiratory rate may be increased appropriately. However, inappropriately high respiratory rates may also lead to harm. Increasing the respiratory rate may lead to dynamic hyperinflation and right ventricular dysfunction [25]. Besides, the respiratory rate is one of the components of the mechanical power of ventilation. A higher respiratory rate increases the mechanical power and may be related to increased hospital mortality [5].

9.4.2 Reduction of Dead Space

Simple interventions to reduce dead space ventilation include connection of the Y-piece of the ventilator circuit directly to the endotracheal tube, without an intervening catheter mount. The heat and moisture exchanger adds to the dead space and may be replaced by a heated humidifier.

9.4.3 Optimization of PEEP Levels

Appropriate titration of PEEP levels is a crucial intervention with the lung-protective ventilation strategy. An adequate level of PEEP results in optimal recruitment of collapsed alveoli. However, excessive PEEP leads to overdistension and an increase in the physiological dead space. The ART trial compared the strategy of a lung recruitment maneuver and titration of PEEP based on the best respiratory system compliance with a low PEEP strategy. The lung recruitment-PEEP titration group revealed a significantly higher 28-day mortality, possibly related to excessive airway pressures [26].

9.4.4 Prone Ventilation

Assuming the prone position enables recruitment of the dorsal areas of the lung, with a more homogenous distribution of ventilation. The lung mass is greater in the dorsal compared to the ventral aspect, enabling greater recruitment of previously collapsed lung. The 28-day survival was higher among patients with ARDS who responded to the prone position with a decrease in PCO_2 levels in a retrospective analysis of one of the early RCTs on prone ventilation [27].

9.4.5 The Use of Buffers

Although controversial at best, buffers have been used to mitigate the effect of hypercapnia-induced acidosis. There are no RCTs that evaluate the effect of buffers in respiratory acidosis. Moderate levels of hypercapnic acidosis are generally well tolerated, if oxygenation is adequate and tissue perfusion is maintained. Following the ARDS network trial, the recommendation was made to administer sodium bicarbonate if hypercapnia resulted in a pH of less than 7.1 [1]. However, alkali therapy is generally not recommended for hypercapnia alone; it may be more appropriate in patients with a mixed acidosis [28].

9.4.6 Extracorporeal Carbon Dioxide Removal

Extracorporeal carbon dioxide removal involves the elimination of carbon dioxide using a gas exchange membrane; there is no significant improvement in oxygenation. The extracorporeal flow for the removal of carbon dioxide is considerably less than that required for oxygenation. Extracorporeal carbon dioxide removal may enable "ultra-lung-protective" ventilation with tidal volumes of 4 mL/kg or less and

P_{plat} of ≤25 cmH_2O [29]. However, currently there is no robust evidence to support improved clinical outcomes with this modality of treatment. Extracorporeal carbon dioxide removal may reduce the requirement for invasive mechanical ventilation in patients with acute exacerbation chronic obstructive pulmonary disease [30]. It may also enable reduction of the work of breathing and facilitate weaning [31].

Key Points

- The use of a lung-protective ventilation strategy often leads to hypercapnic acidosis.
- Earlier studies had suggested no significant adverse impact and possible beneficial effect from hypercapnia. This led to the concept of "permissive hypercapnia"; however, hypercapnia may not be entirely benign.
- Hypercapnia may increase pulmonary artery pressure and overload the right ventricle; besides, it may lead to intracranial hypertension, affect diaphragmatic function, and cause intracellular acidosis.
- Hypercapnic acidosis has been shown to be an independent predictor of hospital mortality among critically ill patients.
- High carbon dioxide levels may have a protective effect in patients ventilated with high tidal volumes; this salutary effect seems to disappear with a lung-protective strategy using low tidal volumes.
- A $PaCO_2$ of more than 50 cmH_2O should raise concern, with consideration of appropriate measures to reduce levels.
- Measures to reduce carbon dioxide levels include increasing the minute ventilation, reduction in the dead space of the ventilator circuit, optimization of PEEP levels, prone ventilation, and the use of extracorporeal carbon dioxide removal.

References

1. Acute Respiratory Distress Syndrome Network, Brower RG, Matthay MA, Morris A, Schoenfeld D, Thompson BT, et al. Ventilation with lower tidal volumes as compared with traditional tidal volumes for acute lung injury and the acute respiratory distress syndrome. N Engl J Med. 2000;342(18):1301–8.
2. Amato MB, Barbas CS, Medeiros DM, Magaldi RB, Schettino GP, Lorenzi-Filho G, et al. Effect of a protective-ventilation strategy on mortality in the acute respiratory distress syndrome. N Engl J Med. 1998;338(6):347–54.
3. Bigatello LM, Patroniti N, Sangalli F. Permissive hypercapnia. Curr Opin Crit Care. 2001;7(1):34–40.
4. Feihl F, Perret C, Permissive hypercapnia. How permissive should we be? Am J Respir Crit Care Med. 1994;150(6 Pt 1):1722–37.
5. Barnes T, Zochios V, Parhar K. Re-examining permissive hypercapnia in ARDS: a narrative review. Chest. 2018;154(1):185–95.

6. Contreras M, Ansari B, Curley G, Higgins BD, Hassett P, O'Toole D, et al. Hypercapnic acidosis attenuates ventilation-induced lung injury by a nuclear factor-κB-dependent mechanism. Crit Care Med. 2012;40(9):2622–30.
7. Takeshita K, Suzuki Y, Nishio K, Takeuchi O, Toda K, Kudo H, et al. Hypercapnic acidosis attenuates endotoxin-induced nuclear factor-[kappa]B activation. Am J Respir Cell Mol Biol. 2003;29(1):124–32.
8. O'Toole D, Hassett P, Contreras M, Higgins BD, McKeown STW, McAuley DF, et al. Hypercapnic acidosis attenuates pulmonary epithelial wound repair by an NF-kappaB dependent mechanism. Thorax. 2009;64(11):976–82.
9. Briva A, Vadász I, Lecuona E, Welch LC, Chen J, Dada LA, et al. High CO2 levels impair alveolar epithelial function independently of pH. PLoS One. 2007;2(11):e1238.
10. Sinclair SE, Kregenow DA, Starr I, Schimmel C, Lamm WJE, Hlastala MP, et al. Therapeutic hypercapnia and ventilation-perfusion matching in acute lung injury: low minute ventilation vs inspired CO2. Chest. 2006;130(1):85–92.
11. Cullen DJ, Eger EI. Cardiovascular effects of carbon dioxide in man. Anesthesiology. 1974;41(4):345–9.
12. Viitanen A, Salmenperä M, Heinonen J. Right ventricular response to hypercarbia after cardiac surgery. Anesthesiology. 1990;73(3):393–400.
13. Kontos HA, Raper AJ, Patterson JL. Analysis of vasoactivity of local pH, PCO2 and bicarbonate on pial vessels. Stroke. 1977;8(3):358–60.
14. Sieker HO, Hickam JB. Carbon dioxide intoxication: the clinical syndrome, its etiology and management with particular reference to the use of mechanical respirators. Medicine (Baltimore). 1956;35(4):389–423.
15. Hickling KG. Permissive hypercapnia. Respir Care Clin N Am. 2002;8(2):155–69. v
16. Nagi MM, Ward ME. Modulation of myogenic responsiveness by CO2 in rat diaphragmatic arterioles: role of the endothelium. Am J Phys. 1997;272(3 Pt 2):H1419–25.
17. Jaitovich A, Angulo M, Lecuona E, Dada LA, Welch LC, Cheng Y, et al. High CO2 levels cause skeletal muscle atrophy via AMP-activated kinase (AMPK), FoxO3a protein, and muscle-specific ring finger protein 1 (MuRF1). J Biol Chem. 2015;290(14):9183–94.
18. Morales-Quinteros L, Camprubí-Rimblas M, Bringué J, Bos LD, Schultz MJ, Artigas A. The role of hypercapnia in acute respiratory failure. Intensive Care Med Exp. 2019;7(S1):39.
19. Orchard CH, Kentish JC. Effects of changes of pH on the contractile function of cardiac muscle. Am J Phys. 1990;258(6 Pt 1):C967–81.
20. Ni Chonghaile M, Higgins BD, Costello JF, Laffey JG. Hypercapnic acidosis attenuates severe acute bacterial pneumonia-induced lung injury by a neutrophil-independent mechanism. Crit Care Med. 2008;36(12):3135–44.
21. Tiruvoipati R, Pilcher D, Buscher H, Botha J, Bailey M. Effects of hypercapnia and Hypercapnic acidosis on hospital mortality in mechanically ventilated patients. Crit Care Med. 2017;45(7):e649–56.
22. Kregenow DA, Rubenfeld GD, Hudson LD, Swenson ER. Hypercapnic acidosis and mortality in acute lung injury. Crit Care Med. 2006;34(1):1–7.
23. Tiruvoipati R, Serpa Neto A, Young M, Marhoon N, Wilson J, Gupta S, et al. An exploratory analysis of the association between hypercapnia and hospital mortality in critically ill patients with sepsis. Ann Am Thorac Soc. 2021;19(2):245–54.
24. Nin N, Muriel A, Peñuelas O, Brochard L, Lorente JA, et al. For the VENTILA group severe hypercapnia and outcome of mechanically ventilated patients with moderate or severe acute respiratory distress syndrome. Intensive Care Med. 2017;43(2):200–8.
25. Vieillard-Baron A, Prin S, Augarde R, Desfonds P, Page B, Beauchet A, et al. Increasing respiratory rate to improve CO2 clearance during mechanical ventilation is not a panacea in acute respiratory failure. Crit Care Med. 2002;30(7):1407–12.

26. Writing Group for the Alveolar Recruitment for Acute Respiratory Distress Syndrome Trial (ART) Investigators, Cavalcanti AB, Suzumura ÉA, Laranjeira LN, de Paisani DM, Damiani LP, et al. Effect of lung recruitment and titrated positive end-expiratory pressure (PEEP) vs low PEEP on mortality in patients with acute respiratory distress syndrome: a randomized clinical trial. JAMA. 2017;318(14):1335–45.
27. Gattinoni L, Vagginelli F, Carlesso E, Taccone P, Conte V, Chiumello D, et al. Decrease in $PaCO_2$ with prone position is predictive of improved outcome in acute respiratory distress syndrome. Crit Care Med. 2003;31(12):2727–33.
28. Adrogué HJ, Madias NE. Alkali therapy for respiratory acidosis: a medical controversy. Am J Kidney Dis. 2020;75(2):265–71.
29. Combes A, Fanelli V, Pham T, Ranieri VM. European Society of Intensive Care Medicine Trials Group and the "strategy of ultra-protective lung ventilation with extracorporeal CO2 removal for new-onset moderate to severe ARDS" (SUPERNOVA) investigators. Feasibility and safety of extracorporeal CO2 removal to enhance protective ventilation in acute respiratory distress syndrome: the SUPERNOVA study. Intensive Care Med. 2019;45(5):592–600.
30. d'Andrea A, Banfi C, Bendjelid K, Giraud R. The use of extracorporeal carbon dioxide removal in acute chronic obstructive pulmonary disease exacerbation: a narrative review. Can J Anaesth. 2020;67(4):462–74.
31. Staudinger T. Update on extracorporeal carbon dioxide removal: a comprehensive review on principles, indications, efficiency, and complications. Perfusion. 2020;35(6):492–508.

Tracheostomy in the ICU: Early or Late? 10

10.1 Introduction

Tracheostomy is performed in critically ill patients when long-term mechanical ventilation is anticipated. Traditionally, tracheostomy was carried out as an open surgical procedure. Percutaneous tracheostomy was first described by Ciaglia et al. in 1985 [1]; since then, this technique has been in widespread use among intensive care physicians with a relatively low incidence of serious complications. The technique of percutaneous tracheostomy has evolved over the years from the use of the Griggs dilatational forceps [2] to a single-stage, tapered dilator using a Seldinger technique [3]. Percutaneous tracheostomy may be carried out by the traditional landmark-based method [4], under bronchoscopic [5] or real-time ultrasound guidance [6].

10.2 Tracheostomy: Pros and Cons

Although tracheostomies are performed much more commonly in recent times [7], considerable debate remains on the optimal timing. The usual practice among most clinicians is to consider the performance of a tracheostomy if weaning and extubation seem unlikely after 5–7 days of endotracheal intubation and mechanical ventilation. Prolonged endotracheal intubation may cause airway stenosis due to tracheal injury at the site of cuff inflation [8]. However, the use of high-volume, low-pressure cuffs may significantly reduce this complication [9]. Most guidelines recommend consideration of tracheostomy after a week of mechanical ventilation through an endotracheal tube [10, 11].

Compared to continued translaryngeal intubation, the performance of a tracheostomy may potentially enable an enhanced level of comfort with a reduced dose of sedative agents, allow more rapid weaning from mechanical ventilation, reduce the incidence of ventilator-associated pneumonia (VAP), and shorten ICU and hospital

J. Chacko et al., *Controversies in Critical Care*,
https://doi.org/10.1007/978-981-19-9940-6_10

stay. The presence of a tracheostomy also allows more efficient management of secretions [12]. The reduced length of the tracheostomy tube offers less resistance to airflow and may reduce the effort of spontaneous breaths and thereby decrease the work of breathing [13]. The shorter tracheostomy tube may also reduce the apparatus dead space [13].

Compared to an endotracheal tube, the performance of a tracheostomy has been shown to improve commonly measured weaning parameters. In a cohort of difficult to wean patients, the performance of a tracheostomy resulted in more favorable ventilation parameters, including a greater maximum negative inspiratory pressure and maximum expiratory pressures. Furthermore, compared to spontaneous breathing through an endotracheal tube, higher tidal volumes, lower rapid shallow breathing index (RSBI), and lower airway resistance were observed following tracheostomy [14].

Switching from an endotracheal tube to a tracheostomy has disadvantages too. The tracheostomy tube may get clogged with secretions leading to ventilation problems. There is a potential for tube dislodgement; reinsertion may not be easy through a poorly matured track. Injury to prominent veins over the neck and hemorrhage, although usually minor, may pose problems. Ultrasonographic identification and real-time guidance may prevent injury to the blood vessels [6]. If subcutaneous emphysema develops, pneumothorax must be considered. The likelihood of posterior tracheal wall injury is also a potential complication [15]. Surgical emphysema can also occur due to air leak around the tracheal stoma with positive pressure ventilation. Complications during the procedure may include loss of PEEP and possible aspiration of airway secretions, resulting in worsening of hypoxia [16]. Hence, tracheostomy is usually delayed until the PEEP level has come down to a reasonable level (10 cmH_2O). Late complications of tracheostomy include tracheal stenosis, tracheomalacia, formation of a tracheoinnominate fistula leading to exsanguinating hemorrhage [17], and development of a tracheoesophageal fistula [18]. Considering these potential complications, a considered decision must be made to choose an optimal time for the performance of a tracheostomy. The potential benefits vs. risks of tracheostomy in critically ill patients are summarized in Table 10.1.

Table 10.1 Potential benefits compared to risks of tracheostomy in critically ill patients

Benefits	Risks
More comfortable, potential for reducing or ceasing sedation; earlier weaning	Procedure-related complications, including bleeding, pneumothorax, worsening of hypoxia, rise in ICP
Reduced risk of VAP, shorter ICU, and hospital stay	Cannula displacement with an immature track may lead to difficulty with reinsertion
Ease of clearance of secretions	Stomal infection
Reduced apparatus dead space, lower resistance compared to translaryngeal intubation, reduced work of breathing	Long-term complications including tracheal stenosis, collapse
Earlier initiation of oral intake	Unnecessary tracheostomies in patients who can be extubated leads to inordinate delays in weaning
Mobilization easier	

10.3 The Evidence: Early Vs. Delayed Tracheostomy

Several randomized controlled trials (RCTs) have been performed to evaluate the optimal timing of tracheostomy. Most of the RCTs are of small sample size, involving heterogeneous groups of patients, and offer conflicting results (Table 10.2).

Table 10.2 Main randomized controlled trials that compared clinical outcomes with early vs. late tracheostomy

Study/year	Population	Early	Late	Outcomes
Rumbak et al. (2004) [19]	Acute respiratory failure with predicted ventilation requirement for >14 days	Within 48 h of intubation	14–16 day after intubation	Lower morality, reduced ICU stay, shorter duration of ventilation lower incidence of VAP with early tracheostomy
Terragini et al. (2010) [20]	Mechanically ventilation for ≥24 h, SAPS score 35–65, SOFA score ≥5	After 6–8 day of intubation	After 13–15 day of intubation	Similar incidence of VAP. More ventilator-free and ICU-free days, likelihood of weaning, 28-day survival with early tracheostomy
Young et al. (TracMan 2013) [21]	Enrolled patients within 4 days of ICU admission, deemed to require at least 7 more days of ventilation	Within 4 days of mechanical ventilation	On day 10 or later if tracheostomy still considered appropriate	53.7% in the late group did not undergo tracheostomy. 30-day all-cause mortality, 2-year mortality, duration of ICU stay, similar. Clinician judgment regarding the need for tracheostomy could be imprecise at an early stage
Trouillet et al. (2011) [25]	Cardiac surgical patients requiring mechanical ventilation at 4 or more days postoperatively	Within 5 days of surgery	Tracheostomy if the duration of ventilation >15 days	Ventilator-free days at 60 days, 28-, 60-, and 90-day mortality, duration of ventilation and hospitalization, incidence of VAP, similar between groups. Reduced IV sedation, less delirium, increased level of comfort, earlier initiation of oral nutrition with early tracheostomy

(continued)

Table 10.2 (continued)

Study/year	Population	Early	Late	Outcomes
Bösel et al. (SETPOINT-2, 2022) [29]	Patients with stroke (ischemic stroke, intracerebral or subarachnoid hemorrhage)	≤5 days of mechanical ventilation	After 10 days if tracheostomy still considered necessary	No significant difference in the number of patients without severe disability at 6 months (modified Rankin score 0–4). Time to commence weaning, duration of ventilation, time to discharge from ICU and hospital similar between groups

An early study by Rumbak et al. suggested that a very early tracheostomy may be advantageous. This RCT included 120 patients admitted to a medical ICU who were intubated for acute respiratory failure with a predicted duration of ventilation of more than 14 days [19]. In the early group, percutaneous tracheostomy was performed within 48 h after intubation, compared to 14–16 days after intubation in the late group. Sixty patients were included in each group. Ten patients in the late group did not undergo tracheostomy; two of these patients died, while eight were extubated before day 14. Early tracheostomy was associated with significantly lower mortality (31.7% vs. 61.7%), reduced ICU stay (4.8 ± 1.4 vs. 16.2 ± 3.8 days), and lower duration of mechanical ventilation (7.6 ± 2.0 vs. 17.4 ± 5.3 days). The cumulative incidence of VAP was also lower with an early tracheostomy. Furthermore, early tracheostomy resulted in less damage to the mouth and larynx and superior airway control compared to late tracheostomy. This RCT supported early tracheostomy within 48 h of intubation. However, the results of subsequent controlled trials have been less promising with an early approach.

Terragni et al. carried out a multicentric RCT in Italy to specifically evaluate the incidence of pneumonia with early compared to late tracheostomy [20]. The study population included patients who were ventilated for at least 24 h for acute respiratory failure with a Simplified Acute Physiology Score (SAPS) of 35–65 and Sequential Organ Failure Assessment (SOFA) score ≥5. There was no evidence of lung infection at the time of enrolment, based on a Clinical Pulmonary Infection Score (CPIS) of <6. The study included 209 patients in the early tracheostomy group and 210 patients in the late tracheostomy group. The primary endpoint, the incidence of VAP, was 14% (95% CI, 10–19%) in the early compared to 21% (95% CI, 15%–26%) in the late group, and not significantly different between groups ($P = 0.07$). Among the secondary outcomes, the number of ventilator-free days and ICU-free days at 28 days was higher in the early tracheostomy group. Besides, the likelihood of successful weaning from mechanical ventilation and survival at day 28 was also greater with early compared to late tracheostomy.

The TracMan trial was conceived against the background of the equivocal results from previous RCTs and observational studies. In the largest RCT so far, this study enrolled patients within 4 days of ICU admission, who were judged by the treating clinician to require at least 7 more days of mechanical ventilation [21]. The multicentric study from the UK included 909 patients from 70 critical care units. In the early group, tracheostomy was performed within 4 days of mechanical ventilation. Patients in the late group underwent tracheostomy on day 10 or later if still considered appropriate by the treating clinician. Four hundred and fifty-five patients were assigned to the early group and 454 to the late group. In the early group, 91.9% of assigned patients underwent tracheostomy. Among the 454 patients assigned to the late group, 244 (53.7%) did not undergo tracheostomy; 19.6% were discharged from the ICU by day 10, and 17.2% were still in the ICU, but off ventilator support, 11.9% had died, and 2.4% were too unstable, or for end of life care alone. The all-cause mortality at 30 days, the primary endpoint, was similar between the two groups (early, 30.8%, vs. late, 31.5%). The duration of ICU stay among survivors and the 2-year mortality were also not significantly different between groups. Besides showing no survival benefit, this study also suggested that clinician judgment regarding the requirement for tracheostomy could be very imprecise at an early stage of mechanical ventilation. A large number of patients who were considered to require tracheostomy and randomized to the late arm could be weaned off ventilator support and extubated.

10.4 Meta-Analyses on Tracheostomy Timing

Two recent meta-analyses have evaluated clinical outcomes with early compared to late tracheostomy. Chorath et al. analyzed data from 17 RCTs, including 3145 patients [22]. Tracheostomy performed within 7 days of initiation of mechanical ventilation was considered early; patients who underwent tracheostomy later or received no tracheostomy were included in the late group. The incidence of VAP was significantly lower with early compared to late tracheostomy. Ventilator-free days were higher in the early tracheostomy group. Some of the included studies had used ventilator days as the outcome; this was not different between the two groups. The duration of ICU stay was lower in the early tracheostomy group; two studies included in the meta-analysis evaluated ICU-free days as the outcome; the number of ICU-free days was higher in the early group. All-cause mortality at 30 days was not different between the two groups.

In another meta-analysis by Deng et al., 15 RCTs were included, comprising of 3003 patients [23]. The definition of early vs. late was based on individual studies. There was no significant difference in the short-term mortality between the early compared to the late tracheostomy group. The incidence of VAP was 10% lower in the early tracheostomy group, but this difference was not statistically significant. The duration of mechanical ventilation and the duration of ICU stay were significantly lower with an early tracheostomy.

10.5 Early Tracheostomy in Specific Subgroups of Patients

10.5.1 Post-Cardiovascular Surgery

Most of the studies conducted so far have compared early with late tracheostomy among heterogeneous groups of patients admitted to general ICUs. A pertinent question is whether specific subgroups of patients might benefit from an early tracheostomy.

Postoperative cardiovascular surgical patients often develop complications, with multiorgan failure, including respiratory failure, and may need prolonged mechanical ventilatory support [24]. Does early tracheostomy benefit patients who require prolonged mechanical ventilation after cardiac surgery? Trouillet et al. randomized postoperative cardiac surgical patients to either early tracheostomy within 5 days of surgery or prolonged intubation and tracheostomy only if the duration of mechanical ventilation exceeded 15 days [25]. The operative procedures performed in this cohort included coronary artery bypass graft, valve surgery, and heart transplantation. There was no significant difference between groups in the number of ventilator-free days at 60 days, the primary endpoint. Among the secondary endpoints, there was no significant difference in the 28-, 60-, and 90-day mortality. Besides, the duration of mechanical ventilation and hospitalization and the incidence of VAP were also similar between groups. The authors observed a reduction in the use of intravenous sedation, a lower incidence of delirium, a higher level of comfort, and a more rapid initiation of oral nutrition with an early tracheostomy.

10.5.2 Patients with Neurological Injury

Patients with neurological injury who require long-term airway protection and tracheal toilet, but able to breathe unsupported, may benefit from an early tracheostomy. They may be weaned rapidly and cared for in a normal ward, thereby reducing the duration of stay in the ICU. Expeditious transfer to a ward or home care could also reduce the overall cost of care. A meta-analysis revealed that early tracheostomy may reduce the duration of mechanical ventilation and ICU and hospital stay in patients with traumatic brain injury (TBI) [26]. In another meta-analysis, early tracheostomy was associated with a reduced duration of mechanical ventilation, ICU stay, and long-term mortality risk in patients who had suffered acute brain injury of varying etiology including TBI, acute ischemic stroke, spontaneous intracerebral hemorrhage, stroke, and hypoxic-ischemic encephalopathy [27]. Specifically, in stroke patients, the duration of hospital stay and the incidence of VAP have also been shown to be less in a meta-analysis, although there was no difference in the duration of mechanical ventilation, ICU stay, or mortality [28].

The SETPOINT-2 RCT evaluated outcomes following an early compared with a late tracheostomy among patients with stroke requiring mechanical ventilation [29].

The study included 382 patients following ischemic stroke, intracerebral, or subarachnoid hemorrhage who were receiving mechanical ventilation. The requirement for tracheostomy was assessed using a previously validated, 15-item score (SETscore) [30]. Patients were randomized to an early tracheostomy at ≤5 days or continued on mechanical ventilation with attempts to wean. A tracheostomy was performed if needed, after 10 days in the late group. A tracheostomy was performed in 95.2% of patients randomized to the early group. However, among patients randomized to the late group, only 67% patients underwent a tracheostomy; 22% of patients were successfully extubated, while 10.8% died prior to consideration of the procedure. The primary outcome, the proportion of patients without severe disability at 6 months, defined as a modified Rankin Scale score 0–4, was not significantly different between the early compared to the late group (43.5% vs. 47.1%; adjusted OR, 0.93 [95% CI, 0.60–1.42]; $p = 0.73$). The time to commence weaning, the duration of mechanical ventilation, and the time to discharge from ICU and hospital were also similar between the two groups. Similar to the TracMan trial, this RCT also showed that a significant number of patients may not require a tracheostomy if a late compared to an early strategy is followed.

Key Points

- The putative advantages of tracheostomy include an increased level of patient comfort with a reduced dose of sedative agents and more rapid weaning from mechanical ventilation. However, these potential benefits must be balanced against the likelihood of short and long-term complications related to tracheostomy.
- Tracheostomy within a week of mechanical ventilation is of no proven benefit and might lead to an unnecessary procedure among patients who could be extubated at a later stage.
- Patients who are on a high PEEP level or hemodynamically unstable are generally not suitable for tracheostomy.
- Early tracheostomy may reduce the duration of mechanical ventilation and ICU stay in selected patients subgroups; however, there is no good evidence of improved survival with an early tracheostomy.
- There is moderate evidence that suggests a lower incidence of VAP in patients who undergo an earlier tracheostomy; however, this effect needs confirmation in future trials.
- In some patient populations, prolonged mechanical ventilation is easily predictable. This includes patients with TBI, stroke, and other underlying causes of neurological injury. Early tracheostomy in this subgroup of patients may reduce the duration of mechanical ventilation and ICU stay.

References

1. Ciaglia P, Firsching R, Syniec C. Elective percutaneous dilatational tracheostomy. A new simple bedside procedure; preliminary report. Chest. 1985;87(6):715–9.
2. Griggs WM, Worthley LI, Gilligan JE, Thomas PD, Myburg JA. A simple percutaneous tracheostomy technique. Surg Gynecol Obstet. 1990;170(6):543–5.
3. Ambesh SP, Pandey CK, Srivastava S, Agarwal A, Singh DK. Percutaneous tracheostomy with single dilatation technique: a prospective, randomized comparison of Ciaglia blue rhino versus Griggs' guidewire dilating forceps. Anesth Analg. 2002;95(6):1739–45.
4. Rudas M, Seppelt I, Herkes R, Hislop R, Rajbhandari D, Weisbrodt L. Traditional landmark versus ultrasound guided tracheal puncture during percutaneous dilatational tracheostomy in adult intensive care patients: a randomised controlled trial. Crit Care. 2014;18(5):514.
5. Fernandez L, Norwood S, Roettger R, Gass D, Wilkins H. Bedside percutaneous tracheostomy with bronchoscopic guidance in critically ill patients. Arch Surg. 1996;131(2):129–32.
6. Chacko J, Gagan B, Kumar U, Mundlapudi B. Real-time ultrasound guided percutaneous dilatational tracheostomy with and without bronchoscopic control: an observational study. Minerva Anestesiol. 2015;81(2):166–74.
7. Cox CE, Carson SS, Holmes GM, Howard A, Carey TS. Increase in tracheostomy for prolonged mechanical ventilation in North Carolina, 1993-2002. Crit Care Med. 2004;32(11):2219–26.
8. Grillo HC, Donahue DM. Post intubation tracheal stenosis. Semin Thorac Cardiovasc Surg. 1996;8(4):370–80.
9. Cooper JD. Tracheal injuries complicating prolonged intubation and tracheostomy. Thorac Surg Clin. 2018;28(2):139–44.
10. Adly A, Youssef TA, El-Begermy MM, Younis HM. Timing of tracheostomy in patients with prolonged endotracheal intubation: a systematic review. Eur Arch Otorhinolaryngol. 2018;275(3):679–90.
11. Holevar M, Dunham JCM, Brautigan R, Clancy TV, Como JJ, Ebert JB, et al. Practice management guidelines for timing of tracheostomy: the EAST practice management guidelines work group. J Trauma. 2009;67(4):870–4.
12. Durbin CG. Tracheostomy: why, when, and how? Respir Care. 2010;55(8):1056–68.
13. Davis K. Changes in respiratory mechanics after tracheostomy. Arch Surg. 1999;134(1):59.
14. Lim CK, Ruan SY, Lin FC, Wu CL, Chang HT, Jerng JS, et al. Effect of tracheostomy on weaning parameters in difficult-to-wean mechanically ventilated patients: a prospective observational study. PLoS One. 2015;10(9):e0138294.
15. Douglas WE, Flabouris A. Surgical emphysema following percutaneous tracheostomy. Anaesth Intensive Care. 1999;27(1):69–72.
16. Durbin CG. Early complications of tracheostomy. Respir Care. 2005;50(4):511–5.
17. Goldenberg D, Ari EG, Golz A, Danino J, Netzer A, Joachims HZ. Tracheotomy complications: a retrospective study of 1130 cases. Otolaryngol Head Neck Surg. 2000;123(4):495–500.
18. Fernandez-Bussy S, Mahajan B, Folch E, Caviedes I, Guerrero J, Majid A. Tracheostomy tube placement: early and late complications. J Bronchol Interv Pulmonol. 2015;22(4):357–64.
19. Rumbak MJ, Newton M, Truncale T, Schwartz SW, Adams JW, Hazard PB. A prospective, randomized, study comparing early percutaneous dilational tracheotomy to prolonged translaryngeal intubation (delayed tracheotomy) in critically ill medical patients*. Crit Care Med. 2004;32(8):1689–94.
20. Terragni PP, Antonelli M, Fumagalli R, Faggiano C, Berardino M, Pallavicini FB, et al. Early vs late tracheotomy for prevention of pneumonia in mechanically ventilated adult ICU patients: a randomized controlled trial. JAMA. 2010;303(15):1483–9.
21. Young D, Harrison DA, Cuthbertson BH, Rowan K, TracMan Collaborators. Effect of early vs late tracheostomy placement on survival in patients receiving mechanical ventilation: the TracMan randomized trial. JAMA. 2013;309(20):2121–9.

22. Chorath K, Hoang A, Rajasekaran K, Moreira A. Association of early vs late tracheostomy placement with pneumonia and ventilator days in critically ill patients: a meta-analysis. JAMA Otolaryngol Head Neck Surg. 2021;147(5):450–9.
23. Deng H, Fang Q, Chen K, Zhang X. Early versus late tracheotomy in ICU patients: a meta-analysis of randomized controlled trials. Medicine (Baltimore). 2021;100(3):e24329.
24. Walts PA, Murthy SC, Arroliga AC, Yared JP, Rajeswaran J, Rice TW, et al. Tracheostomy after cardiovascular surgery: an assessment of long-term outcome. J Thorac Cardiovasc Surg. 2006;131(4):830–7.
25. Trouillet JL, Luyt CE, Guiguet M, Ouattara A, Vaissier E, Makri R, et al. Early percutaneous tracheotomy versus prolonged intubation of mechanically ventilated patients after cardiac surgery: a randomized trial*. Ann Intern Med. 2011;154(6):373.
26. de Franca SA, Tavares WM, Salinet ASM, Paiva WS, Teixeira MJ. Early tracheostomy in severe traumatic brain injury patients: a meta-analysis and comparison with late tracheostomy. Crit Care Med. 2020;48(4):e325–31.
27. McCredie VA, Alali AS, Scales DC, Adhikari NKJ, Rubenfeld GD, Cuthbertson BH, et al. Effect of early versus late tracheostomy or prolonged intubation in critically ill patients with acute brain injury: a systematic review and meta-analysis. Neurocrit Care. 2017;26(1):14–25.
28. Araujo de Franca S, Tavares WM, ASM S, Paiva WS, Teixeira MJ. Early tracheostomy in stroke patients: a meta-analysis and comparison with late tracheostomy. Clin Neurol Neurosurg. 2021;203:106554.
29. Bösel J, Niesen WD, Salih F, Morris NA, Ragland JT, Gough B, et al. Effect of early vs standard approach to tracheostomy on functional outcome at 6 months among patients with severe stroke receiving mechanical ventilation: the SETPOINT2 randomized clinical trial. JAMA. 2022;327(19):1899–909.
30. Schönenberger S, Al-Suwaidan F, Kieser M, Uhlmann L, Bösel J. The SETscore to predict tracheostomy need in cerebrovascular neurocritical care patients. Neurocrit Care. 2016;25(1):94–104.

Diaphragmatic Dysfunction in Critical Illness

11

11.1 Introduction

Although limb muscle weakness associated with critical illness-related polyneuromyopathy raises concern among clinicians, there may be a relative lack of awareness regarding diaphragmatic weakness among critically ill patients. The difficulty encountered in the monitoring of diaphragm function by the bedside may have contributed to the relative lack of focus on the diaphragm. The incidence of diaphragm dysfunction in critically ill patients undergoing mechanical ventilation remains high [1, 2]. In fact, diaphragmatic weakness may be twice as common as limb muscle weakness in ICU patients [3].

11.2 Clinical Signs of Diaphragm Dysfunction

During an inspiratory effort, the diaphragm moves in a caudal direction, with a decrease in the intrathoracic pressure and an increase in the intra-abdominal pressure, resulting in an outward movement of the abdominal wall. When the diaphragm is paralyzed, during the inspiratory phase, the intercostal muscles contract leading to a fall in the intrathoracic pressure. The flaccid diaphragm moves cephalad as it is "sucked in," leading to a drop in the intra-abdominal pressure. The fall in intra-abdominal pressure leads to the inward movement of the abdominal wall during inspiration, resulting in the typical "paradoxical" breathing pattern. It is important to confirm diaphragmatic weakness as excessive expiratory muscle activity can also lead to a similar clinical finding.

J. Chacko et al., *Controversies in Critical Care*,
https://doi.org/10.1007/978-981-19-9940-6_11

11.3 Causes of Diaphragm Dysfunction

11.3.1 Electrolyte and Endocrine Abnormalities

Hypophosphatemia, hypomagnesemia, and hypocalcemia may result in significant diaphragmatic weakness and should be actively sought for and corrected. Severe hypothyroidism often causes diaphragmatic dysfunction leading to respiratory failure. Prolonged hyperglycemia, and severe malnutrition, and renal failure may also cause diaphragmatic weakness.

11.3.2 Sedatives, Neuromuscular Blocking Drugs, and Corticosteroids

Excessive sedation in patients undergoing mechanical ventilation may lead to disuse atrophy of the diaphragm. Specifically, there may be a dose-related association of propofol use with diaphragmatic weakness [2]. Prolonged use of corticosteroids may also lead to diaphragmatic weakness, depending on the duration and the specific agent used [4]. The use of neuromuscular blocking agents for an extended duration has also been associated with disuse atrophy of the diaphragm. The impact of neuromuscular blockade-associated diaphragmatic weakness may be exacerbated by the concomitant use of corticosteroids [4]. Compared to the aminosteroid class of neuromuscular blockers (rocuronium, vecuronium), benzylisoquinoline esters (atracurium, cisatracurium) may be associated with a lower incidence of diaphragmatic impairment [5].

11.3.3 Ventilator-Induced Diaphragm Dysfunction (VIDD)

Atrophy and reduction in the contractile force of the diaphragm have been observed within a few hours of commencement of controlled mechanical ventilation in animal models [6]. Total mechanical inactivity and controlled ventilation may lead to rapid disuse atrophy. In a study of 14 brain-dead organ donors, 18–69 h of diaphragmatic inactivity with controlled mechanical ventilation resulted in marked atrophy of the diaphragm myofibers [7].

11.3.4 Sepsis

Infection and sepsis are leading causes of diaphragmatic dysfunction in critically ill patients [8]. In particular, sepsis may be associated with diaphragmatic weakness in more than 50% of mechanically ventilated patients [9]. Besides ischemia to the muscle fibers, inflammatory mediator release in sepsis may induce detrimental effects on diaphragmatic contractility [10].

11.3.5 Primary Neuromyopathic Syndromes

Patients with a primary neuromyopathic syndrome may occasionally present with hypercapnic respiratory failure with no previous history of lung disease and without parenchymal lesions in the lung. Common clinical conditions that may present with hypercapnic respiratory failure include Guillain-Barre syndrome, myasthenia gravis, hypothyroidism, amyotrophic lateral sclerosis, and muscle disorders.

11.4 Monitoring of Diaphragm Activity

As the diaphragm contracts, it thickens, shortens, and displaces caudally. Ultrasonography enables the evaluation of the diaphragmatic thickening and displacement during a spontaneous inspiratory effort. During ultrasonographic evaluation, the patient must be breathing at the lowest level of respiratory support feasible, preferably on continuous positive airway pressure set to zero or a T-piece. Evaluation is performed in the supine position.

11.4.1 Ultrasonographic Evaluation of Thickening Fraction

The maximal increase in diaphragm thickness from the expiratory to the inspiratory position is measured to determine the thickening fraction. To assess diaphragmatic thickening during inspiration, a high frequency (8–12 MHz) linear probe is used. The probe is placed between the seventh to ninth intercostal spaces in the midaxillary line. The diaphragm is viewed in the zone of apposition, where it meets the costal margin laterally. It is seen as a three-layered structure: the pleural line above, the peritoneal line below, and the muscle layer sandwiched in between. Thickness at end-expiration and end-inspiration are measured on the B or M mode [11] (Fig. 11.1).

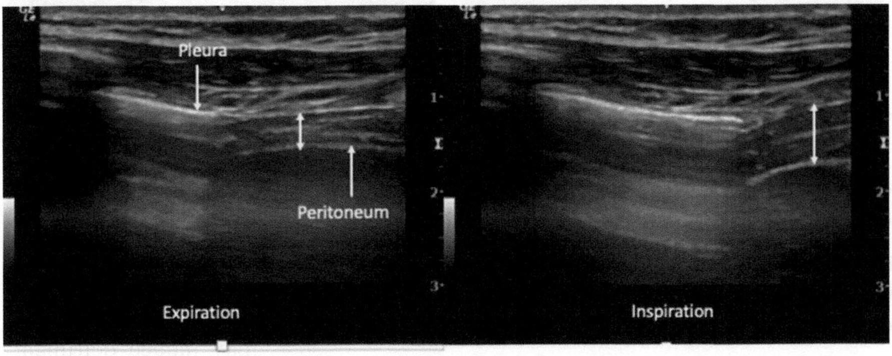

Fig. 11.1 Diaphragmatic thickening. The diaphragm consists of the pleural and peritoneal layers with the muscular layer (double-headed arrow) in between. Thickening occurs during inspiration

$$\text{Thickening fraction} = \frac{\text{end-inspiratory thickness} - \text{end-expiratory thickness}}{\text{end-expiratory thickness}}$$

There is a wide range in the thickening fraction observed with reasonably intact diaphragmatic function. The thickening fraction ranges between 20 and 50% in spontaneously breathing patients, soon after extubation [12]. A thickening fraction of <29% may reliably identify diaphragmatic dysfunction [13]. In a systematic review, a cutoff range between 30 and 36% predicted successful extubation [14]. A thickening fraction of less than 20% is associated with severe diaphragmatic weakness [15].

11.4.2 Ultrasonographic Evaluation of Diaphragmatic Excursion

The diaphragm displaces caudally during inspiration. The extent of caudal displacement as assessed by ultrasonography is termed diaphragmatic excursion. A low-frequency curvilinear probe (2–5 MHz) is used to evaluate diaphragmatic excursion. An anterior subcostal approach is used on the right side; the probe is placed just below the costal margin between the midclavicular and anterior axillary lines. The probe is placed in the longitudinal plane with the probe marker pointing cranially. The diaphragm is visualized as a curved, thick, hyperechoic line (Fig. 11.2). The distance by which it displaces during inspiration is measured on M-mode. A diaphragmatic excursion of less than 11 mm on quiet breathing is strongly suggestive of diaphragmatic dysfunction [16]. In complete paralysis of the diaphragm, there is no perceptible diaphragmatic excursion, or it may move paradoxically during normal breathing or sniffing [17].

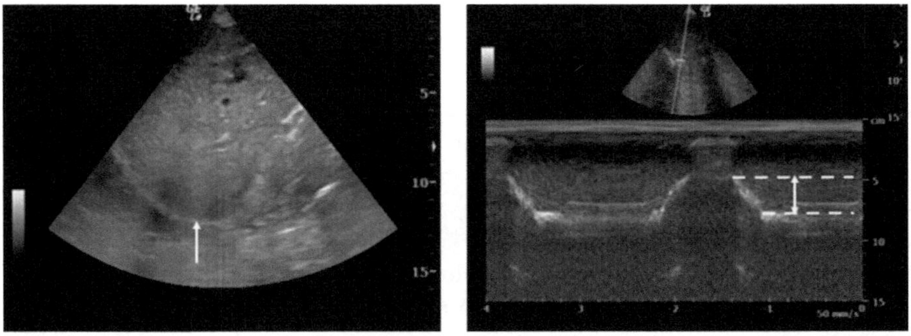

Fig. 11.2 Diaphragmatic excursion. Left: B-mode. The diaphragm is visualized as a curved, thick, hyperechoic line (white arrow). Right: M-mode. The double-headed arrow indicates diaphragmatic excursion during inspiration

11.5 Other Techniques

11.5.1 Transdiaphragmatic Pressure

The force-generating capacity of the diaphragm may be measured by the transdiaphragmatic pressure (Pdi) as it contracts. Pdi represents the pressure gradient across the diaphragm. During an inspiratory effort, the abdominal viscera is pushed down and out, while the chest expands, reducing the pleural pressure and inflation of the lungs. The pressure generated by the diaphragm is [18]:

$$\text{Pdi} = \text{Pleural pressure} - \text{abdominal pressure}$$

Twitch stimulation of the diaphragm is carried out by magnetic stimulation of both phrenic nerves in the neck. Balloon-tipped catheters are inserted transnasally into the stomach and the esophagus. The esophageal pressure is taken as the surrogate for the pleural pressure and the gastric pressure for the abdominal pressure. The transdiaphragmatic twitch pressure (Pdi, tw) is given by:

$$\text{Pdi, tw} = \text{Esophageal pressure} - \text{gastric pressure}$$

The twitch pressure generated at the proximal end of the endotracheal tube (Pet, tw) may be a close approximation of Pdi, tw and easier to perform, without the requirement for esophageal and gastric balloons [19]. A Pet, tw of less than – 11 cm H_2O represents diaphragmatic dysfunction.

11.5.2 Diaphragm Electromyography

Electromyography (EMG) may be used to assess diaphragmatic activity and is often used in conjunction with NAVA (neurally adjusted ventilatory assist). Esophageal electrodes are passed through a nasogastric tube, with continuous monitoring of the electrical activity of the diaphragm (EAdi). However, EAdi values need further investigation to define normal levels and are difficult to interpret [20].

11.6 Diaphragmatic Weakness and Clinical Outcomes

Diaphragmatic weakness is akin to dysfunction of other organs and is associated with increased mortality [9]. In a prospective observational study, diaphragmatic dysfunction was observed in the large majority of critically ill patients who were mechanically ventilated for more than 5 days. The onset of diaphragmatic dysfunction was variable; besides, diaphragmatic dysfunction improved in many patients in spite of continued mechanical ventilation [21]. Delayed-onset diaphragmatic weakness is an important risk factor for weaning failure [22]. It is important to note that diaphragmatic dysfunction may persist, leading to ICU and hospital readmission [23] and delayed mortality, even after a year [24].

11.7 Prevention

The extent of diaphragm atrophy and dysfunction may be reduced by allowing spontaneous respiratory efforts as much as possible during mechanical ventilation. Maintenance of the contractile activity of the diaphragm has been shown to preserve diaphragm thickness [25]. Patient-ventilator asynchrony should be reduced by titrating the dose of sedative agents. In patients with acute respiratory distress syndrome, vigorous spontaneous respiratory efforts may worsen lung injury; deep sedation and neuromuscular blockade are appropriate in these patients. Once the underlying illness has improved, an assisted mode of ventilation is appropriate [26]. Use of the NAVA mode enables monitoring of respiratory muscle activity and provides support adjusted to patient effort [27].

11.8 Management of Diaphragm Dysfunction

Methylxanthines may have a therapeutic role in ventilated patients who develop diaphragmatic dysfunction and are difficult to wean, although there is no robust evidence to support their use [28]. Electrolyte abnormalities including hypophosphatemia and endocrine dysfunction including hypothyroidism need to be addressed. Levosimendan has been shown to improve diaphragm contractility in experimental studies [29]. However, in a clinical study that evaluated the efficacy in reducing the severity of organ dysfunction in sepsis, levosimendan-treated patients were less likely to wean from ventilator support compared to the control group [30].

Key Points

- Diaphragmatic dysfunction commonly occurs in mechanically ventilated patients and may lead to weaning failure and adverse clinical outcomes including mortality.
- Limb muscle weakness due to critical illness-related polyneuromyopathy is usually obvious; however, the diagnosis of diaphragm dysfunction may remain elusive.
- The pressure-generating capacity of the diaphragm may be monitored by measurement of the transdiaphragmatic pressure or changes in tracheal pressure following magnetic stimulation of the phrenic nerves in the neck.
- Bedside ultrasonography is a reliable tool in the evaluation of diaphragm dysfunction by measurement of diaphragmatic excursion and the thickening fraction.
- Maintenance of spontaneous respiratory efforts through appropriate titration of sedative agents may help preserve diaphragm thickness and function.
- Early switch to an assisted mode of ventilation once the underlying illness has improved enables preservation of diaphragm activity.
- Electrolyte and endocrine abnormalities that may impair diaphragm function must be actively sought for and corrected.

References

1. Laghi F, Cattapan SE, Jubran A, Parthasarathy S, Warshawsky P, Choi YSA, et al. Is weaning failure caused by low-frequency fatigue of the diaphragm? Am J Respir Crit Care Med. 2003;167(2):120–7.
2. Hermans G, Agten A, Testelmans D, Decramer M, Gayan-Ramirez G. Increased duration of mechanical ventilation is associated with decreased diaphragmatic force: a prospective observational study. Crit Care. 2010;14(4):R127.
3. Dres M, Dubé BP, Mayaux J, Delemazure J, Reuter D, Brochard L, et al. Coexistence and impact of limb muscle and diaphragm weakness at time of liberation from mechanical ventilation in medical intensive care unit patients. Am J Respir Crit Care Med. 2017;195(1):57–66.
4. Kress JP, Hall JB. ICU-acquired weakness and recovery from critical illness. N Engl J Med. 2014;371(3):287–8.
5. Testelmans D, Maes K, Wouters P, Powers SK, Decramer M, Gayan-Ramirez G. Infusions of rocuronium and cisatracurium exert different effects on rat diaphragm function. Intensive Care Med. 2007;33(5):872–9.
6. Powers SK, Shanely RA, Coombes JS, Koesterer TJ, McKenzie M, Van Gammeren D, et al. Mechanical ventilation results in progressive contractile dysfunction in the diaphragm. J Appl Physiol (1985). 2002;92(5):1851–8.
7. Levine S, Nguyen T, Taylor N, Friscia ME, Budak MT, Rothenberg P, et al. Rapid disuse atrophy of diaphragm fibers in mechanically ventilated humans. N Engl J Med. 2008;358(13):1327–35.
8. Supinski GS, Callahan LA. Diaphragm weakness in mechanically ventilated critically ill patients. Crit Care. 2013;17(3):R120.
9. Demoule A, Jung B, Prodanovic H, Molinari N, Chanques G, Coirault C, et al. Diaphragm dysfunction on admission to the intensive care unit. Prevalence, risk factors, and prognostic impact-a prospective study. Am J Respir Crit Care Med. 2013;188(2):213–9.
10. Shindoh C, Hida W, Ohkawara Y, Yamauchi K, Ohno I, Takishima T, et al. TNF-alpha mRNA expression in diaphragm muscle after endotoxin administration. Am J Respir Crit Care Med. 1995;152(5 Pt 1):1690–6.
11. Supinski GS, Morris PE, Dhar S, Callahan LA. Diaphragm dysfunction in critical illness. Chest. 2018;153(4):1040–51.
12. Vivier E, Mekontso Dessap A, Dimassi S, Vargas F, Lyazidi A, Thille AW, et al. Diaphragm ultrasonography to estimate the work of breathing during non-invasive ventilation. Intensive Care Med. 2012;38(5):796–803.
13. Dubé BP, Dres M, Mayaux J, Demiri S, Similowski T, Demoule A. Ultrasound evaluation of diaphragm function in mechanically ventilated patients: comparison to phrenic stimulation and prognostic implications. Thorax. 2017;72(9):811–8.
14. Zambon M, Greco M, Bocchino S, Cabrini L, Beccaria PF, Zangrillo A. Assessment of diaphragmatic dysfunction in the critically ill patient with ultrasound: a systematic review. Intensive Care Med. 2017;43(1):29–38.
15. Gottesman E, McCool FD. Ultrasound evaluation of the paralyzed diaphragm. Am J Respir Crit Care Med. 1997;155(5):1570–4.
16. Kim WY, Suh HJ, Hong SB, Koh Y, Lim CM. Diaphragm dysfunction assessed by ultrasonography: influence on weaning from mechanical ventilation. Crit Care Med. 2011;39(12):2627–30.
17. Matamis D, Soilemezi E, Tsagourias M, Akoumianaki E, Dimassi S, Boroli F, et al. Sonographic evaluation of the diaphragm in critically ill patients. Technique and clinical applications. Intensive Care Med. 2013;39(5):801–10.
18. Brochard L. Transdiaphragmatic Pressure. In: Benito, S., Net, A. (eds) Pulmonary Function in Mechanically Ventilated Patients. Update in Intensive Care and Emergency Medicine, vol 13. Springer, Berlin, Heidelberg; 1991. https://doi.org/10.1007/978-3-642-84209-2_5.
19. Watson AC, Hughes PD, Louise Harris M, Hart N, Ware RJ, Wendon J, et al. Measurement of twitch transdiaphragmatic, esophageal, and endotracheal tube pressure with bilateral anterolateral magnetic phrenic nerve stimulation in patients in the intensive care unit. Crit Care Med. 2001;29(7):1325–31.

20. Piquilloud L, Beloncle F, Richard JCM, Mancebo J, Mercat A, Brochard L. Information conveyed by electrical diaphragmatic activity during unstressed, stressed and assisted spontaneous breathing: a physiological study. Ann Intensive Care. 2019;9(1):89.
21. Demoule A, Molinari N, Jung B, Prodanovic H, Chanques G, Matecki S, et al. Patterns of diaphragm function in critically ill patients receiving prolonged mechanical ventilation: a prospective longitudinal study. Ann Intensive Care. 2016;6(1):75.
22. Jung B, Moury PH, Mahul M, de Jong A, Galia F, Prades A, et al. Diaphragmatic dysfunction in patients with ICU-acquired weakness and its impact on extubation failure. Intensive Care Med. 2016;42(5):853–61.
23. Adler D, Dupuis-Lozeron E, Richard JC, Janssens JP, Brochard L. Does inspiratory muscle dysfunction predict readmission after intensive care unit discharge? Am J Respir Crit Care Med. 2014;190(3):347–50.
24. Medrinal C, Prieur G, Frenoy É, Robledo Quesada A, Poncet A, Bonnevie T, et al. Respiratory weakness after mechanical ventilation is associated with one-year mortality - a prospective study. Crit Care. 2016;20(1):231.
25. Goligher EC, Fan E, Herridge MS, Murray A, Vorona S, Brace D, et al. Evolution of diaphragm thickness during mechanical ventilation. Impact of inspiratory effort. Am J Respir Crit Care Med. 2015;192(9):1080–8.
26. Sassoon CSH, Zhu E, Caiozzo VJ. Assist-control mechanical ventilation attenuates ventilator-induced diaphragmatic dysfunction. Am J Respir Crit Care Med. 2004;170(6):626–32.
27. Sinderby C, Navalesi P, Beck J, Skrobik Y, Comtois N, Friberg S, et al. Neural control of mechanical ventilation in respiratory failure. Nat Med. 1999;5(12):1433–6.
28. Aubier M. Effect of theophylline on diaphragmatic muscle function. Chest. 1987;92(1 Suppl):27S–31S.
29. van Hees HWH, Dekhuijzen PNR, Heunks LMA. Levosimendan enhances force generation of diaphragm muscle from patients with chronic obstructive pulmonary disease. Am J Respir Crit Care Med. 2009;179(1):41–7.
30. Gordon AC, Perkins GD, Singer M, McAuley DF, Orme RML, Santhakumaran S, et al. Levosimendan for the prevention of acute organ dysfunction in sepsis. N Engl J Med. 2016;375(17):1638–48.

12 Weaning and Liberation from Mechanical Ventilation: Is My Patient Ready?

Although a crucial life-support intervention, mechanical ventilation may lead to complications. Delays in liberation from ventilator support can result in complications including ventilator-associated lung injury (VILI), pneumonia, and diaphragmatic dysfunction. In contrast, premature weaning and extubation may lead to adverse outcomes including airway compromise, pulmonary aspiration, and respiratory muscle fatigue. Hence, appropriate timing of extubation is of paramount importance in patients who undergo mechanical ventilation. Extubation failure occurs in approximately 10% of planned extubations and may increase up to 20% in high-risk patients [1]. Failed extubation leading to reintubation leads to significantly higher mortality compared to successful extubation [1]. Common causes of extubation failure are summarized in Fig. 12.1.

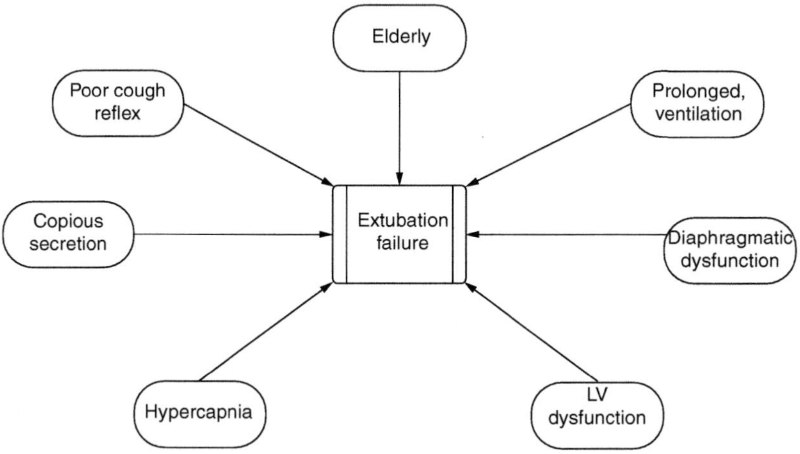

Fig. 12.1 Predisposing factors that may contribute to extubation failure

J. Chacko et al., *Controversies in Critical Care*, https://doi.org/10.1007/978-981-19-9940-6_12

12.1 The Spontaneous Breathing Trial (SBT)

How may readiness for extubation be assessed?

Critically ill patients on invasive mechanical ventilation need to undergo an assessment of the ability to generate adequate spontaneous respiratory efforts before they are extubated. Ely et al., in a pioneering trial, demonstrated that daily assessment of spontaneous respiratory efforts, followed by an SBT reduces the duration of mechanical ventilation, results in fewer complications and reduces the cost of care [2].

In contrast to the previously held paradigm of gradual weaning down of sedation and ventilator support, the current approach is to awaken the patient and liberate from mechanical ventilatory support as early as possible. Once the patient has recovered sufficiently from the underlying illness, regular SBTs are performed as a screening tool to assess readiness for liberation from mechanical ventilatory support. The SBT seeks to subject the patient to conditions akin to breathing through the natural airways after extubation. The SBT is a crucial phase prior to extubation as spontaneous breathing efforts can precipitate complications including left ventricular failure (LVF) in vulnerable subjects. Switching from a controlled to a spontaneous mode of breathing may precipitate left ventricular dysfunction due to an increase in the cardiac preload and afterload [3]. The SBT aims to evaluate whether respiratory mechanics are favorable to consider liberation from mechanical ventilation. It is a safe and effective technique to assess readiness for liberation from mechanical ventilation compared to a gradual reduction in support.

12.2 Techniques of SBT

The two common modalities of SBT are pressure support ventilation (PSV) with low levels of inspiratory support and breathing through a T-piece. The airway resistance offered by the endotracheal tube may unfavorably impact unassisted breathing through a T-piece [4]. Hence, a modest level of pressure support is often preferred to counter the resistance of the endotracheal tube. The work of breathing on PSV is less compared to T-piece breathing. However, breathing through a T-piece may more closely represent the physiological conditions after extubation [5].

PSV may be a less demanding weaning process compared to T-piece breathing as the work of breathing is less with the former. Hence, a successful SBT may tend to be higher with PSV, leading to a higher likelihood of extubation compared to T-piece [6].

Cabello et al. conducted a physiological study in 14 patients, who underwent 3 different modalities of SBT, including PSV with zero PEEP (PSV-ZEEP), PSV with added PEEP (PSV-PEEP), and T-piece. The SBT was successful in most patients with PSV-ZEEP and PSV-PEEP; however, all patients failed with the T-piece trial. Patient effort was greater, with a high incidence of LVF (11 of 14 patients). The pulmonary artery pressure and respiratory rate were higher with T-piece compared to PSV-ZEEP and PSV-PEEP. This study demonstrated significantly different respiratory and hemodynamic parameters with PSV modes compared to T-piece [7].

12.3 The Evidence

Current guidelines support SBT with PSV compared to spontaneous breathing through a T-piece [8]. Several studies have evaluated the preferred mode of SBT. In an early randomized controlled trial (RCT), Esteban et al. observed a higher rate of extubation using an SBT with pressure support of 7 cm H_2O compared to T-piece [1]. Subsequently, several RCTs have been performed to evaluate the optimal modality of SBT.

Subirà et al. compared a 2-h SBT through a T-piece with a less strenuous approach of PSV-ZEEP of 8 cm of H_2O in a multicenter RCT [9]. The study population included patients who underwent mechanical ventilation for 24 h and fulfilled prespecified weaning criteria. Patients who failed the SBT according to prespecified criteria were recommenced on an adequate level of support. The modality of respiratory support after extubation included noninvasive ventilation (NIV) and high-flow nasal cannula (HFNC), decided by the clinician prior to randomization. A total of 1153 patients were included, 575 in the PSV-ZEEP group and 578 in the T-piece arm. A significantly larger number of patients were extubated after PSV-ZEEP compared to T-piece (92.5 vs. 84.1%). Successful extubation, defined as remaining free of invasive mechanical ventilation for 72 h post-extubation, was significantly higher with PSV-ZEEP compared to T-piece according to Kaplan-Meier probability curves (hazard ratio, 1.54; 95% CI, 1.19–1.97; $P < 0.001$). The rate of reintubation within 72 h of extubation was not significantly different between the two groups. The 90-day mortality, one of the secondary outcomes, was lower in the PSV-ZEEP group. This study demonstrated a higher rate of extubation using a PSV-ZEEP strategy without an increase in the reintubation rates. One of the limitations of the study was the lack of a protocolized approach to post-extubation respiratory support with either NIV or HFNC.

Does the weaning strategy matter in patients who are at high risk of extubation failure?

In a recent RCT, Thille et al. compared SBTs using PSV with T-piece among patients who were > 65 years old with underlying chronic cardiac or respiratory disease [10]. In the PSV arm, inspiratory support of 8 cm of H_2O with zero PEEP and FiO_2 of ≤ 0.4 was employed; in the T-piece arm, supplemental oxygen of up to 6 l/min was administered at an FiO_2 of 0.4 or less. SBTs were performed for up to 1 h. Prespecified criteria were used to define failure of SBT. In both groups of patients, extubation was performed as soon as feasible after a 1-h period of resuming ventilator support using the same settings prior to commencement of SBT as a measure to avoid fatigue.

A total of 969 patients were included in the final analysis, including 484 patients in the PSV group and 485 in the T-piece group. The primary outcome, the median ventilator-free days at day 28, was similar between the two groups [PSV vs. T-piece: 27 (24–27) vs. 27 (23–27) days; $p = 0.31$]. Among the secondary outcomes, the number of patients extubated within 24 h and within 7 days after the initial SBT was similar. A similar number of patients were extubated with no reintubation within 72 h following a single SBT. Reintubation within 7 days of extubation was also similar between the two groups. Besides, there was no significant difference in the median length of stay in the ICU, the 28-day, 90-day, and ICU mortality. This RCT revealed no difference in important clinical outcomes with the mode of SBT in patients at high risk of extubation failure.

Prior to extubation, would it be beneficial to reconnect the patient back to full ventilator support for a brief period after a successful SBT? Fernandez et al. hypothesized that such a strategy may offer a period of rest after a demanding SBT and enhance the likelihood of successful extubation [11]. Patients who received at least 12 h of mechanical ventilation were included in this RCT. The modality of SBT included T-piece, PSV, or CPAP alone for a duration of 30, 60, or 90 min according to clinician judgment. Patients randomized to the standard care group were extubated directly after a successful SBT; patients in the "rest" group were switched back to the ventilator setting prior to the commencement of SBT for a 1-h period before extubation. The rest group included 227 patients and the control group, 243 patients. The primary outcome, reintubation within 48 h after extubation, was significantly lower in the rest compared with the control group (5% vs. 14%, $p < 0.001$). Among the secondary outcomes, the median duration of ICU and hospital stay were not different between the two groups. This study suggested that switching back to a full support mode for a 1-h period after a successful SBT resulted in a lower requirement for reintubation.

A post hoc analysis of a multicenter trial compared a PSV modality of SBT with T-piece in patients at high risk of extubation failure based on clinician judgment [12]. The median level of PSV was 7 cm H_2O without PEEP. The extubation rate after initial SBT was significantly higher with PSV compared to T-piece; however, the reintubation rates at 72 h did not differ between groups. A significantly higher number of patients remained successfully extubated at 72 h after PSV compared to a T-piece SBT (67 vs. 56%, $p = 0.0076$). This post hoc analysis of a large multicentric trial also suggests that extubation may be possible earlier in patients at a high risk of failure using a PSV compared to a T-piece strategy of SBT, with no increase in reintubation rates.

Several meta-analyses have been performed comparing PSV with T-piece as the SBT strategy, with conflicting results. Burns et al. included 31 randomized or quasi-randomized trials; a PSV approach was more likely to result in successful extubation [13]. In another meta-analysis including 16 studies, the respiratory effort was 30% lower with PSV compared to T-piece. However, the authors concluded that a CPAP level of 0 cm H_2O with no inspiratory support and T-piece reflected the physiological conditions after extubation more precisely compared with PSV [14].

12.4 SBT with Automatic Tube Compensation (ATC)

A low level of PSV during SBT is meant to overcome the airflow resistance of the endotracheal tube. However, an arbitrary level of PSV may overcompensate and thereby reduce the work of breathing. ATC has been devised to precisely compensate for the increase in the work of breathing imposed by the resistance of the artificial airway device. The target pressure required to overcome this resistance is calculated from continuous measurement of the airway pressure and the flow rate across the tube. ATC aims to simulate physiological conditions of flow and resistance after removal of the artificial airway. It facilitates a variable level of support commensurate with the ventilatory drive and airflow that may vary considerably during the course of the SBT.

Guérin et al. compared the level of support offered with low-level PSV and ATC in a crossover trial [15]. Twenty patients who were ready to wean were crossed over between PSV and ATC for 30 min each to compare the breathing power, an indication of the level of support (a higher breathing power denotes a lower level of support). During the period of ATC, the pressure support was set at 0 cm H_2O with a PEEP of 4 cm H_2O; the ATC was set according to the internal diameter of the endotracheal tube with 100% compensation for the inspiratory flow resistance. With PSV, the inspiratory support was set a 7 cm H_2O above PEEP. The breathing power was calculated from the esophageal and airway pressures, flow rates, and the volume generated. The key finding of this study was that the breathing power was significantly higher with ATC compared with low-level PSV, suggesting that even low levels of PSV may provide more respiratory assistance than required to overcome the resistance of the endotracheal tube.

ATC was associated with a lower failure rate with SBT compared to PSV in an RCT, although the difference was not statistically significant. The reintubation rates were not significantly different between the two modalities of weaning [16]. In another RCT, the SBT was equally successful with ATC compared to PSV; besides, ATC was associated with higher PaO_2/FIO_2 ratios, dynamic compliance, and lower airway resistance [17]. Compared to CPAP alone, ATC combined with CPAP results may result in better tolerance of the SBT and a higher rate of successful extubation. In a three-armed trial, among patients who failed a breathing trial with PSV or T-piece, a subsequent SBT with ATC resulted in successful extubation [18]. Future studies are needed to further evaluate ATC as a viable option for SBT and successful extubation. Controlled trials that compare different modes of SBT prior to extubation are summarized in Table 12.1.

Table 12.1 Controlled trials that compare different modes of SBT

Study/year	Population/ design	Group 1	Group 2	Outcomes
Esteban et al. [1] (1997)	Ventilated for >48 h, RCT	T-piece	PS 7 cm H_2O	SBT failure higher with T-piece. Extubation failure similar
Subirà et al. [9] (2019)	Ventilated for ≥24 h, RCT	T-piece	PS 8 cm H_2O-ZEEP	Extubation rates higher, failed extubation lower with PS-ZEEP. 90-day mortality lower with PS-ZEEP

(continued)

Table 12.1 (continued)

Study/year	Population/ design	Group 1	Group 2	Outcomes
Fernandez et al. [11] (2017)	Ventilated for ≥12 h, RCT	SBT with T-piece, PS, or CPAP. Extubated if successful	Back to the level of support prior to SBT for a 1-h rest period followed by extubation	Reintubation rates lower in the rest group. No difference in ICU or hospital stay
Thille et al. [12] (2020)	Ventilated for ≥24 h, post hoc analysis of a multicenter study	T-piece	PS at low levels	Extubation rates higher with PS; reintubation rates not different. More patients remained successfully extubated at 72 h with PS
Batanouny et al. [17] (2017)	Nonrandomized study; patients who met weaning criteria	ATC with PEEP 5 cm H_2O	PS 7, PEEP 5 cm H_2O	Extubation success similar. ATC associated with higher PaO_2/FiO_2 ratio, dynamic compliance, and lower airway resistance
Thille et al. [10] (2022)	RCT; patients at high risk of extubation failure	PS 8 cm H_2O, PEEP 0, $FiO_2 \leq 0.4$	T-piece with supplemental oxygen, $FiO_2 \leq 0.4$	Median ventilator-free days at day 28 similar between the two groups. Number of patients extubated within 24 h and within 7 days after the initial SBT were similar. Similar number of patients extubated with no reintubation within 72 h following a single SBT. Reintubation rates within 7 days of extubation similar. No difference in the median length of stay in the ICU, the 28-day, 90-day, and ICU mortality

RCT randomized controlled trial, *PS* pressure support, *SBT* spontaneous breathing trial, *ZEEP* zero end-expiratory pressure, *ATC* automatic tube compensation

Key Points

- The current paradigm in critical care is to awaken the patient and liberate from mechanical ventilatory support as early as possible once the patient is on the road to recovery from the underlying illness. This contrasts with the previous practice of gradually weaning down sedation and ventilator support that may lead to unnecessary prolongation of mechanical ventilation.
- The timing of extubation is of crucial importance in mechanically ventilated patients. While premature extubation and reinstitution of ventilator support lead to a high incidence of complications including mortality, delaying extubation may result in ventilator-associated lung injury (VILI), pneumonia, and diaphragmatic dysfunction. SBTs are routinely employed to evaluate readiness for extubation.
- Commonly used modalities of SBT include T-piece breathing, CPAP alone, CPAP with inspiratory pressure support, or PS with zero PEEP.
- Although T-piece breathing may more closely represent the physiological conditions after extubation, PSV with low levels of inspiratory support is a less demanding SBT modality compared to T-piece. A low level of inspiratory support is aimed to overcome flow resistance imposed by the endotracheal tube and, thereby, reduce the work of breathing.
- A reasonably large body of evidence suggests that SBTs with inspiratory pressure support are better tolerated, with higher rates of extubation compared with T-piece trials. The reintubation rates appear to be similar with PSV and T-piece SBT.
- Switching back to a full support mode for a brief period after a successful SBT may reduce the requirement for reintubation.
- Instead of setting an arbitrary level of inspiratory support with PSV, ATC titrates the level of inspiratory support to compensate for the increase in the work of breathing imposed by the resistance of the artificial airway. Early studies have demonstrated a lower level of support with ATC compared to PSV during SBT, with a similar likelihood of extubation success.

References

1. Esteban A, Alía I, Gordo F, Fernández R, Solsona JF, Vallverdú I, et al. Extubation outcome after spontaneous breathing trials with T-tube or pressure support ventilation. Am J Respir Crit Care Med. 1997;156(2):459–65.
2. Ely EW, Baker AM, Dunagan DP, Burke HL, Smith AC, Kelly PT, et al. Effect on the duration of mechanical ventilation of identifying patients capable of breathing spontaneously. N Engl J Med. 1996;335(25):1864–9.
3. Buda AJ, Pinsky MR, Ingels NB, Daughters GT, Stinson EB, Alderman EL. Effect of intrathoracic pressure on left ventricular performance. N Engl J Med. 1979;301(9):453–9.
4. Dhand R. Special problems in aerosol delivery: artificial airways. Respir Care. 2000;45(6):636–45.

5. Straus C, Louis B, Isabey D, Lemaire F, Harf A, Brochard L. Contribution of the endotracheal tube and the upper airway to breathing workload. Am J Respir Crit Care Med. 1998;157(1):23–30.
6. Ezingeard E, Diconne E, Guyomarc'h S, Venet C, Page D, Gery P, et al. Weaning from mechanical ventilation with pressure support in patients failing a T-tube trial of spontaneous breathing. Intensive Care Med. 2006;32(1):165–9.
7. Cabello B, Thille AW, Roche-Campo F, Brochard L, Gómez FJ, Mancebo J. Physiological comparison of three spontaneous breathing trials in difficult-to-wean patients. Intensive Care Med. 2010;36(7):1171–9.
8. Schmidt GA, Girard TD, Kress JP, Morris PE, Ouellette DR, Alhazzani W, et al. Official executive summary of an American Thoracic Society/American College of Chest Physicians Clinical Practice Guideline: liberation from mechanical ventilation in critically ill adults. Am J Respir Crit Care Med. 2017;195(1):115–9.
9. Subirà C, Hernández G, Vázquez A, Rodríguez-García R, González-Castro A, García C, et al. Effect of pressure support vs T-piece ventilation strategies during spontaneous breathing trials on successful Extubation among patients receiving mechanical ventilation: a randomized clinical trial. JAMA. 2019;321(22):2175–82.
10. Thille AW, Gacouin A, Coudroy R, Ehrmann S, Quenot JP, Nay MA, et al. Spontaneous-breathing trials with pressure-support ventilation or a T-piece. N Engl J Med. 2022;387(20):1843–54.
11. Fernandez MM, González-Castro A, Magret M, Bouza MT, Ibañez M, García C, et al. Reconnection to mechanical ventilation for 1 h after a successful spontaneous breathing trial reduces reintubation in critically ill patients: a multicenter randomized controlled trial. Intensive Care Med. 2017;43(11):1660–7.
12. Thille AW, Coudroy R, Nay MA, Gacouin A, Demoule A, Sonneville R, et al. Pressure-support ventilation vs T-piece during spontaneous breathing trials before Extubation among patients at high risk of Extubation failure. Chest. 2020;158(4):1446–55.
13. Burns KEA, Soliman I, Adhikari NKJ, Zwein A, Wong JTY, Gomez-Builes C, et al. Trials directly comparing alternative spontaneous breathing trial techniques: a systematic review and meta-analysis. Crit Care. 2017;21(1):127.
14. Sklar MC, Burns K, Rittayamai N, Lanys A, Rauseo M, Chen L, et al. Effort to breathe with various spontaneous breathing trial techniques. A physiologic meta-analysis. Am J Respir Crit Care Med. 2017;195(11):1477–85.
15. Guérin C, Terzi N, Mezidi M, Baboi L, Chebib N, Yonis H, et al. Low-pressure support vs automatic tube compensation during spontaneous breathing trial for weaning. Ann Intensive Care. 2019;9(1):137.
16. Cohen J, Shapiro M, Grozovski E, Fox B, Lev S, Singer P. Prediction of extubation outcome: a randomised, controlled trial with automatic tube compensation vs. pressure support ventilation. Crit Care. 2009;13(1):R21.
17. ELBatanouny M, Abdelbary AM. Use of automatic tube compensation (ATC) for weaning from mechanical ventilation in acute respiratory failure. Egypt J Chest Dis Tuberc. 2017;66(4):699–701.
18. Haberthür C, Mols G, Elsasser S, Bingisser R, Stocker R, Guttmann J. Extubation after breathing trials with automatic tube compensation, T-tube, or pressure support ventilation. Acta Anaesthesiol Scand. 2002;46(8):973–9.

When to Decannulate a Tracheostomy? 13

13.1 Introduction

Patients who undergo prolonged invasive mechanical ventilation and those with the inability to maintain airway and clear secretions require tracheostomy. A tracheostomy becomes necessary in approximately 10% of critically ill patients who require invasive mechanical ventilation [1]. Once the underlying illness has resolved, the patient must be evaluated for decannulation of the tracheostomy. The ability to maintain adequate spontaneous breathing and protect the airway must be carefully assessed before deciding on decannulation. Premature decannulation can lead to serious complications including inadequate spontaneous respiratory efforts, loss of airway, and pulmonary aspiration. Inordinate delays in decannulation can also be counterproductive and predispose to late complications, including tracheal stenosis, hemorrhage, tracheomalacia, fistula formation, and infections [2]. In an international survey of physicians and respiratory therapists from 118 centers across 10 countries, the key criteria for decannulation were an adequate level of consciousness, tolerance to capping of the tracheostomy tube, effectiveness of cough, oxygenation, and the quantity and character of secretions [3]. Decannulation improves physical comfort, facilitates speech, and may lead to improved swallowing function [4]. The approach to decannulation is the key initial step toward the rehabilitation of the patient who is on the way to recovery from critical illness and strongly influences long-term clinical outcomes.

13.2 Weaning and Liberation from Mechanical Ventilation

Prior to the consideration of decannulation, it is important to ensure the adequacy of respiratory efforts. This may be accomplished by gradually increasing the duration of unsupported breathing. Adequate humification must be ensured during this

J. Chacko et al., *Controversies in Critical Care*,
https://doi.org/10.1007/978-981-19-9940-6_13

period, especially in patients with thick, tenacious secretions. A protocol-driven approach may hasten the weaning process and allow earlier liberation from mechanical ventilation [5]. A gradual weaning strategy should be followed in patients with diaphragmatic dysfunction, multiorgan failure, and impaired left ventricular function [6]. In a prospective cohort study, Mah et al. evaluated the efficacy of a bundled approach to post-tracheostomy care on decannulation success and improved swallowing function [7]. Compared to a historical control group, a bundled approach executed by a dedicated tracheostomy service led to significantly improved decannulation rates and earlier commencement of oral diet.

13.3 Decannulation Strategies

Several techniques have been conventionally followed for the removal of tracheostomy tubes. One method involves downsizing the tracheostomy tube to a suitable size and capping it with the cuff deflated for a variable period ranging from 12 to 48 h [8]. However, if uncapping is required, spontaneous breathing through a narrow tracheostomy tube may cause distress as the resistance is inversely proportional to the fourth power of the radius of the tube. Hence, an alternate option is single-stage decannulation without downsizing. Cohen et al. conducted a retrospective observational study that compared a single-stage decannulation protocol with a control group that underwent gradual downsizing of the tube or capping [9]. Twenty-nine patients underwent single-stage decannulation, while 20 underwent traditional decannulation with downsizing and capping of the tube. There was no decannulation failure in the single-stage decannulation group; four patients in the control group experienced failure of decannulation. The duration of hospitalization was also less in patients who underwent single-stage decannulation. The authors proposed that a single-stage decannulation strategy may be safe and feasible.

13.3.1 Capping Techniques

Successful decannulation requires the demonstration of the ability to breathe around the tracheostomy tube, through the natural airways. This is commonly tested by capping the tracheostomy tube after deflation of the cuff. Tolerance to capping demonstrates patency of the glottis, vocal cords, and subglottic space. The inability to phonate, development of stridor, or breathing difficulty may point toward an upper airway obstruction and necessitate endoscopic examination of the airway. If the airway appears patent on endoscopy, downsizing the tube to a suitable size will facilitate improved airflow around the capped tube.

The alternative option is to use a one-way speaking valve at the proximal end of the tracheostomy tube, with the cuff fully deflated. During inspiration, air flows in through the speaking valve; during expiration, the speaking valve closes and airflow occurs around the tracheostomy tube through the upper airways, thus enabling speech (Fig. 13.1).

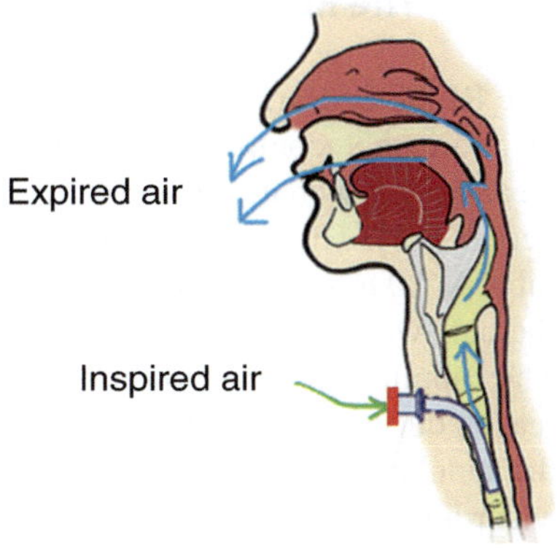

Fig. 13.1 Speaking valve attached to the tracheostomy tube. The one-way valve allows inspired air to pass through the tracheostomy tube; during expiration, the valve remains closed. Expired air passes through the upper airways and larynx enabling speech

13.4 Capping vs. Single-Stage Decannulation: The Evidence

Protocol-based capping trials have been tested in observational studies. A capping protocol was evaluated as a quality improvement project among inpatients of a tertiary academic hospital in the USA [10]. The protocol was executed by a multidisciplinary team that included head and neck surgeons, anesthesiologists, respiratory therapists, and nurse practitioners. Eligible patients were screened for a capping trial and subsequent decannulation. A tracheostomy tube of size 4.0 mm internal diameter (ID) was used during the capping trial. If a 24-h capping trial was successful, decannulation was performed. If the patients failed to tolerate the capping trial, the tracheostomy tube was opened, and recapping was attempted on the following day. During a 12-month period, 54 patients underwent the capping trial. All 50 patients who underwent a successful capping trial were decannulated successfully. In this study, the tracheostomy capping trial predicted successful decannulation with a high degree of sensitivity and specificity. Furthermore, there was a decrease in the incidence of safety concerns raised after the implementation of the protocol.

A prospective study of patients with severe traumatic brain injury compared a downsizing and capping strategy with a single-stage approach to decannulation [11]. In this study of 118 patients, 68 underwent downsizing and capping followed by decannulation, while 50 underwent single-stage decannulation. Patients were evaluated at the end of 1 month; decannulation was considered successful among those who did not require re-tracheostomy or intubation during the follow-up period. There was no significant difference in decannulation success between the two groups (capping vs. single-stage decannulation: 98.5% vs. 94%). This study suggested that single-stage decannulation may not be inferior to downsizing and capping strategy.

A retrospective study of 450 patients from an acute care setting in Australia also revealed similar findings [12]. This study compared cuff deflation trials, downsizing and capping with decannulation after 24–48 h of cuff deflation. The incidence of recannulation was less than 3% in both groups. However, decannulation could be performed 5–6 days earlier among patients who did not undergo downsizing and capping.

13.4.1 The REDECAP Randomized Controlled Trial

The REDECAP trial was a multicenter randomized controlled trial from five ICUs in Spain that compared two different methods of decannulation. Patients were weaned off mechanical ventilation and did not require ventilator support for a 24-h period [13]. High-flow oxygen therapy was provided through the tracheostomy tube. A 7.0 mm ID tracheostomy tube was used in all patients. In the control group, the cuff was deflated and the tracheostomy tube capped, followed by a 24-h trial. The capping trial was considered to have failed if uncapping was required for any reason during the trial period. Patients in the intervention group were assessed for decannulation based on the requirement for suctioning of the tracheostomy tube according to predefined indications. Decannulation was performed if the frequency of suctioning was no more than twice in 8 h during a 24-h period. Capping was not carried out in this group. The control group (capping trial) included 161 patients with 169 patients in the intervention group (decannulation based on suctioning frequency). Patients who underwent decannulation based on suctioning frequency were decannulated significantly earlier compared to those who underwent the capping trial [median time to decannulation: 6 (5–7) days vs. 13 (11–14 days)]. Among the secondary outcomes, the incidence of pneumonia and tracheobronchitis was lower and the duration of hospital stay shorter among patients who underwent decannulation based on the suctioning frequency. There was no difference between groups in ICU or hospital mortality, duration of stay in ICU or hospital, and the incidence of sepsis or multiorgan failure.

The REDECAP trial excluded patients with anatomical abnormalities of the airway. Hence, the findings of this study are questionable among patients who have vocal cord pathology, airway narrowing, and swallowing impairment. Narrowed airways following tracheostomy may be unrecognized and lead to complications including stridor and pulmonary aspiration if abrupt decannulation is carried out with no capping trial.

13.5 Endoscopic Evaluation Before Decannulation

There is a relatively high incidence of tracheal narrowing of 20% or more in patients who undergo long-term mechanical ventilation. Formation of granulation tissue, tracheomalacia, tracheal stenosis, and vocal cord abnormalities may lead to airway obstruction following decannulation [14]. Hence, a routine endoscopic inspection of the airway prior to decannulation is sometimes advocated [15]. A fiberoptic bronchoscope may be introduced through a partially withdrawn tracheostomy tube and retroflexed to visualize the vocal cords from below and the trachea above the stoma. The trachea distal to the stoma is also inspected through the tracheostomy tube. The bronchoscope is inserted through the nose to visualize the vocal cords from above and the trachea above the stoma.

Rumbak et al., in a prospective observational study, performed a capping trial with an 8.0 or 7.0 mm ID tracheostomy tube after deflation of the cuff [16]. All patients underwent a bronchoscopic evaluation of the airway—above the stoma by partial tube withdrawal and retroflexion and distally through the tracheostomy tube. The airway above the stoma was assessed by passing the bronchoscope through the nose. Patients who successfully completed the capping trial could be decannulated uneventfully. Those who failed had significant narrowing identified on bronchoscopy that required definitive management including tracheal resection. Although milder grades of narrowing may be observed on bronchoscopy, they are likely to be clinically relevant only if >50% of the cross-sectional area of the tracheal lumen is involved. Table 13.1 summarizes important studies that evaluated the technique of decannulation.

Table 13.1 Important studies evaluating the technique of decannulation

Study/year	Population/ design	Intervention	Control	Outcomes
Cohen et al. [9] (2016)	Retrospective observational	Single-stage decannulation	Downsizing or capping	Single-stage decannulation was successful in all 29 patients; 4/20 patients in the control group failed decannulation. Duration of hospitalization less with single-stage decannulation
Pandian et al. [10] (2014)	Adult patients who were ready for decannulation; part of a quality improvement project	Capping trial with a 4.0 mm ID tracheostomy tube. Decannulation if 24-h capping trial successful. If unsuccessful, tracheostomy tube was opened and capping attempted the following day	No control group	All 50 patients who underwent the capping trial were successfully decannulated. Tracheostomy capping predicted successful decannulation with a high degree of sensitivity and specificity
Shrestha et al. [11] (2012)	TBI, prospective observational study	Single-stage decannulation	Downsizing and capping followed by decannulation	Decannulation success similar between groups
Thompson-Ward et al. [12] (1999)	Tracheostomy patients in an acute care setting. Retrospective observational study	Deflation trials, downsizing and capping	Decannulation after 24–48 h of cuff deflation	Recannulation rates similar and less than 3% in both groups. Decannulation performed 5–6 days earlier in the group that did not undergo downsizing and capping

(continued)

Table 13.1 (continued)

Study/year	Population/ design	Intervention	Control	Outcomes
Hernández Martínez et al. [13] (REDECAP, 2020)	ICU patients, ventilation-free for 24 h and eligible for decannulation. RCT	Decannulation if frequency of suctioning not more than twice in 8 h during a 24-h period. No capping. HF oxygen through a 7.0 mm ID tracheostomy tube	Tracheostomy tube capped for 24 h after cuff deflation. Capping trial considered to have failed if uncapping required during trial period. HF oxygen through a 7.0 mm ID tracheostomy tube	Decannulation based on suction frequency resulted in more rapid decannulation compared to the group who underwent capping. Incidence of VAP, tracheobronchitis lower, hospital stay shorter with suction frequency-based decannulation. No difference in ICU or hospital mortality, duration of ICU stay, sepsis, or multiorgan failure

ID internal diameter, *VAP* ventilator-associated pneumonia, *TBI* traumatic brain injury

13.6 Cuff Deflation During Weaning

Deflation of the tracheostomy cuff during weaning trials allows airflow around the tube and increases the effective cross-sectional area of the airway. The breathing effort required for airflow through the natural airway depends on the size of the tracheostomy tube. A smaller ID offers less resistance to flow around the tube, through the natural airway. Peak flow and forced vital capacity have been shown to increase with the cuff deflated [17]. Intermittent deflation of the tracheostomy cuff during spontaneous breathing trials may shorten the weaning time. Besides, the incidence of respiratory infections may be lower with improvement in swallowing function when cuff deflation is carried out during spontaneous breathing trials [18].

Key Points

- Most patients who have recovered from the underlying illness may be safely decannulated if they are fully awake, have minimal secretions, and cough effectively. However, if the situation is unclear, with the likelihood of airway narrowing, it may be safer to consider a capping trial.
- Narrowed airways following tracheostomy may be difficult to identify; complications including stridor and pulmonary aspiration may ensue if abrupt decannulation is performed in this situation.

- The normal tracheal diameter is 16–18 mm; resistance to airflow usually does not occur unless the diameter is narrowed to less than 50%. Hence, a capped tracheostomy tube of 7.0 mm ID or less would not normally lead to stridor unless there is tracheal narrowing.
- A capping trial may enhance the safety of decannulation; in case of distress, uncapping may be carried out and ventilator support provided if necessary.
- If a single-stage decannulation is carried out without a capping trial, difficulty may be encountered if reinsertion of the tracheostomy tube is required for respiratory distress. This may be particularly important in situations outside the ICU, where emergency airway access may be difficult to obtain. However, reinsertion is usually straightforward if the track is mature (beyond 2 weeks).
- Routine bronchoscopic evaluation of the airway may not be necessary if a capping trial is carried out. A successful 24-hour capping trial usually excludes a significant degree of tracheal narrowing.
- Deflation of the cuff of the tracheostomy tube may shorten the weaning time, reduce the incidence of respiratory infections, and improve swallowing function.

References

1. Fischler L, Erhart S, Kleger GR, Frutiger A. Prevalence of tracheostomy in ICU patients. A nation-wide survey in Switzerland. Intensive Care Med. 2000;26(10):1428–33.
2. Epstein SK. Late complications of tracheostomy. Respir Care. 2005;50(4):542–9.
3. Stelfox H, Crimi C, Berra L, Noto A, Schmidt U, Bigatello LM, et al. Determinants of tracheostomy decannulation: an international survey. Crit Care. 2008;12(1):R26.
4. O'Connor HH, Kirby KJ, Terrin N, Hill NS, White AC. Decannulation following tracheostomy for prolonged mechanical ventilation. J Intensive Care Med. 2009;24(3):187–94.
5. de Medeiros GC, Sassi FC, Lirani-Silva C, de Andrade CRF. Criteria for tracheostomy decannulation: literature review. Codas. 2019;31(6):e20180228.
6. Shaikh H, Morales D, Laghi F. Weaning from mechanical ventilation. Semin Respir Crit Care Med. 2014;35(4):451–68.
7. Mah JW, Staff II, Fisher SR, Butler KL. Improving decannulation and swallowing function: a comprehensive, multidisciplinary approach to post-tracheostomy care. Respir Care. 2017;62(2):137–43.
8. Mitchell RB, Hussey HM, Setzen G, Jacobs IN, Nussenbaum B, Dawson C, et al. Clinical consensus statement: tracheostomy care. Otolaryngol Head Neck Surg. 2013;148(1):6–20.
9. Cohen O, Tzelnick S, Lahav Y, Stavi D, Shoffel-Havakuk H, Hain M, et al. Feasibility of a single-stage tracheostomy decannulation protocol with endoscopy in adult patients: Immediate Decannulation: Feasibility and Safety. Laryngoscope. 2016;126(9):2057–62.
10. Pandian V, Miller CR, Schiavi AJ, Yarmus L, Contractor A, Haut ER, et al. Utilization of a standardized tracheostomy capping and decannulation protocol to improve patient safety: Tracheostomy Capping and Decannulation Protocol. Laryngoscope. 2014;124(8):1794–800.

11. Shrestha KK, Mohindra S, Mohindra S. How to decannulate tracheostomised severe head trauma patients: a comparison of gradual vs. abrupt technique. Nepal Med Coll J. 2012;14(3):207–11.
12. Thompson-Ward E, Boots R, Frisby J, Bassett L, Timm M. Evaluating suitability for tracheostomy decannulation: A critical evaluation of two management protocols. J Med Speech Language Pathol. 1999;7(4):273–81.
13. Hernández Martínez G, Rodriguez ML, Vaquero MC, Ortiz R, Masclans JR, Roca O, et al. High-flow oxygen with capping or suctioning for tracheostomy decannulation. N Engl J Med. 2020;383(11):1009–17.
14. Law JH, Barnhart K, Rowlett W, de la Rocha O, Lowenberg S. Increased frequency of obstructive airway abnormalities with long-term tracheostomy. Chest. 1993;104(1):136–8.
15. O'Connor HH, White AC. Tracheostomy Decannulation. Respir Care. 2010;55(8):6.
16. Rumbak MJ, Graves AE, Scott MP, Sporn GK, Walsh FW, Anderson WM, et al. Tracheostomy tube occlusion protocol predicts significant tracheal obstruction to air flow in patients requiring prolonged mechanical ventilation. Crit Care Med. 1997;25(3):413–7.
17. Hernández G, Ortiz R, Pedrosa A, Cuena R, Vaquero Collado C, González Arenas P, et al. The indication of tracheotomy conditions the predictors of time to decannulation in critical patients. Med Intensiva. 2012;36(8):531–9.
18. Hernandez G, Pedrosa A, Ortiz R, del Cruz Accuaroni M, del Mar Cruz Accuaroni M, Cuena R, Collado CV, Plaza SG, Arenas PG, Fernandez R, et al. The effects of increasing effective airway diameter on weaning from mechanical ventilation in tracheostomized patients: a randomized controlled trial. Intensive Care Med. 2013;39(6):1063–70.

Thrombolytic Therapy in Acute Pulmonary Embolism

14

14.1 Introduction

The history of thrombolytic therapy dates back to the isolation of a fibrinolytic agent from Group A beta-hemolytic streptococci [1]. The first study of intravenous streptokinase in acute myocardial infarction was published in 1958 [1]. Thrombolytic therapy for acute pulmonary embolism (PE) was first reported in 1968. In this series, 13 patients with angiographically confirmed pulmonary embolism were treated with urokinase, with favorable clinical outcomes [2].

Thrombolytic agents activate plasminogen to generate plasmin. The plasmin degrades fibrin resulting in clot lysis. In acute pulmonary embolism, thrombolysis enables rapid reduction of the clot burden and improvement in the hemodynamic and respiratory status. Thrombolytic therapy also carries the potential to result in catastrophic hemorrhage. Hence, it is crucial to weigh the balance of risk with potential benefit and individualize therapy based on the clinical status.

14.2 Pathophysiology of Acute Pulmonary Embolism (PE)

Impedance to pulmonary blood flow due to mechanical obstruction by the thrombus, combined with vasoconstriction mediated by humoral factors, and hypoxia leads to an increase in the right ventricular (RV) afterload. The RV fails to compensate for the fairly abrupt rise in the afterload leading to progressive dilatation and severe impairment of function. RV overload triggers a shift of the interventricular septum as it bows out into the left ventricular (LV) lumen (Fig. 14.1). The septal shift results in impaired LV filling in diastole and reduced systemic flow. Increased RV pressure leads to constriction of the right coronary artery, compromise of subendocardial perfusion, and microinfarction with the elevation of cardiac biomarkers. Hypoxia occurs due to a mismatch of ventilation to perfusion; redistribution of

J. Chacko et al., *Controversies in Critical Care*,
https://doi.org/10.1007/978-981-19-9940-6_14

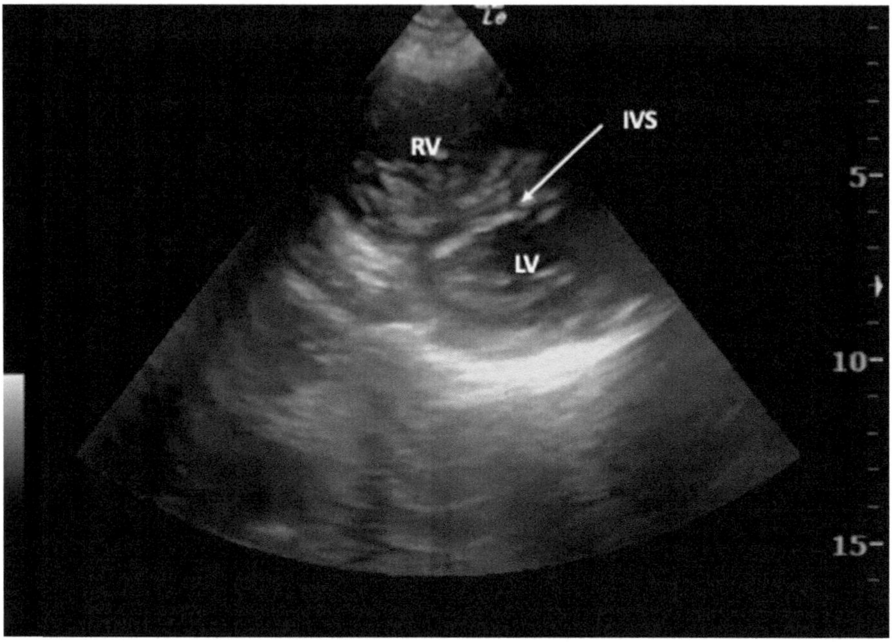

Fig. 14.1 Acute pulmonary embolism, parasternal short-axis view on echocardiography. The RV is dilated, with shift of the interventricular septum toward the left, giving the left ventricle a typical "D" shape. *RV* right ventricle, *LV* left ventricle, *IVS* interventricular septum

pulmonary blood flow occurs leading to areas of high perfusion compared to ventilation, creating a shunt within the lung. Intracardiac right to left shunting may also occur through a patent foramen ovale as right-sided pressures rise acutely.

Thrombolytic therapy relieves obstruction to blood flow across the lung and unloads the RV leading to improved function. Consequently, the interventricular septum shifts back toward the RV with an increase in the LV diameter and filling, resulting in improved cardiac output.

14.3 Risk Stratification of PE

Acute PE is classified into high, intermediate, or low risk based on the hemodynamic status, RV function, and rise in the level of biomarkers [3].

14.3.1 High-Risk (Massive) PE

Presence of shock or hypotension (systolic BP <90 mmHg or a decrease of ≥40 mmHg from the baseline) and RV dysfunction

14.3.2 Intermediate-Risk (Submassive) PE

No shock or hypotension. Presence of RV dysfunction or elevated cardiac biomarkers.

14.3.3 Low-Risk (Non-massive) PE

No shock or hypotension; no evidence of RV dysfunction.

14.4 Contraindications to Thrombolysis in PE

Thrombolysis is contraindicated in the presence of intracranial trauma and tumors, following recent intracranial or spinal surgery, in the presence of a hemorrhagic stroke, or a recent ischemic stroke within the previous 3 months. Any active bleeding is also a contraindication. Hypertension, nonhemorrhagic stroke more than 3 months previously and recent surgical procedures are relative contraindications that need judicious decision-making depending on the clinical scenario [4].

14.5 Early Clinical Trials of Thrombolysis

The first randomized controlled trial (RCT) evaluated a combination of thrombolytic therapy with urokinase followed by heparin and compared it with heparin alone. Although this study demonstrated evidence of clot lysis, no mortality benefit was observed, probably due to a low incidence of hemodynamic compromise (9%) prior to therapy [5]. Subsequent follow-up studies corroborated the findings of clot lysis and hemodynamic improvement but raised questions regarding bleeding complications [6, 7]. Jerjes-Sanchez et al. evaluated the efficacy of intravenous thrombolytic therapy with streptokinase 1,500,000 IU over a 1-h period followed by heparin infusion in four patients. The control group included four patients who received heparin alone. All patients in the heparin alone group died within 3 h of admission to hospital; in contrast, all patients in the streptokinase group were alive at the 2-year follow-up [8]. Although this pioneering study included just eight patients, it was a strong pointer toward possible clinical benefit of thrombolytic therapy in acute PE.

14.6 Thrombolysis in Acute Massive (High-Risk) PE

What is the real-world experience with thrombolytic therapy in acute massive pulmonary embolism?

A database study was performed on patients in shock or mechanically ventilated with acute massive PE between 1999 and 2008 [9]. In this study, 21,390 of 72,230

(30%) patients underwent thrombolytic therapy. The all-cause in-hospital mortality rate was significantly lower in patients who received thrombolysis compared to those who did not (15% vs. 47%, $p = 0.0001$). Patients who received a combination of thrombolysis and vena caval filters experienced the lowest mortality in this cohort. A mortality benefit with thrombolysis was also observed in eight trials that included 1775 patients with intermediate-risk PE [10]. Although used only in a minority of patients, this study reinforced the evidence for thrombolytic therapy in PE, particularly in patients with hemodynamic compromise.

Marti et al. performed a meta-analysis of 15 RCTs that compared intravenous thrombolysis and heparin with heparin alone in acute PE [11]. The overall mortality was significantly lower with thrombolysis compared to heparin alone (OR, 0.59, 95% CI: 0.36–0.96). However, the mortality benefit was not evident after the exclusion of studies consisting of patients with high-risk PE suggesting a lack of benefit in low- and intermediate-risk PE. The composite endpoint of death or treatment escalation was also significantly lower with thrombolytic therapy. The incidence of major hemorrhage was more common with thrombolysis; intracranial hemorrhage and hemorrhage-related mortality were also higher with thrombolysis.

14.7 Thrombolysis in Submassive (Intermediate-Risk) PE

While decision-making in acute massive PE is usually straightforward, there is considerable ambiguity in the optimal therapeutic modality in the patient with acute PE and RV dysfunction with no hemodynamic instability. A fine balance has to be struck between the potential for clot lysis with improved RV function and the risk of catastrophic bleeding. What is the evidence for the safety and efficacy of thrombolytic treatment in acute submassive PE (Table 14.1)?

Goldhaber et al. evaluated the effect of intravenous thrombolysis in patients with acute PE with RV dysfunction on echocardiography and stable hemodynamic parameters [12]. Patients were randomized to receive recombinant tissue plasminogen activator (rt-PA) combined with heparin or heparin alone. The RV function improved in significantly more patients who received rt-PA compared to those who received heparin alone (39% vs. 17%, $p = 0.005$). Improvement in pulmonary flow on perfusion scans occurred in a significantly larger number of patients who received rt-PA (14.6% vs. 1.5%). Recurrent PE was not observed among patients who received rt-PA. However, 5/55 patients in the heparin alone group developed recurrent PE—two were fatal. This early study suggested potential benefit with thrombolytic therapy in acute submassive PE.

The MAPPET trial evaluated the efficacy of thrombolytic therapy among patients with acute PE who had pulmonary hypertension or RV dysfunction, without arterial hypotension or shock [13]. In the thrombolysis group, patients received heparin combined with alteplase 100 mg; the control group received placebo with heparin. The mortality rate was low and similar in both groups. However, the need for treatment escalation including vasopressor infusion, secondary thrombolysis, mechanical ventilation, cardiopulmonary resuscitation, pulmonary embolectomy, or

Table 14.1 Studies evaluating the efficacy of thrombolysis in acute submassive pulmonary embolism

Study/year	Design	Population	Intervention	Control	Outcomes
Goldhaber et al. [12] (1993)	RCT	Acute PE with RV dysfunction and stable hemodynamic parameters	rt-PA with heparin	Heparin alone	Improved RV function, improved pulmonary flow; no recurrent PE with rt-PA vs. 5 in the control group
Konstantinides et al. [13] (2002) (MAPPET)	RCT	Acute PE with pulmonary hypertension or RV dysfunction, without systemic hypotension or shock	Alteplase with heparin	Placebo with heparin	Need for treatment escalation lower in the alteplase-heparin group. Low mortality in both groups with no significant difference
Fasullo et al. [14] (2011)	RCT	Acute PE with RV dysfunction on echocardiography	Alteplase with heparin	Heparin alone	RV function better at 24 h, hospital mortality lower with alteplase
Meyer et al. [15] (2014) (PEITHO)	RCT	Intermediate-risk PE with RV dysfunction, high troponin levels	Tenecteplase with heparin	Placebo with heparin	Higher risk of major extracranial hemorrhage and stroke. Similar 30-day mortality

RCT randomized controlled trial, *RV* right ventricle, *PE* pulmonary embolism

catheter-directed treatment was lower in the alteplase-heparin group compared to the placebo-heparin group (10.2% vs. 24.6%, $P = 0.004$). Treatment with heparin alone was associated with three times the risk of death or escalation of treatment compared to treatment with the combination of alteplase and heparin. The incidence of bleeding complications was low and similar in both groups. This study suggested that hemodynamically stable patients with RV dysfunction or pulmonary hypertension have a lower incidence of clinical deterioration with thrombolytic treatment compared to treatment with heparin alone, although there was no difference in mortality.

Fasullo et al. used a similar dose of alteplase in patients with acute PE and RV dysfunction and compared it with heparin alone. RV function at 24 h was significantly better and hospital mortality significantly lower following treatment with alteplase in this RCT [14].

The PEITHO trial studied patients with intermediate-risk PE with evidence of RV dysfunction and elevated troponin levels, suggestive of myocardial injury [15]. Patients were randomized to receive intravenous tenecteplase in a dose range of 30–50 mg, based on body weight or placebo. Intravenous heparin was administered in both groups of patients. The primary outcome was death or hemodynamic decompensation within 7 days of randomization. Among 506 patients in the tenecteplase group, 13 (2.6%) experienced the primary outcome compared to 28 of 499 (5.6%) in the placebo group (OR, 0.44; 95% confidence interval, 0.23 to 0.87; $P = 0.02$). A significantly higher risk of major extracranial hemorrhage and stroke was observed in the tenecteplase group. The 30-day mortality was similar between the two groups. Considering the modest beneficial effect on the hemodynamic status with no difference in survival and the tenfold higher incidence of intracranial hemorrhage, this study did not support the use of tenecteplase in submassive PE.

A meta-analysis including 16 RCTs comprising 2115 patients with acute PE compared thrombolytic therapy with anticoagulation alone. Thrombolytic treatment reduced the all-cause mortality compared to anticoagulation alone (OR, 0.53, 95% CI: 0.32–0.88). Major bleeding was more common with thrombolysis; however, the incidence was not higher in patients below 65 years. The risk of recurrent PE was also lower with thrombolytic therapy. Among patients with PE, including those who were hemodynamically stable with right ventricular dysfunction, thrombolytic therapy was associated with lower rates of all-cause mortality and increased risks of major bleeding and ICH [10].

Although thrombolytic therapy may improve outcomes in submassive PE, identifying patients who might benefit often presents a clinical conundrum. This is particularly relevant considering the relatively low risk of mortality in submassive compared to massive PE. Reduction of pulmonary artery pressures and reversal of RV dilatation with improved function are often considered to be advantages of thrombolytic therapy; however, these putative benefits need to be balanced against the risk of morbidity and mortality due to bleeding. It is also important to reckon with the fact that the RV systolic pressure has been shown to normalize in 93% of patients at 6 months following submassive PE treated with anticoagulation alone [16]. The choice of therapy based on risk stratification is presented in Table 14.2.

Table 14.2 Choice of therapy in acute PE based on risk stratification

Risk category	Treatment
• Low risk	• Anticoagulation, preferably with direct oral anticoagulants. Low-risk patients may be discharged early
• Intermediate/ high risk	• Anticoagulation with unfractionated heparin • Intravenous thrombolysis • If the risk of bleed is high, administer low-dose intravenous thrombolysis • Catheter-directed therapy or surgical embolectomy are alternatives • In PE with cardiogenic shock mechanical support may be required; intravenous thrombolysis, catheter-directed therapy, and surgical embolectomy are other therapeutic options

PE pulmonary embolism

14.8 Low-Dose Thrombolysis

Despite the established efficacy of thrombolytic therapy in clot lysis with improved pulmonary blood flow and augmentation of RV function, there is concern regarding adverse outcomes related to major bleeding complications. The question arises, compared to the standard regimen of rt-PA of 100 mg over 2 h, would a reduced dose be equally effective, with a lower incidence of bleeding?

Wang et al. compared the safety and efficacy of half the conventional dose of rt-PA, at 50 mg over 2 h with the standard dose of 100 mg over 2 h in patients with acute PE [17]. The study patients were hemodynamically unstable or had evidence of massive obstruction of the pulmonary artery as evident on the CT pulmonary angiogram or a V/Q scan. RV function and lung perfusion assessed by echocardiography, V/Q scans, and CT pulmonary angiogram improved similarly in both groups of patients. The incidence of bleeding, including major bleeding, was higher with the 100 mg dose although the difference fell short of statistical significance. On subgroup analysis, among patients with a bodyweight <65 kg, the number of bleeding episodes was lower in the 50 mg arm.

Sharifi et al. randomized 121 patients with moderate PE to undergo thrombolytic therapy with low-dose rt-PA of 50 mg for patients weighing ≥50 kg and 0.5 mg/kg for those weighing <50 kg. In the control arm, patients received anticoagulation alone. The composite outcome of death and recurrent PE at 28 months was significantly lower in the low-dose thrombolysis group compared to anticoagulation alone (1.6% vs. 10%, $p = 0.0489$). The individual components of the primary outcome, death, and recurrent PE were not significantly different between the two groups. A significant reduction in the pulmonary artery pressure was maintained at 28 months with low-dose thrombolysis [18].

A meta-analysis including five RCTs that compared standard-dose rt-PA with a lower dose also revealed a lower incidence of major bleeding in the low-dose group. No significant difference was observed in the all-cause mortality and the incidence of recurrent PE [19]. A lower half-dose rt-PA has been also shown to be safe and effective in two controlled studies [19, 20].

Low-dose thrombolytic therapy may have similar efficacy in reducing pulmonary artery pressure and improving RV function compared to a conventional dose. Particularly, among patients who present with contraindications, half-dose thrombolytic therapy may offer a safer, effective option.

Commonly used thrombolytic agents and dosing are presented in Table 14.3.

Table 14.3 The dose of commonly used fibrin specific thrombolytic agents in acute PE

Drug	Dose
Alteplase	100 mg IV over 2 h
Reteplase	10 units IV bolus, two doses, 30 min apart
Tenecteplase	Less than 60 kg: 30 mg 60–70 kg: 35 mg 70–80 kg: 40 mg 80–90 kg: 45 mg More than 90 kg: 50 mg (all: over 5 s)

14.9 Catheter-Directed Thrombolysis (CDT)

Thrombolytic therapy may be delivered directly to the clot obstructing the pulmonary artery with the potential for greater efficacy besides enabling a lower dose of the thrombolytic agent, with a lower risk of bleeding. Systemic therapy may lead to a disproportionately higher dose being delivered to unobstructed regions of the lung, thus reducing efficacy. The most studied technique is ultrasound-assisted, catheter-directed thrombolysis (USAT) [21]. The ultrasound transducer enables disruption of the clot allowing penetration of the thrombolytic agent into the core of the clot.

CDT offers a viable alternative to systemic thrombolysis, transcatheter or surgical embolectomy in patients with hemodynamic instability and at high risk of complications. CDT has been associated with a lower risk of bleeding compared to systemic therapy [22]. It may be superior to anticoagulation alone in reducing RV dilatation and dysfunction, with alleviation of pulmonary hypertension and reduction of the clot load [23].

Key Points

- Thrombolytic therapy in acute PE enables rapid reduction of the clot burden, thereby relieving obstruction to pulmonary blood flow. A reduction in the pulmonary artery pressure results in reduced afterload, thereby improving RV function.
- Thrombolytic therapy may also lead to bleeding complications with adverse outcomes including mortality. Hence, it is crucial to weigh the benefits of early clot lysis with the likelihood of harm from catastrophic bleeding.
- In acute massive PE, the efficacy of thrombolysis is well established, with improvement in hemodynamic parameters and overall survival.
- In submassive PE, in the absence of systemic hypotension or shock, the potential for benefit may be more contentious.

- Among patients with a high risk for bleeding or other relative contraindications, a low-dose thrombolytic therapy may be a reasonable, equally effective option compared to conventional doses.
- Catheter-directed therapy has the potential to deliver an enhanced dose of the thrombolytic agent at the site of the clot with a lower dose; future investigations need to evaluate the clinical efficacy of catheter-directed therapies, including the use of ultrasonographic clot disruption.

References

1. Sherry S. The origin of thrombolytic therapy. J Am Coll Cardiol. 1989;14(4):1085–92.
2. Sautter RD, Emanuel DA, Fletcher FW, Wenzel FJ, Matson JI. Urokinase for the treatment of acute pulmonary thromboembolism. JAMA. 1967;202(3):215–8.
3. Konstantinides SV, Meyer G, Becattini C, Bueno H, Geersing GJ, Harjola VP, et al. ESC Guidelines for the diagnosis and management of acute pulmonary embolism developed in collaboration with the European Respiratory Society (ERS): The Task Force for the diagnosis and management of acute pulmonary embolism of the European Society of Cardiology (ESC). Eur Respir J. 2019;54(3):1901647. Available from: https://erj.ersjournals.com/content/54/3/1901647
4. Kearon C, Akl EA, Comerota AJ, Prandoni P, Bounameaux H, Goldhaber SZ, et al. Antithrombotic therapy for VTE disease: antithrombotic therapy and prevention of thrombosis, 9th ed: American College of Chest Physicians Evidence-Based Clinical Practice Guidelines. Chest. 2012;141(2 Suppl):e419S–96S.
5. Urokinase pulmonary embolism trial. Phase 1 results: a cooperative study. JAMA. 1970;214(12):2163–72.
6. Dotter CT, Seaman AJ, Rösch J, Porter JM. Streptokinase and heparin in the treatment of pulmonary embolism: a randomized comparison. Vasc Surg. 1979;13(1):42–52.
7. Ly B, Arnesen H, Eie H, Hol R. A controlled clinical trial of streptokinase and heparin in the treatment of major pulmonary embolism. Acta Med Scand. 1978;203(6):465–70.
8. Jerjes-Sanchez C, Ramírez-Rivera A, de Lourdes GM, Arriaga-Nava R, Valencia S, Rosado-Buzzo A, et al. Streptokinase and heparin versus heparin alone in massive pulmonary embolism: a randomized controlled trial. J Thromb Thrombol. 1995;2(3):227–9.
9. Stein PD, Matta F. Thrombolytic therapy in unstable patients with acute pulmonary embolism: saves lives but underused. Am J Med. 2012 May;125(5):465–70.
10. Chatterjee S, Chakraborty A, Weinberg I, Kadakia M, Wilensky RL, Sardar P, et al. Thrombolysis for pulmonary embolism and risk of all-cause mortality, major bleeding, and intracranial hemorrhage: a meta-analysis. JAMA. 2014;311(23):2414–21.
11. Marti C, John G, Konstantinides S, Combescure C, Sanchez O, Lankeit M, et al. Systemic thrombolytic therapy for acute pulmonary embolism: a systematic review and meta-analysis. Eur Heart J. 2015;36(10):605–14.
12. Goldhaber SZ, Haire WD, Feldstein ML, Miller M, Toltzis R, Smith JL, et al. Alteplase versus heparin in acute pulmonary embolism: randomised trial assessing right-ventricular function and pulmonary perfusion. Lancet. 1993;341(8844):507–11.
13. Konstantinides S, Geibel A, Heusel G, Heinrich F, Kasper W. Management strategies and prognosis of pulmonary Embolism-3 trial investigators. Heparin plus alteplase compared with heparin alone in patients with submassive pulmonary embolism. N Engl J Med. 2002;347(15):1143–50.

14. Fasullo S, Scalzo S, Maringhini G, Ganci F, Cannizzaro S, Basile I, et al. Six-month echocardiographic study in patients with submassive pulmonary embolism and right ventricle dysfunction: comparison of thrombolysis with heparin. Am J Med Sci. 2011;341(1):33–9.
15. Meyer G, Vicaut E, Danays T, Agnelli G, Becattini C, Beyer-Westendorf J, et al. Fibrinolysis for patients with intermediate-risk pulmonary embolism. N Engl J Med. 2014;370(15):1402–11.
16. Kline JA, Steuerwald MT, Marchick MR, Hernandez-Nino J, Rose GA. Prospective evaluation of right ventricular function and functional status 6 months after acute submassive pulmonary embolism: frequency of persistent or subsequent elevation in estimated pulmonary artery pressure. Chest. 2009;136(5):1202–10.
17. Wang C, Zhai Z, Yang Y, Wu Q, Cheng Z, Liang L, et al. Efficacy and safety of low dose recombinant tissue-type plasminogen activator for the treatment of acute pulmonary thromboembolism: a randomized, multicenter, controlled trial. Chest. 2010;137(2):254–62.
18. Sharifi M, Bay C, Skrocki L, Rahimi F, Mehdipour M. "MOPETT" investigators. Moderate pulmonary embolism treated with thrombolysis (from the "MOPETT" trial). Am J Cardiol. 2013;111(2):273–7.
19. Zhang Z, Zhai Z-g, Rong LL, Fang LF, Hua YY, Wang C. Lower dosage of recombinant tissue-type plasminogen activator (rt-PA) in the treatment of acute pulmonary embolism: a systematic review and meta-analysis. Thromb Res. 2014;133(3):357–63.
20. Yilmaz ES, Uzun O. Low-dose thrombolysis for submassive pulmonary embolism. J Investig Med. 2021;69(8):1439–46.
21. Halaby R, Giri J. Keep it simple? Half-dose systemic thrombolysis or catheter-directed thrombolysis for pulmonary embolism. Vasc Med. 2019;24(2):110–1.
22. Kuo WT, Banerjee A, Kim PS, DeMarco FJ, Levy JR, Facchini FR, et al. Pulmonary embolism response to fragmentation, embolectomy, and catheter thrombolysis (PERFECT): initial results from a prospective multicenter registry. Chest. 2015;148(3):667–73.
23. Kucher N, Boekstegers P, Müller OJ, Kupatt C, Beyer-Westendorf J, Heitzer T, et al. Randomized, controlled trial of ultrasound-assisted catheter-directed thrombolysis for acute intermediate-risk pulmonary embolism. Circulation. 2014;129(4):479–86.

Part II

Shock and Circulatory Support

Corticosteroids in Sepsis: The Enduring Debate

15

15.1 Introduction

The use of corticosteroids as adjunctive therapy in septic shock has captivated intensive care physicians for over five decades. Many of the early studies used industrial doses of synthetic glucocorticoids and, predictably, led to poor clinical outcomes [1]. The concept of corticosteroid insufficiency related to critical illness (CIRCI) has arisen more recently [2]. The CIRCI paradigm is based on the hypothesis that even maximal stimulation of the hypothalamic-pituitary-adrenal axis in disease states such as sepsis results in insufficient corticosteroid levels. Besides, there may be tissue resistance to corticosteroids in the presence of sepsis. Based on this theory, the use of more physiological doses of corticosteroids as adjuvant therapy in sepsis was conceptualized, with several small randomized controlled studies (RCTs) demonstrating improvement in hemodynamic parameters and a trend toward improved survival [3, 4]. Many large RCTs have been carried out since then, evaluating the effect of low-dose corticosteroids to replenish insufficient endogenous activity. What does the current evidence suggest regarding the efficacy of corticosteroids in septic shock?

15.2 The Pathophysiological Basis of Steroid Effect in Sepsis

The nuclear factor kappa B (NF-Kβ) system is the key trigger for the intense inflammatory reaction in sepsis. This proinflammatory effect is balanced by the anti-inflammatory effect mediated by the glucocorticoid-glucocorticoid receptor α (G-GRα) interaction. Corticosteroids suppress the NF-Kβ activity, thereby attenuating the inflammatory response [5]. Glucocorticoid receptors are present in the endothelium and vascular smooth muscle; they augment the effect of catecholamines and angiotensin II leading to enhanced responsiveness to vasopressor agents [6]. Besides, glucocorticoids inhibit the synthesis of vasodilator agents

J. Chacko et al., *Controversies in Critical Care*,
https://doi.org/10.1007/978-981-19-9940-6_15

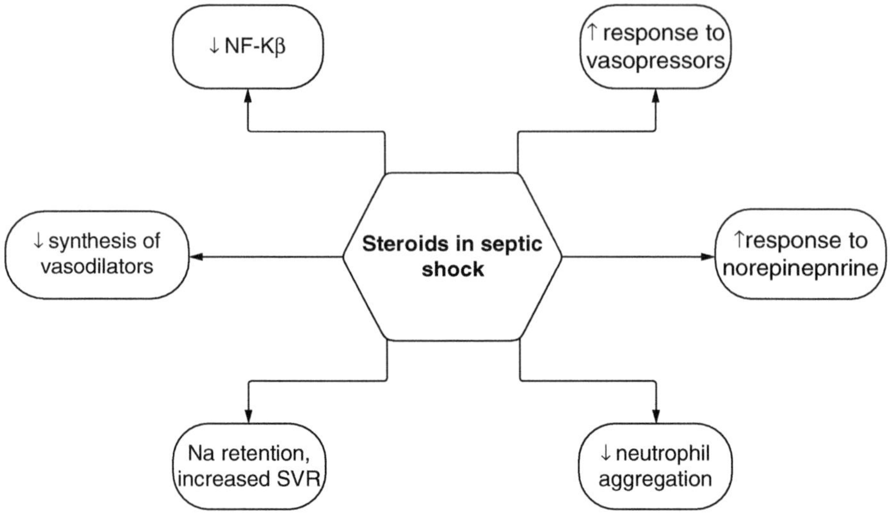

Fig. 15.1 Potential mechanisms of beneficial effect of corticosteroids in septic shock

including inducible nitric oxide (iNO) and cyclooxygenase 2 (COX-2) [7]. The inhibitory effect on the generation of vasodilator agents results in a reduced requirement for vasopressor support [8]. Glucocorticoids may potentiate the vasoconstrictor effect of norepinephrine through increased alpha-receptor gene expression [9]. Furthermore, sodium retention through the mineralocorticoid effect may raise the systemic vascular resistance and increase the mean arterial pressure [10] (Fig. 15.1).

15.3 Earlier Randomized Controlled Trials

Annane et al. conducted the first, adequately powered RCT to evaluate the efficacy of corticosteroids in septic shock. The combination of intravenous hydrocortisone 50 mg every 6 h intravenously and fludrocortisone 50 μg once daily by the enteral route was administered for a week and compared with placebo. A short corticotrophin test was performed in all patients to test adrenal function. Patients with a rise in cortisol level of less than 9 μg/dl in response to corticotrophin were considered "nonresponders." The 28-days survival, the primary outcome, was significantly higher among nonresponders who received corticosteroid therapy, suggesting that exogenous administration of corticosteroids leads to improved survival in patients with relative adrenal insufficiency. The time to cessation of vasopressors was also significantly less among nonresponders who were treated with corticosteroids [11]. This was followed by the CORTICUS trial, which included 499 patients; in this study, intravenous hydrocortisone alone was administered as adjunctive therapy (fludrocortisone was not used) and compared with placebo [12]. No difference was observed in the 28-days mortality in this study; however, a reduced time to shock reversal was noted in corticosteroid-treated patients. The patients in the CORTICUS trial were less severely ill, compared to the Annane et al. study, with relatively fewer patients who fulfilled the criteria for septic shock.

15.4 Recent Randomized Controlled Trials

Considering the contrasting results of these two studies, the Adjunctive Corticosteroid Treatment in Critically Ill Patients with Septic Shock (ADRENAL) study was carried out by the Australian-New Zealand Intensive Care Society Clinical Trials Group [13]. The ADRENAL study, the largest RCT to address this question, recruited 3800 patients involving 69 medical-surgical ICUs in Australia, the UK, New Zealand, Saudi Arabia, and Denmark. Patients were on invasive or noninvasive ventilation and vasopressor therapy for more than 4 h at randomization. In the intervention arm, hydrocortisone was administered as an intravenous infusion of 200 mg/day for 7 days or until death or discharge from the ICU. No difference was observed in the 90-days mortality, the primary outcome, for which the study was powered. Among the secondary outcomes, the investigators observed significantly less time to shock resolution, reduced time to initial of discontinuation of mechanical ventilation, less time to ICU discharge, and fewer patients who received a blood transfusion in the hydrocortisone treated group. The 28-day mortality, shock recurrence, use of renal replacement therapy, number of days alive and out of ICU, the median time to hospital discharge, and the number of days alive and out of hospital were not different between groups.

The combination of hydrocortisone, 50 mg/kg intravenously, and 50 μg fludrocortisone once daily was evaluated in a French multicentric study (APROCCHSS) among patients with septic shock who were on vasopressor therapy for at least 6 h [14]. The study was originally designed to assess the efficacy of the combination of drotrecogin alfa and corticosteroids. However, during the course of the study, drotrecogin alfa was withdrawn from the market; thereafter, the study was continued with corticosteroids alone and compared with placebo. In contrast to ADRENAL, a statistically significant difference was observed in the 90-day mortality, the primary endpoint. The all-cause mortality at ICU and hospital discharge and at 180 days were also significantly lower among corticosteroid-treated patients. Earlier shock reversal was observed, with more patients alive and off vasopressor support at 28 days with corticosteroids. Table 15.1 summarizes the main RCTs that have evaluated the effect of corticosteroids in sepsis.

Table 15.1 Randomized controlled trials evaluating the effect of corticosteroids in sepsis

Study/year	Population	Corticosteroid group	Control	Outcomes
Annane et al. [11] (2002)	Septic shock	Hydrocortisone 50 mg/6 h IV; fludrocortisone 50 μg daily enterally for 7 days	Placebo	28-day mortality significantly less among nonresponders who received corticosteroids. No difference in the overall mortality at 28 days. vasopressors ceased earlier in the treatment group
Sprung et al. [12] (CORTICUS, 2008)	Septic shock	Hydrocortisone 50 mg/6 h IV for 7 days	Placebo	No difference in the 28-day mortality. Earlier shock reversal with hydrocortisone
Venkatesh et al. [13] (ADRENAL, 2018)	Septic shock, on vasopressors for >4 h	Hydrocortisone as a continuous infusion of 200 mg/day for 7 days	Placebo	90-day mortality similar. Earlier shock resolution, discontinuation of mechanical ventilation, and ICU discharge with hydrocortisone. No difference in the 28-day mortality, shock recurrence, RRT requirement, time to hospital discharge, number of days alive and out of hospital
Annane et al. [14] (APROCCHSS, 2018)	Septic shock, on vasopressors for ≥6 h	Hydrocortisone 50 mg/6 h IV; fludrocortisone 50 μg daily enterally for 7 days	Placebo	90-day mortality, all-cause mortality at ICU and hospital discharge and at 180 days significantly lower with corticosteroids. Earlier shock reversal with corticosteroids
Keh et al. [15] (HYPRESS, 2016)	Patients with severe sepsis, not in septic shock	Hydrocortisone as a continuous infusion of 200 mg/days for 5 days, followed by a tapered dose until day 11	Placebo	Development of septic shock not different between groups. 28-day, 90-day, 180-day, ICU, and in-hospital mortality similar. Neuromuscular weakness, nosocomial infections similar

RRT renal replacement therapy

15.5 APROCCHSS vs. ADRENAL: Why the Difference?

A relatively large number of patients were excluded in the ADRENAL trial; 21,818 patients were screened, out of which 8263 patients were excluded. The exclusion of a large number of subjects may represent a bias in RCTs. In contrast, in the APROCCHSS trial, 1671 patients with septic shock were screened, and 1241 patients were included in the study. Patients in the APROCCHSS trial may have been more severely ill. They were on higher doses of norepinephrine and had higher lactate levels, and renal replacement therapy was more frequent, all suggesting a more severe illness at baseline. In the ADRENAL study, patients were enrolled later compared to APROCCHSS, suggesting that earlier administration of corticosteroids may be more efficacious. Administration of hydrocortisone as an infusion may not be optimal, considering that achievement of adequate blood levels may be delayed without an initial bolus. Furthermore, it may be illogical to administer hydrocortisone as an infusion considering its relatively long half-life (8–12 h). Did fludrocortisone make a difference to the final outcome? It is difficult to answer this question based on the current level of evidence. Vasopressin use was much more common in the ADRENAL trial; however, the impact of a combination of vasopressin and corticosteroids needs more detailed evaluation in patients with septic shock.

15.6 Corticosteroids in Severe Sepsis Without Septic Shock

Does hydrocortisone administration in patients with severe sepsis prevent the development of septic shock? The HYPRESS study evaluated this question in an RCT including 353 patients across 34 centers in Germany [15]. The study subjects had an underlying infection with at least two systemic inflammatory response syndrome (SIRS) criteria and the presence of organ dysfunction for less than 48 h. Hydrocortisone was administered as a continuous infusion of 200 mg/day for 5 days and tapered off thereafter. Patients in the control arm received a placebo infusion. The primary endpoint was the development of septic shock within 14 days of randomization, defined as a mean arterial pressure < 65 or systolic blood pressure < 90 mm Hg, or the requirement for vasopressors despite adequate volume resuscitation. The incidence of septic shock did not differ between patients who received hydrocortisone compared to those who received placebo (21.2% vs. 22.9%, $p = 0.7$). Among the secondary outcomes, there was no difference between the hydrocortisone and placebo arms in the mortality at 28 days (8.8% vs. 8.2%), 90 days (16.7 vs. 19.9%), 180 days (26.8% vs. 22.2%), in the ICU (7.6% vs. 8.1%), or in hospital (13.5% vs. 12.8%). No significant difference was observed between the two groups in the ventilation- and renal replacement-free days. The incidence of neuromuscular weakness and nosocomial infections were also similar between the two groups. This study demonstrated that among patients with severe sepsis, hydrocortisone administration did not lower the incidence of septic shock.

15.7 Meta-Analysis on the Efficacy of Corticosteroids in Septic Shock

Two recent meta-analyses have evaluated the effect of corticosteroid administration in patients with sepsis. Fang et al. analyzed 37 RCTs including 9564 patients; corticosteroid administration was associated with a reduced 28-day, ICU, and hospital mortality. Besides, shock reversal was significantly greater with corticosteroid use. The time to shock resolution was also lower with more vasopressor-free days with corticosteroid use [16].

In another meta-analysis of 50 RCTs including 12,304 patients, corticosteroid use in sepsis was associated with a lower ICU and in-hospital mortality; however, there was no difference in longer-term survival at 28 days or longer [17]. A higher incidence of hypernatremia and hyperglycemia was observed with corticosteroid use; however, there was no increase in the incidence of gastrointestinal bleed or nosocomial infections.

Key Points

- There is a strong physiological rationale for the use of corticosteroids as adjunctive treatment in septic shock.
- All major RCTs and several meta-analyses that evaluated the use of corticosteroids in septic shock have shown earlier shock reversal and more rapid weaning down of vasopressors.
- Corticosteroid administration may lead to a shorter duration of mechanical ventilation and length of stay in the intensive care unit.
- Considering the available evidence, it may be appropriate to administer corticosteroids in patients with septic shock. The benefit of corticosteroid therapy may be greater in more severe disease.
- Administration of corticosteroids in severe sepsis may not prevent the development of septic shock.
- Low-dose corticosteroid therapy has not been associated with an increase in the incidence of nosocomial infections.
- Future studies need to be designed to evaluate whether (1) corticosteroids are more efficacious in the more severely ill and (2) addition of fludrocortisone would make a difference.

References

1. Lefering R, Neugebauer EA. Steroid controversy in sepsis and septic shock: a meta-analysis. Crit Care Med. 1995;23(7):1294–303.
2. Annane D, Pastores SM, Arlt W, Balk RA, Beishuizen A, Briegel J, et al. Critical illness-related corticosteroid insufficiency (CIRCI): a narrative review from a multispecialty task force of the Society of Critical Care Medicine (SCCM) and the European Society of Intensive Care Medicine (ESICM). Intensive Care Med. 2017;43(12):1781–92.
3. Bollaert PE, Charpentier C, Levy B, Debouverie M, Audibert G, Larcan A. Reversal of late septic shock with supraphysiologic doses of hydrocortisone. Crit Care Med. 1998;26(4):645–50.
4. Briegel J, Forst H, Haller M, Schelling G, Kilger E, Kuprat G, et al. Stress doses of hydrocortisone reverse hyperdynamic septic shock: a prospective, randomized, double-blind, single-center study. Crit Care Med. 1999;27(4):723–32.
5. Klaitman V, Almog Y. Corticosteroids in sepsis: a new concept for an old drug. Isr Med Assoc J. 2003;5(1):51–5.
6. Lambden S, Creagh-Brown BC, Hunt J, Summers C, Forni LG. Definitions and pathophysiology of vasoplegic shock. Crit Care Lond Engl. 2018;22(1):174.
7. Radomski MW, Palmer RM, Moncada S. Glucocorticoids inhibit the expression of an inducible, but not the constitutive, nitric oxide synthase in vascular endothelial cells. Proc Natl Acad Sci U S A. 1990;87(24):10043–7.
8. Keh D, Boehnke T, Weber-Cartens S, Schulz C, Ahlers O, Bercker S, et al. Immunologic and hemodynamic effects of "low-dose" hydrocortisone in septic shock: a double-blind, randomized, placebo-controlled, crossover study. Am J Respir Crit Care Med. 2003;167(4):512–20.
9. Levy B, Fritz C, Tahon E, Jacquot A, Auchet T, Kimmoun A. Vasoplegia treatments: the past, the present, and the future. Crit Care Lond Engl. 2018;22(1):52.
10. Fadel F, André-Grégoire G, Gravez B, Bauvois B, Bouchet S, Sierra-Ramos C, et al. Aldosterone and vascular mineralocorticoid receptors in murine endotoxic and human septic shock. Crit Care Med. 2017;45(9):e954–62.
11. Annane D, Sébille V, Charpentier C, Bollaert PE, François B, Korach JM, et al. Effect of treatment with low doses of hydrocortisone and fludrocortisone on mortality in patients with septic shock. JAMA. 2002;288(7):862–71.
12. Sprung CL, Annane D, Keh D, Moreno R, Singer M, Freivogel K, et al. Hydrocortisone therapy for patients with septic shock. N Engl J Med. 2008;358(2):111–24.
13. Venkatesh B, Finfer S, Cohen J, Rajbhandari D, Arabi Y, Bellomo R, et al. Adjunctive glucocorticoid therapy in patients with septic shock. N Engl J Med. 2018;378(9):797–808.
14. Annane D, Renault A, Brun-Buisson C, Megarbane B, Quenot JP, Siami S, et al. Hydrocortisone plus fludrocortisone for adults with septic shock. N Engl J Med. 2018;378(9):809–18.
15. Keh D, Trips E, Marx G, Wirtz SP, Abduljawwad E, Bercker S, et al. Effect of hydrocortisone on development of shock among patients with severe sepsis: the HYPRESS randomized clinical trial. JAMA. 2016;316(17):1775–85.
16. Fang F, Zhang Y, Tang J, Lunsford LD, Li T, Tang R, et al. Association of Corticosteroid Treatment with Outcomes in adult patients with sepsis: a systematic review and meta-analysis. JAMA Intern Med. 2019;179(2):213–23.
17. Liang H, Song H, Zhai R, Song G, Li H, Ding X, et al. Corticosteroids for treating sepsis in adult patients: a systematic review and meta-analysis. Front Immunol. 2021;12:709155.

Hyperlactatemia in Critical Illness: Time for Reappraisal?

16

16.1 Introduction

Lactic acidosis commonly occurs in the critically ill, especially among patients with shock of varying etiology. High lactate levels are uniformly associated with poor clinical outcomes, including mortality [1, 2]. However, there has been considerable interest and contradictory views regarding the clinical value of using lactate levels to guide resuscitation in critically ill patients. Although generally considered to be a marker of tissue hypoxia, the etiology of hyperlactatemia in the critically ill may be multifactorial.

16.2 Lactate Production and Metabolism

Lactate is generated at the rate of 0.8 mmol/kg/h (1300 mmol/day), with a normal plasma level between 0.3 and 1.3 mmol/l. Lactate production occurs in the skeletal muscle, intestines, brain, and erythrocytes. In the glycolytic pathway, glucose is oxidized to pyruvate with the generation of NADH from NAD. The pyruvate is metabolized in the mitochondria by the aerobic pathway through the Krebs cycle. The metabolism of each molecule of pyruvate results in the generation of 36 molecules of ATP. Under anaerobic conditions, the pyruvate does not enter the mitochondria; instead, it is converted to lactate by the lactate dehydrogenase enzyme in the cytosol, with the regeneration of NAD from NADH. The concentrations of lactate and pyruvate are maintained at a 10:1 equilibrium by lactate dehydrogenase. The lactate thus generated is transported to the liver, where it is oxidized to pyruvate. The pyruvate is converted back to glucose through gluconeogenesis and reenters the glycolytic pathway (Fig. 16.1). The liver clears 70% of the generated lactate, mainly through gluconeogenesis and partly by oxidation to carbon dioxide and water.

J. Chacko et al., *Controversies in Critical Care*,
https://doi.org/10.1007/978-981-19-9940-6_16

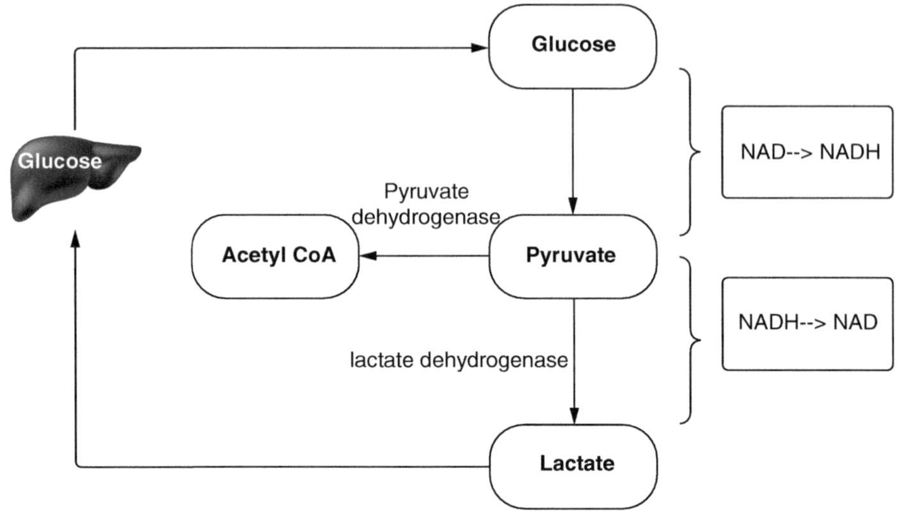

Fig. 16.1 In the glycolytic pathway, glucose is oxidized to pyruvate. The pyruvate is metabolized by the aerobic pathway through the Krebs cycle. Under anaerobic conditions, pyruvate is converted to lactate by the enzyme lactate dehydrogenase. The lactate thus generated oxidized to pyruvate in the liver. The pyruvate is converted back to glucose in the liver through gluconeogenesis and reenters the glycolytic pathway

Tissues rich in mitochondria, including skeletal and cardiac muscle, and the proximal tubular tubules of the kidney eliminate the remaining lactate by conversion to pyruvate. The kidneys excrete less than 5% of the lactate produced.

16.3 Why Do Lactate Levels Rise in the Critically Ill?

Being the predominant metabolic pathway of lactate, impairment of liver function results in raised lactate levels. Any increase in the rate of glycolysis results in the generation of high levels of pyruvate. The pyruvate dehydrogenase enzyme may be overwhelmed by excessive pyruvate levels. As the pyruvate levels rise excessively, it is converted to lactate by the lactate dehydrogenase enzyme. Accelerated glycolysis occurs in hypermetabolic states, including fever, thyrotoxicosis, and the use of beta-agonist drugs such as adrenaline. This may be the mechanism of causation of lactic acidosis in patients with acute severe asthma who are treated with high-dose beta-adrenergic bronchodilators. Thus, lactate levels may continue to rise in a patient with severe asthma who is clinically improving with the alleviation of bronchospasm. Mitochondrial dysfunction leads to the failure of the aerobic pathway of metabolism. Thiamine is a crucial cofactor in the conversion of pyruvate to acetyl CoA. Thiamine deficiency can inhibit this reaction and lead to the conversion of pyruvate to lactate. Ischemic tissues, including gut ischemia, may lead to the generation of high levels of lactate. Toxins that poison the mitochondria, including cyanide and carbon monoxide, can lead to failure of the aerobic pathway and result in lactic acidosis. Biguanides may also lead to excessive lactate levels through inhibition of hepatic gluconeogenesis. Respiratory alkalosis may lead to the movement of intracellular lactate to the extracellular fluid and lead to elevated lactate levels in the plasma [3].

16.4 Does Hyperlactatemia Occur Due to Impaired Oxygen Delivery in Sepsis?

In patients with various types of shock, elevated lactate levels were considered to be due to oxygen delivery failing to meet tissue demand, leading to anaerobic metabolism [4]. The Surviving Sepsis Guidelines (2017) recommended resuscitation aimed to normalize lactate levels based on the hypothesis of oxygen debt [5]. However, there is scant evidence to support oxygen debt in septic shock.

In septic patients, the partial pressure of oxygen in the skeletal muscle was found to be higher than normal and increased with the severity of sepsis [6]. In an animal model of sepsis, elevated plasma lactate levels were observed despite high PO_2 values in the intestinal and bladder mucosa. This suggests that lactate generation occurs through mechanisms unrelated to cellular hypoxia in sepsis [7, 8].

Mitochondrial dysfunction has long been considered to be the underlying mechanism for the failure of oxygen utilization leading to anaerobic metabolism and the generation of lactate in sepsis. Mitochondrial function is evaluated by measurement of the levels of high-energy phosphates, including ATP, phosphocreatine, and intracellular pH. Using this technique, no evidence of mitochondrial dysfunction was observed in animal experiments and studies on human subjects with sepsis [9, 10].

16.5 Is There a Mismatch Between Oxygen Consumption and Delivery in Sepsis?

Ronco et al. studied critical O_2 delivery and O_2 extraction ratio among septic and non-septic patients. Tissue oxygen delivery was maintained in these patients, and the ability of tissues to extract oxygen remained unaffected. However, hyperlactatemia was observed, suggesting that tissue dysoxia was not the underlying mechanism [11]. A recent randomized controlled trial evaluated the administration of esmolol infusion in patients with septic shock. Despite reduced oxygen delivery, a significant decrease in lactate levels was observed, suggesting that lactate levels were unrelated to oxygen delivery among these patients [12].

16.6 What Is the Source of Lactate in Sepsis?

If tissue hypoxia leading to anaerobic metabolism is not the primary source of raised lactate levels in sepsis, what may be the mechanisms of hyperlactatemia in septic shock (Fig. 16.2)?

16.6.1 Impaired Pyruvate Dehydrogenase Activity

There may be an inhibition of the mitochondrial pyruvate dehydrogenase activity in sepsis, the enzyme that converts pyruvate to acetyl CoA prior to its entry into the Krebs cycle. This results in the selective conversion of pyruvate to lactate by the lactate dehydrogenase enzyme, leading to hyperlactatemia. The administration of dichloroacetate, a drug that enhances pyruvate dehydrogenase activity, has been shown to reduce lactate levels in animal models and human studies [13]. Besides, accelerated aerobic glycolysis occurs in sepsis, leading to the generation of excessive pyruvate. High pyruvate levels coupled with impaired pyruvate dehydrogenase activity lead to a predominance of the alternate pathway, with the conversion of pyruvate to lactate.

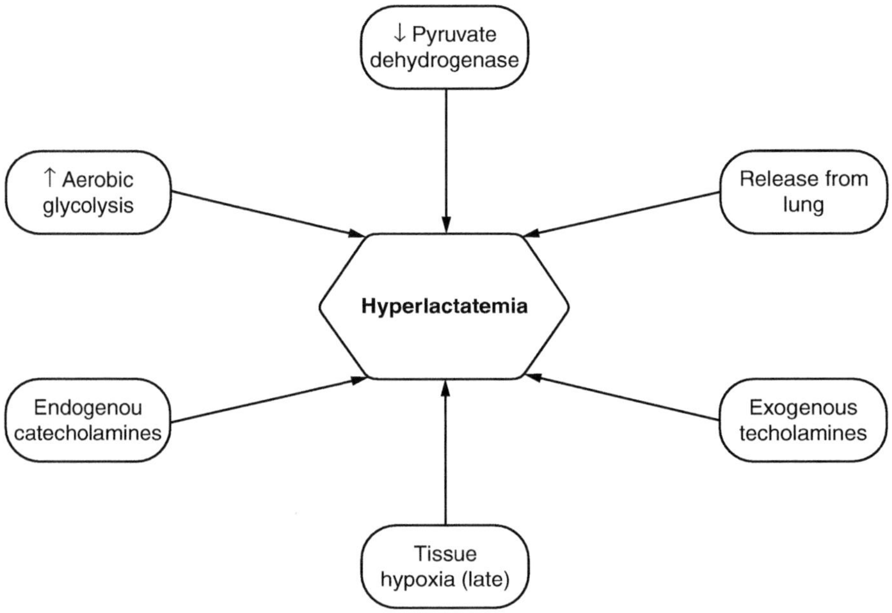

Fig. 16.2 Mechanisms of hyperlactatemia in sepsis

16.6.2 Lactate Release from the Lung

Opdam et al. performed an observational study among patients who underwent cardiopulmonary bypass and in patients with septic shock. They measured pulmonary oxygen consumption and lactate release from the lung. In this study, a substantial release of lactate was observed from the lung related to inflammation associated with cardiopulmonary bypass and sepsis [14]. Thus, the lung may be the source of hyperlactatemia in patients with severe sepsis.

16.6.3 Hypermetabolic State

Excessive endogenous release of catecholamines or their administration for pharmacological support of the circulation may lead to hyperlactatemia through increased activity of the Na^+/K^+–ATPase pump due to β2-receptor stimulation. This results in cyclic AMP release, with stimulation of accelerated glycogenolysis and glycolysis, leading to excessive pyruvate generation. When pyruvate levels continue to rise, increased conversion to lactate occurs, leading to hyperlactatemia. A hypermetabolic state characterized by excessive release of catecholamines may be the trigger for hyperlactatemia in sepsis [15].

16.6.4 Exogenous Catecholamines

We often see lactate levels rise with the use of catecholamine support, particularly with epinephrine infusion. However, the hyperlactatemia induced by catecholamine support does not appear to lead to worse outcomes. A retrospective analysis evaluated the survival of patients in shock in relation to the rise in lactate levels following the commencement of epinephrine infusion. Survivors had a greater increase in lactate levels following the initiation of epinephrine support compared to non-survivors. Thus, failure of lactate levels to rise significantly following epinephrine infusion may be associated with poor outcomes [16].

16.6.5 Tissue Hypoxia

Although not the sole reason for hyperlactatemia, tissue hypoxia may occur in sepsis leading to stimulation of anaerobic metabolism and a rise in lactate levels. Besides, failure of microcirculatory flow may also occur in sepsis. Indeed, studies on animal models suggest that inhibition of oxygen transport in early sepsis may likely result from microcirculatory dysfunction [17].

16.7 Lactate Clearance: A Misnomer in Sepsis

Lactate "clearance" has been suggested as a target to guide resuscitation in septic patients. However, it is important to note that the clearance of a substance denotes the extent of its removal from a unit volume over unit time. Clearly, in severe sepsis, lactate levels may decrease through mechanisms unrelated to its removal, including decreased generation or dilution consequent to fluid resuscitation.

16.8 Lactate-Guided Resuscitation

Should we pursue lactate levels as a resuscitation target in critically ill patients with sepsis? There are very few controlled studies that have compared a lactate-guided resuscitation with a conventional approach to resuscitation.

The time taken for normalization of lactate levels was compared to the normalization of other perfusion-related variables among patients with septic shock in a prospective observational study [18]. Among survivors, the central venous oxygen saturation, capillary refill time, and the PCO_2 gap (difference between the central venous and arterial CO_2 levels) normalized much earlier compared to lactate levels. Only 52% of patients had attained normal lactate levels at 24 h; this was in contrast to more than 70% of patients who had achieved normalization of other perfusion-related parameters at 6 h. This study suggested that lactate levels may take longer to normalize compared to other measures of perfusion. Persisting with resuscitation efforts aiming to normalize lactate levels may thus be counterproductive.

Jansen et al. compared a protocolized approach aiming to decrease lactate by 20% or more during the first 8 h of ICU admission among critically ill patients [1]. This was compared to standard care in a control group with clinicians unaware of lactate levels except for the initial value. On adjusted analysis, the hospital mortality was lower in the lactate-targeted group. However, the change in lactate levels remained similar in both groups during the 8-h study period and until 72 h after randomization. This study suggested that the lower mortality in the experimental group may not be related to a lactate-guided resuscitation strategy.

Other studies have been performed comparing lactate-guided resuscitation with heterogeneous protocols in the control group. In a three-arm study, Tian et al. targeted lactate clearance of 10% or 30% and compared it with early goal-directed therapy among patients with pneumonia and sepsis [19]. No significant difference was observed in the 7-day mortality; however, the 28-day mortality was significantly lower in both groups that targeted lactate clearance. Jones et al., in their RCT, compared a lactate-guided to $SCVO_2$-guided strategy of resuscitation in patients with severe sepsis and hypoperfusion or septic shock. The $SCVO_2$ target was set at 70%; a minimum lactate clearance of 10% was aimed for. The hospital mortality did not differ significantly between the lactate-guided compared to the $SCVO_2$-guided group [20].

16.9 The ANDROMEDA-SHOCK Trial

The ANDROMEDA-SHOCK trial included patients in septic shock defined as the presence of infection, raised lactate levels ≥2.0 mmol/l, and vasopressor requirement for a target mean arterial pressure of 65 mm Hg following initial fluid resuscitation with 20 ml/kg over 60 min. Patients were randomized to undergo resuscitation targeted to normalize capillary refill time (3 s or less) or a decrease in serum lactate level by 20% every 2 h [21]. The lactate level was measured 2 h, and the capillary refill time was evaluated every 30 min for a total duration of 8 h in all patients. The 28-day mortality was higher in the lactate-guided resuscitation group compared to the capillary refill time-guided group, although the difference fell short of statistical significance (hazard ratio, 0.75 [95% CI, 0.55 to 1.02]; $P = 0.06$). The sample size, calculated on the basis of a mortality difference of 15%, may have been too small to achieve statistical significance. The authors observed a significant reduction in organ dysfunction at 72 h in the capillary refill time-guided group.

In a post hoc analysis published later, patients in whom the capillary refill time had normalized following 2 h of resuscitative interventions were further evaluated [22]. Among patients in whom the capillary refill time had normalized at 2 h, those who underwent lactate-guided resuscitation had a higher mortality and organ dysfunction compared to patients who were randomized to the capillary refill time-guided resuscitation. Patients in the lactate-guided group also received more resuscitative interventions with fluid boluses, higher doses of norepinephrine, and inodilator therapy with dobutamine and milrinone. This post hoc analysis suggested that continued interventions aimed to normalize lactate levels in patients with normal capillary refill time at 2 h may lead to adverse clinical outcomes. In light of recent evidence, the recent iteration of the Surviving Sepsis Guidelines no longer recommend normalization of lactate levels in patients with sepsis; instead they suggest targeting decreasing levels of lactate [23]. Table 16.1. Summarizes recent studies that have evaluated the efficacy of a lactate-guided resuscitation strategy in critically ill patients.

Table 16.1 Studies evaluating the impact of lactate-guided resuscitation in critically ill patients

Study/year	Design/ population		Findings	Comments
Hernandez et al. [18] (2014)	Prospective observational study of patients in septic shock	Time to normalization of perfusion-related parameters, including $SCVO_2$, capillary refill time, PCO_2 gap, and lactate levels	Only 52% of patient had normal lactate levels at 24 h compared to 70% who attained normalization of perfusion parameters	Persistent resuscitation efforts directed toward normalization of lactate may not be appropriate
Jansen et al. [1] (2010)	RCT; critically ill patients with lactate level > 3.0 mEq/l	Protocolized approach to decrease lactate levels by 20% within 8 h of ICU admission. Standard care in the control group—clinicians unaware of the lactate levels	Hospital mortality lower in the lactate-guided resuscitation group. However, lactate levels decreased similarly in both groups in the 8-h study period and until 72 h	The lower mortality in the intervention group may not be have been related to a lactate-directed resuscitation strategy
Jones et al. [20] (2010)	RCT; patients with severe sepsis and hypoperfusion or septic shock	$SCVO_2$ group: resuscitation targeted to normalize CVP, MAP, and $SCVO_2$ of at least 70%. Lactate clearance group: Normalize CVP, MAP, and lactate clearance $\geq$10%	Hospital mortality similar between the $SCVO_2$ and the lactate-guided groups	Addition of lactate clearance as a target did not result in improved survival compared to CVP and MAP-guided resuscitation

Table 16.1 (continued)

Study/year	Design/ population		Findings	Comments
Hernández et al. [21] (ANDROMEDA-SHOCK, 2019)	RCT; patients with septic shock	Resuscitation targeted to normalization of CRT (≤3 s) or decrease in lactate level by 20% every 2 h	Trend toward higher 28-day mortality in the lactate-guided resuscitation group. Significant reduction in organ dysfunction at 72 h in the CRT-guided resuscitation group	The sample size, based on a mortality difference of 15%, may have been too small to achieve statistical significance
Kattan et al. [22] (2020)	Post hoc analysis of the ANDROMEDA-SHOCK RCT [21]	The study further evaluated the subgroup of patients who had normalized CRT by 2 h of resuscitative interventions. Compared patients who underwent further resuscitative efforts to normalize lactate with those in whom resuscitative interventions were ceased based on CRT (≤3 s)	Continued resuscitative efforts to normalize lactate levels among patients in whom the CRT had normalized resulted in higher mortality. More fluid boluses, higher doses of norepinephrine, and more inodilator therapy were used in those who underwent additional resuscitation aimed to normalize lactate levels	In septic shock, persisting with resuscitative efforts aimed to normalize lactate levels in those who had already attained normal CRT may be associated with adverse outcomes

$SCVO_2$ central venous oxygen saturation, *RCT* randomized controlled trial, *CVP* central venous pressure, *MAP* mean arterial pressure, *CRT* capillary refill time

Key Points

- High lactate levels in critically ill patients correlate with the severity of illness and strongly predict mortality.
- However, contrary to popular belief, the main reason for lactate rise in patients with severe sepsis is not tissue dysoxia and stimulation of anaerobic metabolism. On the contrary, in most patients with sepsis, tissue dysoxia does not occur.
- The origin of hyperlactatemia in sepsis is multifactorial, including accelerated glycolysis, a hypermetabolic state, and impaired activity or relative deficiency of pyruvate dehydrogenase. The lung may also be a lactate generator in sepsis.
- Under situations of stress, lactate acts as metabolic fuel through oxidation and conversion to pyruvate and glucose in the liver.
- The use of serum lactate levels as an endpoint to guide resuscitation may not represent the ideal approach in septic patients.
- Recognizing a clinical pattern of hypoperfusion-related hyperlactatemia is important since optimizing systemic blood flow in this setting could reverse ongoing hypoperfusion and improve prognosis. Consideration must be given to other parameters of tissue perfusion including the capillary refill time.
- Persistence with resuscitation efforts aimed at normalization of lactate levels in the absence of other manifestations of tissue hypoperfusion is likely to be futile and lead to adverse effects resulting from over-resuscitation.

References

1. Jansen TC, van Bommel J, Schoonderbeek FJ, Sleeswijk Visser SJ, van der Klooster JM, Lima AP, et al. Early lactate-guided therapy in intensive care unit patients: a multicenter, open-label, randomized controlled trial. Am J Respir Crit Care Med. 2010;182(6):752–61.
2. Dettmer M, Holthaus CV, Fuller BM. The impact of serial lactate monitoring on emergency department resuscitation interventions and clinical outcomes in severe sepsis and septic shock: an observational cohort study. Shock. 2015;43(1):55–61.
3. Sandoval DM. Hyperlactatemia in hyperventilation and respiratory alkalosis: report of three cases and literature review. Med Crítica. 2016;30(3):204–8.
4. Nguyen HB, Rivers EP, Knoblich BP, Jacobsen G, Muzzin A, Ressler JA, et al. Early lactate clearance is associated with improved outcome in severe sepsis and septic shock. Crit Care Med. 2004;32(8):1637–42.
5. Rhodes A, Evans LE, Alhazzani W, Levy MM, Antonelli M, Ferrer R, et al. Surviving sepsis campaign: international guidelines for Management of Sepsis and Septic Shock: 2016. Intensive Care Med. 2017;43(3):304–77.
6. Boekstegers P, Weidenhöfer S, Kapsner T, Werdan K. Skeletal muscle partial pressure of oxygen in patients with sepsis. Crit Care Med. 1994;22(4):640–50.

7. VanderMeer TJ, Wang H, Fink MP. Endotoxemia causes ileal mucosal acidosis in the absence of mucosal hypoxia in a normodynamic porcine model of septic shock. Crit Care Med. 1995;23(7):1217–26.
8. Rosser DM, Stidwill RP, Jacobson D, Singer M. Oxygen tension in the bladder epithelium rises in both high and low cardiac output endotoxemic sepsis. J Appl Physiol (1985). 1995;79(6):1878–82.
9. Alamdari N, Constantin-Teodosiu D, Murton AJ, Gardiner SM, Bennett T, Layfield R, et al. Temporal changes in the involvement of pyruvate dehydrogenase complex in muscle lactate accumulation during lipopolysaccharide infusion in rats. J Physiol. 2008;586(6):1767–75.
10. Brealey D, Brand M, Hargreaves I, Heales S, Land J, Smolenski R, et al. Association between mitochondrial dysfunction and severity and outcome of septic shock. Lancet Lond Engl. 2002;360(9328):219–23.
11. Ronco JJ, Fenwick JC, Tweeddale MG, Wiggs BR, Phang PT, Cooper DJ, et al. Identification of the critical oxygen delivery for anaerobic metabolism in critically ill septic and nonseptic humans. JAMA. 1993;270(14):1724–30.
12. Morelli A, Ertmer C, Westphal M, Rehberg S, Kampmeier T, Ligges S, et al. Effect of heart rate control with esmolol on hemodynamic and clinical outcomes in patients with septic shock: a randomized clinical trial. JAMA. 2013;310(16):1683–91.
13. Stacpoole PW, Nagaraja NV, Hutson AD. Efficacy of dichloroacetate as a lactate-lowering drug. J Clin Pharmacol. 2003;43(7):683–91.
14. Opdam H, Bellomo R. Oxygen consumption and lactate release by the lung after cardiopulmonary bypass and during septic shock. Crit Care Resusc. 2000;2(3):181–7.
15. Revelly JP, Tappy L, Martinez A, Bollmann M, Cayeux MC, Berger MM, et al. Lactate and glucose metabolism in severe sepsis and cardiogenic shock. Crit Care Med. 2005;33(10):2235–40.
16. Wutrich Y, Barraud D, Conrad M, Cravoisy-Popovic A, Nace L, Bollaert PE, et al. Early increase in arterial lactate concentration under epinephrine infusion is associated with a better prognosis during shock. Shock. 2010;34(1):4–9.
17. Ellis CG, Bateman RM, Sharpe MD, Sibbald WJ, Gill R. Effect of a maldistribution of microvascular blood flow on capillary O(2) extraction in sepsis. Am J Physiol Heart Circ Physiol. 2002;282(1):H156–64.
18. Hernandez G, Luengo C, Bruhn A, Kattan E, Friedman G, Ospina-Tascon GA, et al. When to stop septic shock resuscitation: clues from a dynamic perfusion monitoring. Ann Intensive Care. 2014;4:30.
19. Tian H-H, Han S-S, Lv C-J, Wang T, Li Z, Hao D, Shang Q-M, Wang X-Z. The effect of early goal lactate clearance rate on the outcome of septic shock patients with severe pneumonia. Zhongguo Wei Zhong Bing Ji Jiu Yi Xue. 2012;24(1):42–5.
20. Jones AE, Shapiro NI, Trzeciak S, Arnold RC, Claremont HA, Kline JA, et al. Lactate clearance vs central venous oxygen saturation as goals of early sepsis therapy: a randomized clinical trial. JAMA. 2010;303(8):739–46.
21. Hernández G, Ospina-Tascón GA, Damiani LP, Estenssoro E, Dubin A, Hurtado J, et al. Effect of a resuscitation strategy targeting peripheral perfusion status vs serum lactate levels on 28-day mortality among patients with septic shock: the ANDROMEDA-SHOCK randomized clinical trial. JAMA. 2019;321(7):654.
22. Kattan E, Hernández G, Ospina-Tascón G, Valenzuela ED, Bakker J, Castro R, et al. A lactate-targeted resuscitation strategy may be associated with higher mortality in patients with septic shock and normal capillary refill time: a post hoc analysis of the ANDROMEDA-SHOCK study. Ann Intensive Care. 2020;10(1):114.
23. Evans L, Rhodes A, Alhazzani W, Antonelli M, Coopersmith CM, French C, et al. Surviving sepsis campaign: international guidelines for Management of Sepsis and Septic Shock 2021. Crit Care Med. 2021;49(11):e1063.

Permissive Hypotension in Severe Trauma

17

17.1 Introduction

Exsanguinating hemorrhage is the most common cause of preventable death following major trauma [1]. The conventional approach to trauma resuscitation is the early administration of large volume crystalloids aimed to restore the circulating volume, maintain blood pressure, and tissue perfusion. This strategy is based on the poor outcomes associated with shock and tissue hypoperfusion in major trauma [2]. Controlled hemorrhage in animals models had lent credence to the concept of filling the extracellular compartment with balanced salt solutions in addition to blood transfusion [3]. The current iteration of the Advanced Trauma Life Support guidelines of the American College of Surgeons also recommend 1 L of initial resuscitation with warm normal saline in patients with up to 30% of estimated blood loss [4].

17.2 Problems with the Conventional Approach

An aggressive approach to early resuscitation may cause significant adverse effects. Large volumes of fluid resuscitation lead to increased hydrostatic pressure with dislodgement of clots resulting in continued hemorrhage. Besides, hypothermia and worsening of trauma-related coagulopathy may occur. Uncontrolled administration of large volumes of crystalloids may provoke the lethal triad of trauma, characterized by hypothermia, coagulopathy, and metabolic acidosis (Fig. 17.1), leading to continued hemorrhage and adverse clinical outcomes including increased mortality [5].

J. Chacko et al., *Controversies in Critical Care*,
https://doi.org/10.1007/978-981-19-9940-6_17

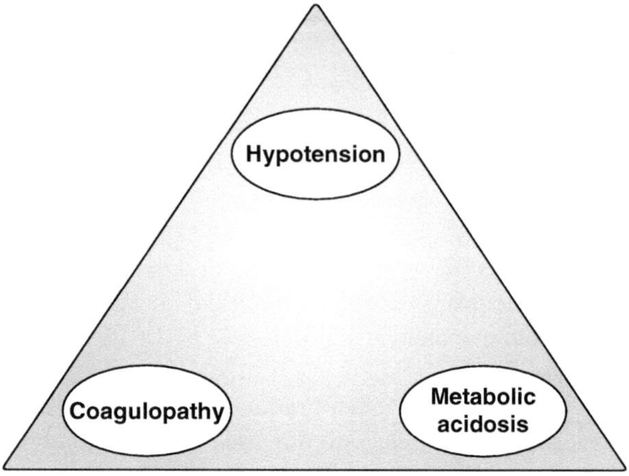

Fig. 17.1 The lethal triad of trauma

17.3 Mechanism of Coagulopathy in Trauma

Major trauma results in the release of factors that trigger the development of a clinically significant coagulopathy. Several cellular and humoral mechanisms are likely to be involved in this process, leading to a consumption coagulopathy, characterized by fibrinolysis, and activation of inflammatory pathways [6]. Tissue injury incites a consumption coagulopathy, with the release of tissue factor, leading to activation of the coagulation pathway [7]. Trauma-associated coagulopathy may be related to high levels of activated protein C, with reduced levels of factors Va and VIIIa [8]. Besides, disruption of the endothelial glycocalyx, fibrinogen depletion, and platelet dysfunction may also contribute significantly to the coagulopathy observed in trauma [8].

17.4 The Concept of Permissive Hypotension in Trauma

More than a century ago, Cannon et al. proposed the concept of a hypotensive resuscitation strategy in battlefield trauma with restriction of crystalloid administration while accepting a lower than normal blood pressure until definitive hemostasis is attained [9]. Later studies from the 1960s suggested that continued attempts at fluid resuscitation in the face of uncontrolled hemorrhage may be detrimental [10]. Over the past two decades or more, questions have been raised against the use of large volumes of crystalloids in the resuscitation of trauma.

Hypotensive resuscitation involves a restrictive approach to the administration of intravenous fluids and blood products, targeting lower than normal blood pressures, aiming to reduce blood loss, and prevent clot disruption and rebleeding. A lower target blood pressure enables less fluid administration, while tissue perfusion and oxygenation are still maintained. The strategy of hypotensive resuscitation involves lower blood pressure targets, restricted use of crystalloids, and the early use of blood products [11].

17.5 What Is the Evidence for Permissive Hypotension in Trauma?

The safety and efficacy of permissive hypotension in severe trauma has been evaluated in controlled clinical trials (Table 17.1).

Bickell et al., in a seminal randomized controlled trial (RCT), compared immediate with delayed resuscitation in 598 patients who had sustained penetrating torso injury with a prehospital systolic BP ≤90 mm Hg [12]. In the immediate resuscitation group, patients received prehospital intravenous fluid resuscitation. Fluid

Table 17.1 Controlled studies that have evaluated the safety and efficacy of permissive hypotension in severe trauma

Study/year	Population	Permissive hypotension	Control	Outcomes
Bickell et al. [12] (1994)	Penetrating torso injury with prehospital systolic BP ≤90 mm Hg	Fluid resuscitation withheld until induction of anesthesia	Prehospital fluid resuscitation, transfusion of red cells at trauma center if systolic BP <100 mm Hg	Survival to hospital discharge significantly higher, hospital stay shorter, with permissive hypotension. Duration of ICU stay, incidence of ARDS, sepsis, AKI, coagulopathy, pneumonia, similar
Dutton et al. [13] (2002)	Trauma with active bleeding and systolic BP of <90 mm Hg	Resuscitation aiming for MAP of 70 mm until hemostasis achieved	Resuscitation aiming for a target systolic BP of 100 mm Hg until hemostasis achieved	Duration of active hemorrhage, mortality, similar
Schreiber et al. [14] (2015)	Blunt or penetrating trauma with out-of-hospital systolic BP ≤90 mm Hg, without severe TBI	Bolus fluid of 250 mL if the systolic BP was <70 mm Hg or radial pulse absent	2 L of IV bolus fluid; additional fluid targeting systolic BP of 110 mm Hg	Lower mortality in the controlled resuscitation group with blunt trauma at 24 h after admission. No difference in AKI, ventilator-free days, ICU-free days
Morrison et al. [15] (2011)	Patients who underwent laparotomy or thoracotomy for blunt or penetrating trauma, with at least one systolic BP reading ≤90 mm Hg	MAP target of 50 mm Hg on arrival to operating room	MAP of 65 mm Hg on arrival to operating room	Higher mortality with continued bleeding due to uncontrolled coagulopathy in the higher MAP group. Trend toward lower mortality in the early postoperative period and at 30 days with lower MAP

ARDS acute respiratory distress syndrome, *AKI* acute kidney injury, *MAP* mean arterial pressure

resuscitation, including transfusion of red cells, was continued at the trauma center if the systolic BP was <100 mm Hg. In the delayed group, fluid resuscitation was withheld until arrival in the operating room and induction of anesthesia. After the initial phase, intravenous crystalloids and red cells were administered to both the groups targeting a systolic BP >100 mm Hg, hematocrit of >25%, and urine output of >50 mL/h. Survival to hospital discharge was significantly higher in the delayed compared to the immediate resuscitation group (70 vs. 62%, $p = 0.04$). A trend toward increased intraoperative blood loss was observed in the immediate resuscitation group. The duration of stay in hospital was also significantly longer in the immediate resuscitation group; however, the duration of ICU stay was similar between groups. The incidence of complications including acute respiratory distress syndrome (ARDS), sepsis, acute renal failure, clotting dysfunction, and pneumonia was not significantly different.

In a later RCT, trauma patients presenting directly from the scene with active bleeding and a systolic BP of <90 mm Hg were included [13]. Patients were fluid resuscitated aiming for a target systolic BP of 100 mm Hg (conventional BP) or 70 mm Hg (low BP) until hemostasis was achieved. A significant difference in the systolic BP was observed between groups (114 vs. 100 mm Hg, $p < 0.001$). However, the duration of active hemorrhage was not different between groups. There were four deaths in each group, with overall survival of 92.7%. The authors hypothesized that similar clinical outcomes in the conventional compared to the low BP group could be due to the heterogeneous nature of injuries sustained and the lack of a precise correlation between systolic BP and tissue oxygen delivery.

Schreiber et al. conducted an RCT to evaluate the feasibility and safety of a strategy of controlled resuscitation compared to standard resuscitation in hypotensive trauma patients [14]. The study included patients who had suffered blunt or penetrating trauma with an out-of-hospital systolic BP of 90 mm Hg or less, without evidence of severe traumatic brain injury. In the standard resuscitation group, a bolus of 2 L of fluid was administered, followed by additional fluid targeting a systolic BP of 110 mm Hg. In the controlled resuscitation group, a fluid bolus of 250 mL was administered if the systolic BP was less than 70 mm Hg or in the absence of a radial pulse. The crystalloid protocol was maintained from the time of enrolment until hemorrhage control or 2 h after arrival to the hospital. The standard resuscitation group received significantly higher volumes of crystalloid during the study period compared to the controlled resuscitation group [2.0 L (±1.4) vs. 1.0 L (±1.5)]. There were fewer deaths in the controlled resuscitation group at 24 h after admission [(5% vs. 25%, adjusted odds ratio: 0.39; 95% CI, 0.12–1.26)]. The difference in the 24-h mortality was evident only among patients who experienced blunt trauma; no difference in mortality was observed among patients who experienced penetrating trauma. There was no difference in renal failure, ventilator-free days, and ICU-free days between the two groups.

Morrison et al. studied patients who underwent laparotomy or thoracotomy for blunt or penetrating trauma, with at least one systolic BP reading ≤90 mm Hg while in hospital [15]. Patients were randomized on arrival to the operating room for a target mean arterial pressure (MAP) of 50 mm Hg (LMAP) or control group with a target MAP of 65 mm Hg (HMAP). The actual MAP measured during the intraoperative period did not differ significantly between groups. Intraoperative transfusion of blood products and intravenous fluids was significantly higher in the HMAP compared to the LMAP group (2898 mL vs. 1594 mL, $p = 0.03$). Death due to continued bleeding due to uncontrolled coagulopathy was more common in the HMAP group. A trend toward lower mortality in the early postoperative period and at 30 days was observed in the LMAP group. Following this interim report of the first 90 patients, the authors published a final analysis that included 168 patients. However, in this final report, no difference in the 24-h or 30-day mortality was observed. The incidence of acute myocardial infarction, stroke, renal failure, and infective complications were also similar between groups [16].

Tran et al. performed a pooled analysis of five RCTs that compared permissive hypotension with conventional resuscitation strategies in trauma-related hemorrhagic shock [17]. A strategy of permissive hypotension resulted in an improved 30-day survival among patients who underwent a strategy of permissive hypotension. Besides, it reduced the administration of crystalloids and red cells with less overall blood loss. There was no significant difference in the incidence of complications including sepsis, coagulopathy, and renal failure.

In another meta-analysis, Owattanapanich et al. included 30 RCTs and cohort studies that reported mortality with a hypotensive resuscitation strategy of limited fluid resuscitation [18]. The hypotensive resuscitation strategy was associated with significantly lower mortality compared with a conventional strategy. Besides, the total volume of fluid administered and transfusion of red cells were also lower with a hypotensive resuscitation strategy. The hypotensive strategy was also associated with a lower incidence of organ dysfunction and ARDS.

17.6 Blood Pressure Target in Traumatic Brain Injury

In traumatic brain injury (TBI), low blood pressures lead to reduced cerebral perfusion pressures [19] and may lead to worsening of ischemic injury. Accordingly, the brain trauma foundation recommends against a target systolic BP <90 mm Hg in TBI. They suggest maintenance of systolic BP ≥100 mm Hg for patients 50–69 years old and ≥110 mm Hg for patients 15–49 and more than 70 years old [20]. A higher target MAP may be appropriate in patients with intracranial hemorrhage with raised intracranial pressure. Intravenous fluids to raise the MAP >80 mm Hg for a cerebral perfusion pressure of >60 mm Hg has been recommended to avoid ischemia [21].

17.7 Transfusion of Blood Products in Trauma

The concept of damage control resuscitation involves rapid hemorrhage control with early administration of blood products in a 1:1:1 ratio of red cells, plasma, and platelets, to approximate the composition of whole blood. The damage control resuscitation strategy has been associated with improved outcomes compared to conventional transfusion strategies in observational studies [22, 23]. The PROPPR RCT compared a 1:1:1 ratio of plasma to platelets to red cells compared to a 1:1:2 ratio in patients with severe trauma predicted to require massive transfusion [24]. There was no significant difference in mortality at 24 h and 30 days between the two transfusion strategies. However, a post hoc analysis revealed that death due to exsanguinating hemorrhage was less common in the 1:1:1 ratio group. Besides, hemostasis was achieved more often with a 1:1:1 ratio of transfusion of blood products.

Key Points

- Large volume fluid resuscitation aimed to target normal blood pressure in the presence of uncontrolled hemorrhage leads to poor clinical outcomes.
- Excessive fluid administration in the bleeding trauma patient may precipitate the lethal triad of trauma, characterized by hypothermia, coagulopathy, and metabolic acidosis.
- Following the seminal paper by Bickell et al., several observational studies and RCTs suggest that a strategy of permissive hypotension with limited fluid and blood product administration is appropriate until control of hemorrhage can be attained.
- No robust evidence exists regarding blood pressure targets to aim for as part of a strategy of permissive hypotension and needs individualization based on the clinical circumstances.
- In TBI, a conventional approach to blood pressure management is recommended considering the importance of maintaining cerebral perfusion pressures.
- Administration of blood products in a 1:1:1 ratio of red cells, plasma, and platelets may improve outcomes in trauma patients who require massive blood transfusion.

References

1. MacLeod JBA, Cohn SM, Johnson EW, McKenney MG. Trauma deaths in the first hour: are they all unsalvageable injuries? Am J Surg. 2007;193(2):195–9.
2. Siegel JH, Fabian M, Smith JA, Kingston EP, Steele KA, Wells MR, et al. Oxygen debt criteria quantify the effectiveness of early partial resuscitation after hypovolemic hemorrhagic shock. J Trauma. 2003;54(5):862–80; discussion 880
3. Shires T, Coln D, Carrico J, Lightfoot S. Fluid therapy in hemorrhagic shock. Arch Surg. 1964;88:688–93.
4. Galvagno SM, Nahmias JT, Young DA. Advanced trauma life support® update 2019. Anesthesiol Clin. 2019;37(1):13–32.
5. Schreiber MA. Coagulopathy in the trauma patient. Curr Opin Crit Care. 2005;11(6):590–7.
6. Godier A, Susen S. Trauma-induced coagulopathy. Ann Fr Anesth Reanim. 2013;32(7–8):527–30.

7. Gando S, Nanzaki S, Sasaki S, Kemmotsu O. Significant correlations between tissue factor and thrombin markers in trauma and septic patients with disseminated intravascular coagulation. Thromb Haemost. 1998;79(6):1111–5.
8. Simmons JW, Powell MF. Acute traumatic coagulopathy: pathophysiology and resuscitation. Br J Anaesth. 2016;117:iii31–43.
9. Cannon WB, Cowell E. The preventive treatment of wound shock. JAMA. 1918;70:618–21.
10. Milles G, Koucky CJ, Zacheis HG. Experimental uncontrolled arterial hemorrhage. Surgery. 1966;60(2):434–42.
11. Kudo D, Yoshida Y, Kushimoto S. Permissive hypotension/hypotensive resuscitation and restricted/controlled resuscitation in patients with severe trauma. J Intensive Care. 2017;20(5):11.
12. Bickell WH, Wall MJ, Pepe PE, Martin RR, Ginger VF, Allen MK, et al. Immediate versus delayed fluid resuscitation for hypotensive patients with penetrating torso injuries. N Engl J Med. 1994;331(17):1105–9.
13. Dutton RP, Mackenzie CF, Scalea TM. Hypotensive resuscitation during active hemorrhage: impact on in-hospital mortality. J Trauma. 2002;52(6):1141–6.
14. Schreiber MA, Meier EN, Tisherman SA, Kerby JD, Newgard CD, Brasel K, et al. A controlled resuscitation strategy is feasible and safe in hypotensive trauma patients: results of a prospective randomized pilot trial. J Trauma Acute Care Surg. 2015;78(4):687–95; discussion 695-697
15. Morrison CA, Carrick MM, Norman MA, Scott BG, Welsh FJ, Tsai P, et al. Hypotensive resuscitation strategy reduces transfusion requirements and severe postoperative coagulopathy in trauma patients with hemorrhagic shock: preliminary results of a randomized controlled trial. J Trauma. 2011;70(3):652–63.
16. Carrick MM, Morrison CA, Tapia NM, Leonard J, Suliburk JW, Norman MA, et al. Intraoperative hypotensive resuscitation for patients undergoing laparotomy or thoracotomy for trauma: early termination of a randomized prospective clinical trial. J Trauma Acute Care Surg. 2016;80(6):886–96.
17. Tran A, Yates J, Lau A, Lampron J, Matar M. Permissive hypotension versus conventional resuscitation strategies in adult trauma patients with hemorrhagic shock: a systematic review and meta-analysis of randomized controlled trials. J Trauma Acute Care Surg. 2018;84(5):802–8.
18. Owattanapanich N, Chittawatanarat K, Benyakorn T, Sirikun J. Risks and benefits of hypotensive resuscitation in patients with traumatic hemorrhagic shock: a meta-analysis. Scand J Trauma Resusc Emerg Med. 2018;26(1):107.
19. Tremblay LN, Rizoli SB, Brenneman FD. Advances in fluid resuscitation of hemorrhagic shock. Can J Surg. 2001;44(3):172–9.
20. Carney N, Totten AM, O'Reilly C, Ullman JS, Hawryluk GWJ, Bell MJ, et al. Guidelines for the management of severe traumatic brain injury, fourth edition. Neurosurgery. 2017;80(1):6–15.
21. Wise R, Faurie M, Malbrain MLNG, Hodgson E. Strategies for intravenous fluid resuscitation in trauma patients. World J Surg. 2017;41(5):1170–83.
22. Borgman MA, Spinella PC, Perkins JG, Grathwohl KW, Repine T, Beekley AC, et al. The ratio of blood products transfused affects mortality in patients receiving massive transfusions at a combat support hospital. J Trauma. 2007;63(4):805–13.
23. Cotton BA, Reddy N, Hatch QM, LeFebvre E, Wade CE, Kozar RA, et al. Damage control resuscitation is associated with a reduction in resuscitation volumes and improvement in survival in 390 damage control laparotomy patients. Ann Surg. 2011;254(4):598–605.
24. Holcomb JB, Tilley BC, Baraniuk S, Fox EE, Wade CE, Podbielski JM, et al. Transfusion of plasma, platelets, and red blood cells in a 1:1:1 vs a 1:1:2 ratio and mortality in patients with severe trauma: the PROPPR randomized clinical trial. JAMA. 2015;313(5):471–82.

Assessment of Volume Responsiveness in the Critically Ill

18

Intravenous fluid administration is one of the most important interventions in the resuscitation of critically ill patients. Titration of fluid resuscitation to optimally fill the intravascular compartment without causing tissue edema from excessive administration holds the key to important clinical outcomes. Injudicious fluid administration without appropriate evaluation of fluid responsiveness has been clearly shown to worsen clinical outcomes, including a longer duration of mechanical ventilation, ICU stay, and mortality [1, 2]. The practice of repeated fluid challenges using blood pressure or urine output as the sole target is fraught with the risk of creating tissue edema with adverse consequences. It is important to note that an increase in the cardiac output occurs only in approximately 50% of critically ill patients after a fluid bolus [3].

18.1 Basic Physiology: The Frank-Starling Curve

The relationship between cardiac preload and stroke volume is depicted by the Frank-Starling curve. If the patient lies along the ascending limb of the Frank-Starling curve, fluid administration would result in myocardial distension, an increase in the preload, and a consequent rise in the stroke volume. If the patient lies in the plateau phase of the curve, fluid administration does not lead to an increase in the stroke volume (Fig. 18.1). Thus, it is important to distinguish between fluid "responders" and "nonresponders" based on their position along the Frank-Starling curve. Phasic changes in preload that occur with respiratory excursions, resulting from a change in intrathoracic pressures, may be utilized to evaluate fluid responsiveness. If the myocardial function is impaired, the curve becomes flatter, with a blunted response to fluid administration.

J. Chacko et al., *Controversies in Critical Care*,
https://doi.org/10.1007/978-981-19-9940-6_18

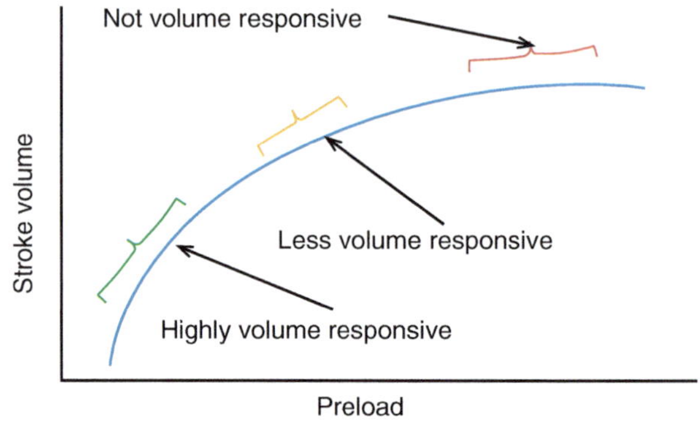

Fig. 18.1 The Frank-Starling curve and fluid responsiveness. Fluid administration would increase the stroke volume only if the patient lies on the ascending limb of the curve

18.2 Techniques to Assess Fluid Responsiveness

18.2.1 Passive Leg Raising

This technique utilizes the increase in preload that occurs with raising both lower limbs passively. Approximately 300 ml of fluid is mobilized from the lower part of the body to augment the cardiac preload during this maneuver. An increase in the stroke volume associated with passive leg raising indicates fluid responsiveness.

The passive leg raising maneuver is commenced with the patient in the propped-up position, with the trunk at an angle of 45°. The baseline cardiac output is measured using the preferred technique. This is followed by returning the trunk to the flat position and raising the legs by adjusting the bed position appropriately. Cardiac output measurement is repeated in this position. The final step is to reposition the patient in the original semi-recumbent position with the reassessment of cardiac output to confirm return to baseline level. A rise in cardiac output of more than 10 ± 2% to passive leg raising was noted to be the best cutoff in a meta-analysis [4]. The passive leg raising test is valid with low tidal volume ventilation and spontaneous or controlled ventilation, in the presence of atrial fibrillation, and in patients with poor lung compliance [4]. It may not be reliable in patients with intra-abdominal hypertension [5].

18.2.2 Pulse Pressure and Stroke Volume Variation

The pulse pressure variation helps identify the location of the patient along the Frank-Starling curve. If a patient lies on the ascending portion of the curve, preload changes associated with phasic changes of the respiratory cycle results in a wide pulse pressure variation (Fig. 18.2). Conversely, on the plateau phase of the curve, the pulse pressure variation becomes narrower.

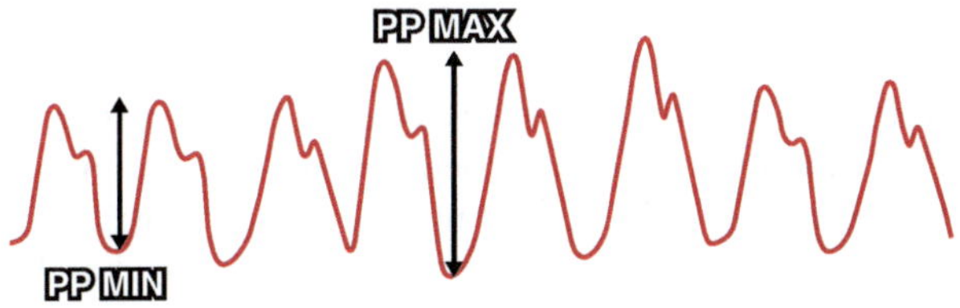

Fig. 18.2 If the patient is fluid-responsive, preload changes associated with the respiratory cycle results in a wide pulse pressure variation; the pulse pressure variation becomes narrower as the patient becomes less fluid-responsive. PPV = ([PPmax − PPmin]/PPmean × 100)

In practice, the highest (PP max) and the lowest (PP min) values of pulse pressure during a respiratory cycle are noted. The mean of these two values is also obtained (PP mean). The pulse pressure variation (PPV) is obtained by the formula (Fig. 18.2):

$$\text{PPV} = \left(\left[\text{PPmax} - \text{PPmin}\right] / \text{PPmean} \times 100\right).$$

A pulse pressure variation of 13% or more has been shown to indicate fluid responsiveness [6]. Myatra et al. performed a "tidal volume challenge" among 20 patients. From a baseline of 6 ml/kg, the tidal volume was increased to 8 ml/kg for a 1-min duration in patients with circulatory failure. An absolute change in pulse pressure variation of 3.5% before and after an increase of tidal volume predicted fluid responsiveness [7].

Stroke volume variation is also based on the reduction in preload and stroke volume that occurs during the inspiratory phase of positive pressure ventilation. If the stroke volume varies between the inspiratory and expiratory phases, it suggests that the patient lies along the preload-dependent part of the Frank-Starling curve. Conventionally, a stroke volume variation of 13% has been used as the threshold level to indicate fluid responsiveness [8]. Using the tidal volume challenge technique described above, an absolute change in the stroke volume variation by more than 2.5% was shown to indicate fluid responsiveness [7].

Pulse pressure variation and stroke volume variation are considered applicable in mechanically ventilated patients with a tidal volume ≥8 ml/kg and no spontaneous respiratory efforts. However, a recent meta-analysis suggests that these parameters may be reliable even at tidal volumes ≤8 ml/kg [9]. Both measurements may be unreliable in patients with lung compliance of less than 30 ml/cm H_2O and in the presence of intra-abdominal hypertension [10].

18.2.3 End-Expiratory Occlusion Test

The end-expiratory occlusion test is performed by interruption of ventilation at the end of expiration for a duration of 15 s, followed by evaluation of the change in cardiac output or surrogate parameters before and after occlusion. This test is based on the principle that in volume-responsive subjects, the cardiac output increases significantly during the expiratory phase of mechanical ventilation.

The test is performed by a baseline measurement of cardiac output or a surrogate parameter. A 15-s expiratory hold is carried out, with repeat measurement during the last 5 s of the expiratory hold. A final measurement is carried out 30 s after the expiratory hold maneuver to assess the return of values to the baseline. An increase in cardiac output of 5% or more following end-expiratory occlusion has been shown to indicate fluid responsiveness [7, 11]. However, another study revealed that the end-expiratory occlusion test was unreliable in predicting volume responsiveness during laparotomy for colorectal, pancreatic, or major gynecological surgery [12].

18.2.4 Respiratory Variation of the Inferior Vena Caval Diameter

The diameter of the inferior vena cava (IVC) is usually evaluated by transthoracic echocardiography. The IVC is viewed from the subxiphoid position in the long axis. The cursor is positioned close to the entry to the right atrium or 1–2 cm downstream to the junction between the hepatic vein and the IVC. The degree of change in the IVC diameter is calculated on the M-mode view. A variation in IVC diameter of 12–18% with fully controlled ventilation and more than 50% in spontaneously breathing patients is suggestive of fluid responsiveness [13].

Although easy to perform by the bedside, the phasic variation in the inferior vena caval diameter (Δ IVC) with respiration has been inconsistent in predicting fluid responsiveness. Ventilation with low tidal volumes, poor lung compliance, and the presence of intra-abdominal hypertension may contribute to relative inaccuracy. In particular, Δ IVC may be a poor indicator of fluid responsiveness in patients with isolated left ventricular dysfunction.

18.2.5 Variation in the End-Tidal Carbon Dioxide Level

An increase in the cardiac output leads to a rise in the pulmonary blood flow, improved perfusion of the alveoli, and a rise in the end-tidal carbon dioxide ($ETCO_2$), provided alveolar ventilation and carbon dioxide production are constant. Thus, in patients who are maintained at a constant level of mechanical ventilation, $ETCO_2$ rise may be used as a simple, noninvasive measure of fluid responsiveness. Fluid responsiveness assessed by an increase in $ETCO_2$ following passive leg raising has been evaluated. An increase by 2 mm Hg [14] or 5% from the baseline level [15] has been proposed to indicate fluid responsiveness. $ETCO_2$ may be superior to other noninvasive surrogates of cardiac output assessment, including pulse pressure variation [16].

18.2.6 The Mini-Fluid Challenge

The conventional fluid challenge of 250–500 ml over approximately 30 min may result in a large volume overload, especially with repeated, injudicious administration. To circumvent this complication, a much smaller fluid volume of 100 ml over a 1 min-period has been proposed [17]. A 6% increase in the cardiac output induced by a mini-fluid challenge has been shown to be superior to pulse pressure variation in the prediction of fluid responsiveness among patients undergoing neurosurgical procedures [18]. A meta-analysis of seven studies revealed a sensitivity of 0.82 (95% CI 0.76–0.88) and a specificity of 0.83 (95% CI 0.77–0.89) for the mini-fluid challenge in identifying fluid responsiveness [19]. It is important to note that continuous, real-time measurements are required during the mini-fluid challenge as the increase in cardiac output is relatively low. Table 18.1 summarizes interventions that enable assessment of fluid responsiveness.

Table 18.1 Methods to assess volume responsiveness

Technique	Intervention	Fluid responsiveness	Comments
Passive leg raising	Start in the propped-up position. Measure baseline cardiac output. Trunk returned to flat position; raise the legs. Repeat cardiac output measurement. Reposition patient in the semi-recumbent position to confirm return of cardiac output to baseline	Rise in cardiac output by more than 10 ± 2% of baseline	Valid with low Vt ventilation, spontaneous and controlled ventilation, in the presence of AF, and in patients with poor lung compliance
PPV	Highest (PPmax) and lowest (PPmin) values of PP noted during a respiratory cycle. The mean of the two values in PPmean. PPV = PPmax − PPmin/PPmean	PPV > 13%	Controlled ventilation with Vt ≥ 8 ml/kg. Unreliable with IAH, and poor lung compliance
SVV	Measure the highest and lowest SV during a respiratory cycle	SVV > 13%	Controlled ventilation with Vt ≥ 8 ml/kg. Unreliable with IAH, and poor lung compliance
End-expiratory occlusion test	Interrupt ventilation for 15 s at end-expiration. Measure cardiac output before and after interruption	Increase in cardiac output ≥5%	Controlled ventilation with Vt ≥ 8 ml/kg

(continued)

Table 18.1 (continued)

Technique	Intervention	Fluid responsiveness	Comments
Respiratory variation of the IVC diameter	IVC diameter measured by TTE in the subxiphoid view. Cursor close to entry of IVC into the RA or 2 cm downstream from the junction of the hepatic vein and the IVC	Variation in IVC diameter of 12–18% with controlled ventilation; 50% with spontaneous breathing	Inconsistent prediction of fluid responsiveness. Low Vt, poor lung compliance and IAH may lead to inaccuracy
$ETCO_2$ variation	Measure $ETCO_2$ before and after passive leg raise	Increase in $ETCO_2$ by 2 mm Hg or by more than 5% from baseline	Initial results suggest superior accuracy compared to PPV
Mini fluid challenge	Fluid bolus of 100 ml over 1 min	Increase in cardiac output by 6%	Change in cardiac output likely to be low; hence, precise, continuous, real-time monitoring of cardiac output required

Abbreviations: *Vt* tidal volume, *AF* atrial fibrillation, *PPV* pulse pressure variation, *PPmax* maximum pulse pressure, *PPmin* minimum pulse pressure, *SVV* stroke volume variation, *IAH* intra-abdominal hypertension, *IVC* inferior vena cava, $ETCO_2$ end-tidal carbon dioxide

Key Points

- Fluid resuscitation is a crucial intervention in the early phase of circulatory shock. Judicious fluid administration based on the assessment of fluid responsiveness is critical, especially in the later phase of resuscitation.
- Injudicious fluid administration based solely on blood pressure or urine output may result in inadvertent hypervolemia and impact clinical outcomes adversely.
- The passive leg raise maneuver is an effective method to assess fluid responsiveness; it is valid in spontaneous or controlled ventilation, with low tidal volumes, in the presence of atrial fibrillation, and in patients with poor lung compliance.
- Pulse pressure and stroke volume variation may be useful primarily in patients who receive mechanical ventilatory support with a tidal volume of ≥8 ml/kg, with no spontaneous respiratory effort.
- $ETCO_2$ rise following a passive leg raise maneuver is yet another noninvasive method that indicates fluid responsiveness.
- If a volume challenge is necessary, it is probably safer and equally effective to use a "mini" volume of 100 ml over 1 min instead of a larger volume.
- It is of paramount importance not to be swayed by a single parameter while assessing fluid responsiveness; decisions must be based on the holistic clinical picture.

References

1. National Heart, Lung, and Blood Institute Acute Respiratory Distress Syndrome (ARDS) Clinical Trials Network, Wiedemann HP, Wheeler AP, Bernard GR, Thompson BT, Hayden D, et al. Comparison of two fluid-management strategies in acute lung injury. N Engl J Med. 2006;354(24):2564–75.
2. van Mourik N, Metske HA, Hofstra JJ, Binnekade JM, Geerts BF, Schultz MJ, et al. Cumulative fluid balance predicts mortality and increases time on mechanical ventilation in ARDS patients: An observational cohort study. PLoS One. 2019;14(10):e0224563.
3. Michard F, Teboul JL. Predicting fluid responsiveness in ICU patients: a critical analysis of the evidence. Chest. 2002;121(6):2000–8.
4. Monnet X, Marik P, Teboul JL. Passive leg raising for predicting fluid responsiveness: a systematic review and meta-analysis. Intensive Care Med. 2016;42(12):1935–47.
5. Beurton A, Teboul JL, Girotto V, Galarza L, Anguel N, Richard C, et al. Intra-abdominal hypertension is responsible for false negatives to the passive leg raising test. Crit Care Med. 2019;47(8):e639–47.
6. Michard F, Boussat S, Chemla D, Anguel N, Mercat A, Lecarpentier Y, et al. Relation between respiratory changes in arterial pulse pressure and fluid responsiveness in septic patients with acute circulatory failure. Am J Respir Crit Care Med. 2000;162(1):134–8.
7. Myatra SN, Prabu NR, Divatia JV, Monnet X, Kulkarni AP, Teboul JL. The Changes in Pulse Pressure Variation or Stroke Volume Variation After a "Tidal Volume Challenge" Reliably Predict Fluid Responsiveness During Low Tidal Volume Ventilation. Crit Care Med. 2017;45(3):415–21.
8. Lee YH, Jang HW, Park CH, An SM, Lee EK, Choi BM, et al. Changes in plasma volume before and after major abdominal surgery following stroke volume variation-guided fluid therapy: a randomized controlled trial. Minerva Anestesiol. 2020;86(5):507–17.
9. Alvarado Sánchez JI, Caicedo Ruiz JD, Diaztagle Fernández JJ, Amaya Zuñiga WF, Ospina-Tascón GA, Cruz Martínez LE. Predictors of fluid responsiveness in critically ill patients mechanically ventilated at low tidal volumes: systematic review and meta-analysis. Ann Intensive Care. 2021;11(1):28.
10. Shi R, Monnet X, Teboul JL. Parameters of fluid responsiveness. Curr Opin Crit Care. 2020;26(3):319–26.
11. Messina A, Montagnini C, Cammarota G, De Rosa S, Giuliani F, Muratore L, et al. Tidal volume challenge to predict fluid responsiveness in the operating room: An observational study. Eur J Anaesthesiol. 2019;36(8):583–91.
12. Weil G, Motamed C, Monnet X, Eghiaian A, Le Maho AL. End-expiratory occlusion test to predict fluid responsiveness is not suitable for Laparotomic surgery. Anesth Analg. 2020;130(1):151–8.
13. Feissel M, Michard F, Faller JP, Teboul JL. The respiratory variation in inferior vena cava diameter as a guide to fluid therapy. Intensive Care Med. 2004;30(9):1834–7.
14. Toupin F, Clairoux A, Deschamps A, Lebon JS, Lamarche Y, Lambert J, et al. Assessment of fluid responsiveness with end-tidal carbon dioxide using a simplified passive leg raising maneuver: a prospective observational study. Can J Anesth. 2016;63(9):1033–41.
15. Monnet X, Bataille A, Magalhaes E, Barrois J, Le Corre M, Gosset C, et al. End-tidal carbon dioxide is better than arterial pressure for predicting volume responsiveness by the passive leg raising test. Intensive Care Med. 2013;39(1):93–100.
16. Lakhal K, Nay MA, Kamel T, Lortat-Jacob B, Ehrmann S, Rozec B, et al. Change in end-tidal carbon dioxide outperforms other surrogates for change in cardiac output during fluid challenge. Br J Anaesth. 2017;118(3):355–62.
17. Muller L, Toumi M, Bousquet PJ, Riu-Poulenc B, Louart G, Candela D, et al. An increase in aortic blood flow after an infusion of 100 ml colloid over 1 minute can predict fluid responsiveness: the mini-fluid challenge study. Anesthesiology. 2011;115(3):541–7.

18. Biais M, de Courson H, Lanchon R, Pereira B, Bardonneau G, Griton M, et al. Mini-fluid challenge of 100 ml of crystalloid predicts fluid responsiveness in the operating room. Anesthesiology. 2017;127(3):450–6.
19. Messina A, Dell'Anna A, Baggiani M, Torrini F, Maresca GM, Bennett V, et al. Functional hemodynamic tests: a systematic review and a metanalysis on the reliability of the end-expiratory occlusion test and of the mini-fluid challenge in predicting fluid responsiveness. Crit Care. 2019;23(1):264.

Getting Rid of Excess Fluid: The Strategy of De-resuscitation

19

19.1 Introduction

The use of intravenous fluid therapy is ubiquitous among critically ill patients to optimize tissue perfusion and oxygen delivery. Apart from intravenous fluids administered during initial resuscitation, fluid accumulation occurs from nutrition, maintenance fluids, and diluents used for intravenous drug therapy. An aggressive resuscitation strategy may be appropriate during the "ebb" phase of septic shock, characterized by widespread vasodilatation, intravascular hypovolemia, and capillary leak, leading to extravasation of fluid into the interstitial compartment. Typically, the "ebb" phase is followed by the "flow" phase, during which the body tries to eliminate excess fluid. However, normal physiological mechanisms may be overwhelmed, especially with the onset of acute kidney injury. In this situation, should we consider a "de-resuscitation" strategy aimed at the active removal of excess fluid?

19.2 Adverse Consequences of Fluid Overload

Excessive fluid accumulation may be the harbinger of multiorgan dysfunction [1]. Interstitial and intra-alveolar edema in the lung may lead to delayed weaning and prolongation of the duration of ventilator support. A rise in the venous pressure may impair renal blood flow, trigger interstitial edema, and result in compromised renal function. Myocardial edema may occur, leading to systolic and diastolic dysfunction. As the intra-abdominal pressure rises due to excessive gastrointestinal fluid accumulation, abdominal perfusion may be compromised. This may trigger increased intestinal permeability and bacterial translocation from the gut. The potential harm arising from injudicious fluid administration has been equated to adverse effects arising from inappropriate drug dosing [1] (Fig. 19.1).

J. Chacko et al., *Controversies in Critical Care*,
https://doi.org/10.1007/978-981-19-9940-6_19

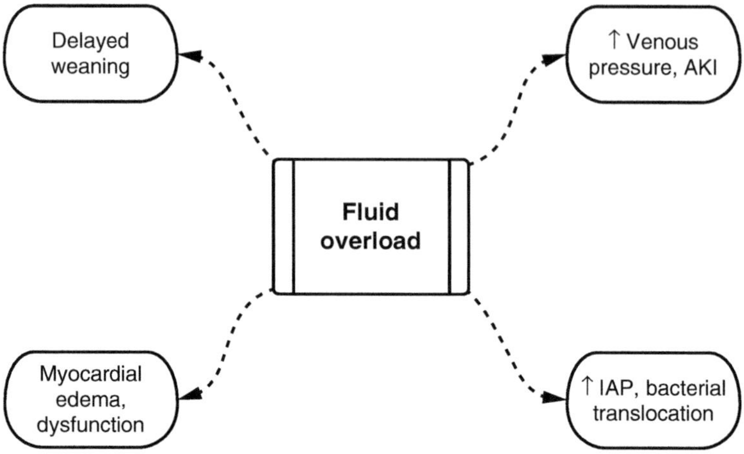

Fig. 19.1 Adverse effects of fluid overload

19.3 What Is De-resuscitation?

Among patients who respond to initial therapeutic interventions, shock resolution and circulatory stabilization typically occur. By this time, a large positive fluid balance develops in critically ill patients, particularly among those with sepsis. In a secondary analysis of the Vasopressin in Septic Shock Trial (VASST), the mean positive fluid balance was 4.2 L at 12 h and 11.0 L on the fourth day of enrollment [2]. It is important to take stock of the net fluid balance after the initial phase of resuscitation. The extent of fluid accumulation may be calculated using the formula [3]:

$$\left[\text{Cumulative fluid balance}\left(\text{liters}\right) / \text{baseline body weight}\left(\text{kg}\right)\right] \times 100.$$

A fluid accumulation of more than 10% has been shown to be associated with poor clinical outcomes [3]. During the "flow" phase, the body attempts to dispose of the accumulated fluid. Therapeutic fluid removal, using diuretics and ultrafiltration with renal replacement therapy, may be appropriate measures during this stage. Aggressive interventions to remove fluid may be combined with a fluid-restrictive strategy.

19.4 What Is the Evidence to Support a De-resuscitative Strategy?

Fluids administered during the early resuscitation phase may constitute only a small fraction of the fluid accumulated over time. A retrospective analysis was performed to evaluate the volume of fluids administered to 14,654 critically ill patients. In this study, maintenance and replacement fluids constituted 24.7% of the daily fluid administered, compared to only 6.5% of resuscitation fluids. Significant volumes of fluid (32.6% of the daily volume administered) were administered as diluents for intravenous or other medication [4].

Silversides et al. conducted a retrospective observational study across 10 ICUs in the UK and Canada to identify outcomes with de-resuscitative strategies and risk factors for positive fluid balance among critically ill patients. Four-hundred adult patients who underwent mechanical ventilation for a minimum period of 24 h were included. Over the first 1–3 days, a positive fluid balance occurred in 87.3% of patients. Medications represented the largest volume of fluid administered (34.5%). The volume of bolus (26.5%) and maintenance fluids (24.4%) were lower compared to fluids administered as medication. A negative balance was observed on day 3 in 123 patients; a spontaneous negative balance, without the use of diuretics or ultrafiltration, occurred in 70 (56.9%) patients and was associated with lower 30-day mortality. De-resuscitative measures were employed in 52.3% of all patients, most frequently on the second or third day. On multivariate logistic regression, the fluid balance on day 3 was an independent predictor of 30-day mortality. A negative fluid balance achieved using active de-resuscitative measures, including frusemide administration and fluid removal using continuous renal replacement therapy, was associated with lower mortality [5].

A meta-analysis of 11 randomized controlled studies, including 2051 adults and children, was performed by Silversides et al. The study included patients with acute respiratory distress syndrome, sepsis, or the systemic inflammatory response syndrome (SIRS). Compared to a liberal approach, the authors found no significant difference in mortality reported at the longest time point between a conservative or de-resuscitative fluid management strategy. However, there was an increase in ventilator-free days and reduced length of stay in the ICU with a conservative or de-resuscitative approach [6].

The FFAKI trial was a pilot randomized controlled trial that tested the feasibility of forced fluid removal compared to standard care among critically ill patients who were at moderate to high risk of acute kidney injury with more than 10% fluid accumulation. Active de-resuscitation was carried out with a bolus dose of furosemide, 40 mg, followed by a continuous infusion of up to 40 mg/h or fluid removal using renal replacement therapy. The investigators aimed for a net negative fluid balance of >1 mL/kg/h (ideal body weight) with a target cumulative fluid balance of less than 1000 mL from the time of ICU admission. The recruitment rate was low, with only 23 included among 1144 patients who were screened. Despite the small sample size, a conspicuous reduction in the cumulative fluid balance was observed with active de-resuscitative measures at 5 days after randomization. The mean difference in the cumulative balance between groups was 5814 mL (95% CI 2063 to 9565, $P = 0.003$). Although not powered to evaluate clinical outcomes, no adverse effects were noted with forced fluid removal in this pilot study [7].

A combination of high PEEP, small volume resuscitation with 20% albumin, and diuretic treatment with furosemide (described as "PAL-treatment") was evaluated among patients with acute lung injury by Cordemans et al., in a retrospective case control study. The PEEP level (cm of H_2O) was set at the level of the intra-abdominal pressure (mm of Hg). This strategy resulted in a lower extravascular lung water index, intra-abdominal pressure, and cumulative fluid balance compared to control patients. The use of the PAL strategy resulted in a shorter duration of mechanical ventilation and ICU stay. The 28-day mortality was also lower with this approach [8]. Table 19.1 summarizes important studies on a de-resuscitation strategy.

Table 19.1 Main studies on a de-resuscitation strategy

Study/year	Design/ population	De-resuscitation group	Control group	Findings
Silversides et al. (2018) [5]	Retrospective observational; mechanically ventilated for ≥24 h	De-resuscitation and negative fluid balance on day 3 of ICU	No de-resuscitation	Positive cumulative fluid balance in 87.3%; most excess fluid from medication and maintenance fluids. Fluid balance on day 3 was an independent risk factor for 30-day mortality. De-resuscitation and negative fluid balance associated with lower mortality
Berthelsen et al. [7] (FAAKI, 2018)	RCT; ICU patients at moderate to high risk of acute kidney injury with 10% fluid accumulation	Fluid removal with furosemide or CRRT aiming for a net negative balance >1 mL/kg/h until cumulative balance from ICU admission less than 1000 mL	Standard care	Significant reduction in cumulative fluid balance 5 days post-randomization with active fluid removal. No harm from a de-resuscitation strategy
Cordemans et al. (2012) [8]	Retrospective matched case control study; mechanically ventilated patients with ALI	High PEEP, small volume resuscitation with 20% albumin, furosemide (PAL strategy)	Historical matched cohort	PAL strategy resulted significantly lower EVLWI, IAP, and cumulative fluid balance. Shorter duration of ventilation, ICU stay, and 28-day mortality with PAL
Silversides et al. (2017) [6]	Meta-analysis of RCTs of patients with ARDS, sepsis, or SIRS	De-resuscitative or conservative fluid strategy	Fluid liberal strategy	More ventilator-free days, reduced ICU LOS with de-resuscitative or conservative strategy. No mortality difference at the longest point of follow-up

Abbreviations: *RCT* randomized controlled trial, *CRRT* continuous renal replacement therapy, *PEEP* positive end-expiratory pressure, *EWLWI* extravascular lung water index, *IAP* intra-abdominal pressure, *ARDS* acute respiratory distress syndrome, *SIRS* systemic inflammatory response syndrome

19.5 Possible Harm from a De-resuscitative Strategy?

The question of choosing the optimal time to commence de-resuscitation can be challenging. Fluid overload may be difficult to recognize in the clinical setting. The central venous pressure is a relatively ineffectual parameter; bedside echocardiography to assess fluid responsiveness vs. overload may not always be practicable due to suboptimal windows among ventilated patients. The clinician may often face the conundrum of when to resort to de-resuscitative measures after the initial stabilization of the hemodynamic status. In a secondary analysis of the Randomized Evaluation of Normal vs. Augmented Level of Renal Replacement Therapy (RENAL) trial, net ultrafiltration of more than 1.75 mL/kg/h was associated with lower 90-day survival compared to ultrafiltration rates of less than 1.01 mL/kg/h [9]. Clearly, more robust evidence from controlled trials is required before the routine adoption of aggressive de-resuscitative measures.

Key Points

- A net positive fluid balance after the initial phase of resuscitation (the "ebb" phase) is strongly associated with mortality.
- Positive fluid balance is an inherently modifiable risk factor that leads to adverse outcomes in critically ill patients.
- After the resuscitation phase, it is appropriate to adopt a conservative fluid strategy and consider active measures of de-resuscitation, including the use of diuretics and fluid removal using renal replacement therapy.
- It may be prudent to aim for a zero or negative balance by day 3 among patients in whom hemodynamic stabilization has been achieved.
- The routine administration of maintenance intravenous fluids to critically ill patients must be strongly discouraged. Besides, the volume of diluents used for intravenous drug administration should also be restricted to the minimum volume possible.

References

1. Malbrain MLNG, Marik PE, Witters I, Cordemans C, Kirkpatrick AW, Roberts DJ, et al. Fluid overload, de-resuscitation, and outcomes in critically ill or injured patients: a systematic review with suggestions for clinical practice. Anaesthesiol Intensive Ther. 2014;46(5):361–80.
2. Boyd JH, Forbes J, Nakada T, Walley KR, Russell JA. Fluid resuscitation in septic shock: a positive fluid balance and elevated central venous pressure are associated with increased mortality. Crit Care Med. 2011;39(2):259–65.
3. O'Connor ME, Prowle JR. Fluid Overload. Crit Care Clin. 2015;31(4):803–21.
4. Van Regenmortel N, Verbrugghe W, Roelant E, Van den Wyngaert T, Jorens PG. Maintenance fluid therapy and fluid creep impose more significant fluid, sodium, and chloride burdens than

resuscitation fluids in critically ill patients: a retrospective study in a tertiary mixed ICU population. Intensive Care Med. 2018;44(4):409–17.
5. Silversides JA, Fitzgerald E, Manickavasagam US, Lapinsky SE, Nisenbaum R, Hemmings N, et al. Deresuscitation of patients with iatrogenic fluid overload is associated with reduced mortality in critical illness. Crit Care Med. 2018;46(10):1600–7.
6. Silversides JA, Major E, Ferguson AJ, Mann EE, McAuley DF, Marshall JC, et al. Conservative fluid management or deresuscitation for patients with sepsis or acute respiratory distress syndrome following the resuscitation phase of critical illness: a systematic review and meta-analysis. Intensive Care Med. 2017;43(2):155–70.
7. Berthelsen RE, Perner A, Jensen AK, Rasmussen BS, Jensen JU, Wiis J, et al. Forced fluid removal in intensive care patients with acute kidney injury: the randomised FFAKI feasibility trial. Acta Anaesthesiol Scand. 2018;62(7):936–44.
8. Cordemans C, De Laet I, Van Regenmortel N, Schoonheydt K, Dits H, Martin G, et al. Aiming for a negative fluid balance in patients with acute lung injury and increased intra-abdominal pressure: a pilot study looking at the effects of PAL-treatment. Ann Intensive Care. 2012;2(Suppl 1):S15.
9. Murugan R, Kerti SJ, Chang C-CH, Gallagher M, Clermont G, Palevsky PM, et al. Association of net ultrafiltration rate with mortality among critically ill adults with acute kidney injury receiving continuous venovenous hemodiafiltration: a secondary analysis of the randomized evaluation of Normal vs augmented level (RENAL) of renal replacement therapy trial. JAMA Netw Open. 2019;2(6):e195418.

Are We Done with Early Goal-Directed Therapy?

20

20.1 Introduction

"Goal-directed therapy" was a concept initially developed in anesthesia, resuscitating patients undergoing major surgery to specific hemodynamic targets, or goals. Shoemaker and colleagues [1] extended this concept into postsurgical intensive care, targeting supranormal cardiac index (CI) and oxygen delivery (DO_2) to match increased oxygen consumption (VO_2), to compensate for increased postoperative metabolism. Using a combination of fluids, blood products, inotropes (particularly dobutamine), vasopressors, and vasodilators, titrated against pulmonary artery catheter (PAC) derived goals, they showed improved clinical outcomes in a single-center study when the PAC was placed preoperatively and used to target these goals in the operating theatre and in the surgical ICU. These results were difficult to replicate; however, 1 trial of 109 patients suggested worse outcomes following this protocol in a treatment group of heterogenous critically ill patients, with the authors concluding "contrary to what might have been expected, our results suggest that in some cases aggressive efforts to increase oxygen consumption may have been detrimental" [2]. While the concept of "goal-directed therapy" remains attractive, it has been difficult to define precisely what goals should be targeted [3].

20.2 Early Goal-Directed Therapy (EGDT) in Sepsis

The concept of early resuscitation to hemodynamic goals was extrapolated to severe sepsis in the emergency department of a major inner-city hospital in Detroit, USA. Critically ill patients with presumed sepsis were resuscitated to achieve goals of cardiac index, central venous pressure (CVP), and superior vena cava oxygen saturation ($ScvO_2$) using a proprietary oximetric catheter developed by Edwards Lifesciences (California). A randomized controlled trial (RCT) evaluated this

J. Chacko et al., *Controversies in Critical Care*,
https://doi.org/10.1007/978-981-19-9940-6_20

approach in 263 patients, where 130 received EGDT according to a specific protocol for 6 h in the emergency department, while 133 received usual care [4]. Subsequent treatment in the ICU was not protocolized, and the intensive care staff were blinded to the treatment allocation as much as possible. There was a spectacular difference in the in-hospital mortality (the primary outcome) from 46.5% in the control group to 30.5%. Patients in the intervention group received more fluid, red cell transfusion, and vasopressors in the first 6 h, and more received mechanical ventilation and PAC insertion. These results led to much discussion. Many institutions, particularly in North America, instituted "sepsis teams" to rapidly implement EGDT protocols, while elsewhere concern was raised about the overall amount of fluid being given [5] and the high baseline mortality in a single-center study, with observational data showing better outcomes elsewhere without the use of an EGDT protocol [6–8].

20.3 The Evidence

This controversy led to three large multicenter RCTs of EGDT in severe sepsis and septic shock, in Australia and New Zealand [9], the UK [10], and the USA [11]. All three evaluated the EGDT protocol published by Rivers et al. [4]. ARISE, in Australia and New Zealand, recruited 1600 patients from 51 hospitals (796 to EGDT and 804 to usual care) with 18.6% vs. 18.8% 90-day mortality, respectively [OR 0.98]. The EGDT group received more fluid, vasopressors, red cell transfusion, and dobutamine. The ProMISe study, conducted in the UK, studied 1260 patients in 56 hospitals (630 assigned to each of EGDT and usual care) with 29.5% 90-day mortality in the EGDT group and 29.2% in the usual care group (risk ratio: 1.01, 95% CI 0.85–1.20). PRoCESS, in the USA, studied 1341 patients in 31 emergency departments using a 3-arm design, where 439 received EGDT, 446 received protocolized "standard therapy," and 456 received usual care alone, with 60-day mortality of 21.0%, 18.2%, and 18.9%, respectively (risk ratio: EGDT vs. protocol-based standard care 1.15, 95% CI 0.88–1.51).

The investigators from the three trials conducted a prespecified individual-patient data meta-analysis (IPDMA) using a predetermined common dataset to look for any subgroup effects that were not apparent in the three primary trials. Overall, they studied 3723 patients in 138 hospitals in 7 countries. The 90-day mortality was similar (24.9% vs 25.4%) between EGDT and usual care (adjusted odds ratio: 0.97, 95%CI 0.82–1.14). EGDT led to greater use of intensive care and greater costs in an economic analysis. There were no subgroup differences, including in the sickest cohort (higher serum lactate level, combined hypotension and hyperlactatemia, or highest predicted risk of death) [12]. Important studies on EGDT are summarized in Table 20.1.

Why did these studies not replicate the findings from Rivers et al. in Detroit? The first word of caution relates to "single-center studies by enthusiasts," where unmeasured differences in treatment may influence the outcomes, potentially demonstrating efficacy but not effective when assessed under "real world" conditions—a

Table 20.1 Important studies that compared early goal-directed therapy with usual care in patients with sepsis

Study/year	Design	Intervention	Control	Outcomes
Rivers et al. (2001) [4]	RCT	EGDT for 6 h	Usual care	In-hospital mortality lower with EGDT (30.5% vs. 46.5%); 28- and 60-day mortality also lower with EGDT. More fluid, vasopressors in the EGDT group
ProMISe (2015) [10]	RCT	EGDT for 6 h	Usual care	All-cause mortality at 90 days, 28 days, and hospital discharge similar. SOFA score at 6 h and median ICU LOS lower with usual care. No difference in the number of days without advanced respiratory, cardiovascular, or renal support. No difference in ICU or hospital stay
ProCESS (2014) [11]	RCT	Three-armed study. EGDT or protocolized standard therapy for 6 h was the intervention arm	Bedside physician-directed usual care	No significant difference in the 60-day, 90-day, and 1-year mortality between the three groups
ARISE (2014) [9]	RCT	EGDT for 6 h	Usual care based on physician discretion	No significant difference in all-cause mortality at 90-day, 28-day, and in hospital. No difference in the ICU or hospital LOS
PRISM (2017) [12]	Individual patient meta-analysis from ProMISe, ProCESS, and ARISE	EGDT	Usual care (excluded patients from the protocol-based standard-therapy group in the ProCESS trial)	90-day mortality similar. EGDT associated with greater use of intensive care and hemodynamic support. Cost of care higher with EGDT. No benefit with EGDT in subgroups of patients with more severe shock or among hospitals that used less vasopressors and fluids with usual resuscitation

Abbreviations: *RCT* randomized controlled trial, *EGDT* early goal-directed therapy, *LOS* length of stay

single-center trial should never lead to widespread change in practice before its findings have been replicated. It has been suggested that the patients in the Rivers et al. trial were sicker at the time of presentation, but even the sickest subgroup in the IPDMA showed no benefit, with mortality of approximately 45% in both arms which was also similar to the mortality in the control group in the Rivers et al. study. It has been suggested that the "usual care" was better in the multicenter studies;

besides, outcomes from sepsis outcomes have progressively improved over time [8]. However, even in emergency departments with the least aggressive usual practice, there was no difference in outcomes. It remains unclear what "goals" should be followed for early resuscitation of sepsis, if CVP and $ScvO_2$ may not be appropriate targets.

The Surviving Sepsis Campaign no longer refers to "EGDT" per se but rather to resuscitation targets including at least 30 ml/kg crystalloid within the first 3 h, using dynamic parameters to guide resuscitation including response to passive leg raise or fluid bolus, using stroke volume, stroke volume variation, pulse pressure variation, or echocardiography where available, while recognizing this is a weak recommendation with very low-quality evidence [13]. Again, the choice of target remains unclear. One recent trial (ANDROMEDA-SHOCK) compared normalization of capillary return time (CRT) with clearance of hyperlactatemia. On day 3, the CRT group had significantly less organ dysfunction as assessed by the SOFA score, with 28-day mortality of 34.9% in the peripheral perfusion group and 43.4% in the lactate group. However, this difference did not reach statistical significance [14].

Sepsis "bundles" have been widely adopted in to practice and since 2013. Hospitals in New York State have been required to deliver 3-h and 6-h "bundles" for sepsis [15]. Hospitals are required to obtain a blood culture, measure the serum lactate level, and administer broad-spectrum antibiotics within 3 h. Within 6 h, hospitals must administer a bolus of 30 ml/kg fluid in patients with hypotension or a serum lactate level of ≥4.0 mmol/l, initiate vasopressors for refractory hypotension, and remeasure the serum lactate level within 6 h. In an analysis of 49,331 patients between 2014 and 2016, the median time to complete the 3-h bundle was 1.3 h, the median time to antibiotics was 0.95 h, and the median time to completion of the fluid bolus was 2.56 h. In those patients with a longer time to completion of the 3-h bundle, the hospital mortality was higher (odds ratio: 1.04/h). However, the increased mortality was associated with a longer time to administration of antibiotics (odds ratio: 1.04/h) but not a longer time to administration of fluids [15].

20.4 Where to Next in Sepsis Resuscitation?

An ongoing area of controversy relates to how *much* fluid to give. The three major EGDT trials all used less fluid than was used in the Rivers et al. study, and there is a growing awareness that fluid overload is associated with worse outcomes in critical illness. In pediatric sepsis in a resource-constrained environment, Maitland et al. demonstrated better outcomes with maintenance fluids alone, rather than 20–40 ml/kg boluses of either 5% albumin or 0.9% saline [16]. The hypothesis that outcomes might be better with less fluid and earlier use of vasopressor drugs compared to usual care is currently being tested in clinical trials. In an observational trial in Australia and New Zealand, there was still wide variation in practice, with patients receiving anything between 1000 and 12,200 ml in the first 24 h (median 4200 ml) with a median of 2000 ml before commencement of vasopressors [17]. The ARISE FLUIDS trial [18] is recruiting patients with septic shock and hyperlactatemia despite a 1000 ml fluid bolus and randomizing them to either restricted fluids and early vasopressor or liberal fluids and delayed vasopressor arm. The CLOVERS trial [19] is testing a similar hypothesis in the USA, where resuscitation practices typically involve a larger initial fluid volume compared to Australia and New Zealand. Recruitment into CLOVERS has recently been ceased.

Key Points

- We may be "done" with EGDT as a specific treatment protocol targeting CVP and $ScvO_2$, after three major international trials failed to show benefit.
- However, the concept of early resuscitation in sepsis continues to hold true. It is self-evident that outcomes will be better with prompt treatment, but it is not at all clear what goals should be targeted. Should we target dynamic indices of volume responsiveness or much simpler goals such as capillary return or blood pressure? (If so, what blood pressure?)
- Current trials are testing the hypothesis that early resuscitation to a hemodynamics target with vasopressors might lead to a better outcome than larger volumes of fluids.
- To date, the only robust evidence is that outcomes are better in septic shock with earlier administration of appropriate antibiotics.

References

1. Shoemaker WC, Appel PL, Kram HB, et al. Prospective trial of supranormal values of survivors and therapeutic goals in high-risk surgical patients. Chest. 1988;94:1176–86.
2. Hayes MA, Timmins AC, Yau EH, et al. Elevation of systemic oxygen delivery in the treatment of critically ill patients. N Engl J Med. 1994;330:1717–22.
3. Pearse R, Dawson D, Fawcett J, et al. Early goal-directed therapy after major surgery reduces complications and duration of hospital stay. A randomized, controlled trial. Crit Care. 2005;9:R687–93.
4. Rivers E, Nguyen B, Havstad S, et al. Early goal-directed therapy in the treatment of severe sepsis and septic shock. N Engl J Med. 2001;345:1368–77.
5. Kelm DJ, Perrin JT, Cartin-Ceba R, et al. Fluid overload in patients with severe sepsis and septic shock treated with early goal-directed therapy is associated with increased acute need for fluid-related medical interventions and hospital death. Shock. 2015;43:68–73.
6. Ho BCH, Bellomo R, McGain F, et al. The incidence and outcome of septic shock patients in the absence of early-goal directed therapy. Crit Care. 2006;10:R80.
7. Peake SL, Bailey M, Bellomo R, et al. Australasian resuscitation of sepsis evaluation (ARISE): a multi-centre, prospective, inception cohort study. Resuscitation. 2009;80:811–8.
8. Kaukonen KM, Bailey M, Suzuki S, Pilcher D, Bellomo R. Mortality related to severe sepsis and septic shock among critically ill patients in Australia and New Zealand, 2000-2012. JAMA. 2014;311:1308–16.
9. The ARISE Investigators and the ANZICS Clinical Trials Group. Goal-directed resuscitation for patients with early septic shock. N Engl J Med. 2014;371:1496–506.

10. Mouncey PR, Osborn TM, Power GS, et al. Trial of early, goal-directed resuscitation for septic shock. N Engl J Med. 2015;372:1301–11.
11. The ProCESS Investigators. A randomized trial of protocol-based care for early septic shock. N Engl J Med. 2014;370:1683–93.
12. The PRISM Investigators. Early goal-directed therapy for septic shock – a patient-level meta-analysis. N Engl J Med. 2017;376:2223–34.
13. Evans L, Rhodes A, Alhazzani W, et al. Surviving sepsis campaign: international guidelines for management of sepsis and septic shock 2021. Intens Care Med. 2021;47:1181–247.
14. Hernandez G, Ospina-Tascon GA, Damiani LP, et al. Effect of a resuscitation strategy targeting peripheral perfusion status vs serum lactate levels on 28-day mortality among patients with septic shock: the ANDROMEDA-SHOCK randomized clinical trial. JAMA. 2019;321:654–64.
15. Seymour CW, Gesten F, Prescott HC, et al. Time to treatment and mortality during mandated emergency care for sepsis. N Engl J Med. 2017;376:2235–44.
16. Maitland K, Kiguli S, Opoka RO, et al. Mortality after fluid bolus in African children with severe infection. N Engl J Med. 2011;364:2483–95.
17. Keijzers G, Macdonald SPJ, Udy AA, et al. The Australasian resuscitation in sepsis evaluation: fluids or vasopressors in emergency department sepsis (ARISE FLUIDS), a multi-centre observational study describing current practice in Australia and New Zealand. Emerg Med Australas. 2020;32:586–98.
18. Australasian Resuscitation in Sepsis Evaluation: FLUid or vasopressors in emergency Department Sepsis, protocol V2.0, 15 Dec 2020. https://clinicaltrials.gov/ct2/show/NCT04569942.
19. The Crystalloid Liberal versus Vasopressors Early (CLOVERS) trial. https://clinicaltrials.gov/ct2/show/NCT03434028.

Normal Saline Versus Balanced Crystalloids Revisited

21

21.1 Introduction

The use of normal saline is ubiquitous in clinical practice. The history of saline resuscitation dates back to 1831 when the cholera epidemic swept across Britain leaving a trail of devastation. Out of sheer desperation, Thomas Latta, a young physician from Leith, near Edinburgh, administered intravenous saline solution to an elderly lady who was on the verge of death from extreme dehydration. He recounted his experience in a letter to The Lancet, "Having inserted a tube into the basilic vein, cautiously - anxiously, I watched the effects; she began to breathe less laboriously, soon the sharpened features, and sunken eye, and fallen jaw, pale and cold, bearing the manifest impress of death's signet, began to glow with returning animation; the pulse, which had long ceased, returned to the wrist; at first small and quick, by degrees it became more and more distinct…" [1]. The solution that Latta administered was different in composition from the normal saline as we know it today. According to later analysis, one of the constituents of the solution he used was sodium bicarbonate. The Latta solution actually contained sodium 134 mmol/L, chloride 118 mmol/L, and bicarbonate 16 mmol/L [2].

21.2 The Possible Adverse Effects of Normal Saline

21.2.1 Hyperchloremia and Acidosis

Normal saline contains 154 mmol/L each of sodium and chloride. The serum chloride levels, normally 96–106 mmol/L, tend to rise with normal saline administration because of the excess chloride load. Hyperchloremia leads to metabolic acidosis, according to the Stewart physicochemical approach. Based on the Stewart equation,

J. Chacko et al., *Controversies in Critical Care*,
https://doi.org/10.1007/978-981-19-9940-6_21

the pH of a solution depends on three variables: the strong ion difference (SID), the partial pressure of carbon dioxide (PCO_2), and the total concentration of weak acids.

$$\text{SID} = (\text{strong cations}) - (\text{strong anions}).$$

$$\text{SID} = \left(\text{Na}^+ + \text{K}^+ + \text{Ca}^{++} + \text{Mg}^{++}\right) - \left(\text{Cl}^- + \text{lactate}^-\right).$$

The normal SID is 40–45 mEq/L. A higher value for SID denotes alkalosis, while a lower value denotes acidosis. How does this happen? As the chloride level rises, the SID decreases; this leads to the dissociation of water molecules to generate H^+ ions to maintain electrical neutrality. The rise in H^+ concentration results in acidosis. Thus, hyperchloremia due to excessive administration of normal saline may lead to metabolic acidosis.

21.2.2 Hyperchloremia and Tubuloglomerular Feedback

Hyperchloremia results in an increase in the chloride ions filtered through the glomeruli. This results in a higher chloride concentration in the distal convoluted tubule. The distal convoluted tubule is lined by specialized cells in the area called macula densa. The macula densa cells sense the high chloride content and trigger vasoconstriction of the adjacent afferent arteriole, thereby reducing glomerular filtration. This phenomenon is known as the tubuloglomerular feedback mechanism [3] (Fig. 21.1). Hyperchloremic afferent arteriolar vasoconstriction and the consequent reduction in glomerular filtration may lead to impairment of renal function [4].

21.2.3 Other Possible Harmful Effects of Hyperchloremia

Excessive chloride levels may lead to splanchnic hypoperfusion [5]. High chloride levels and the consequent metabolic acidosis may also explain the increased blood

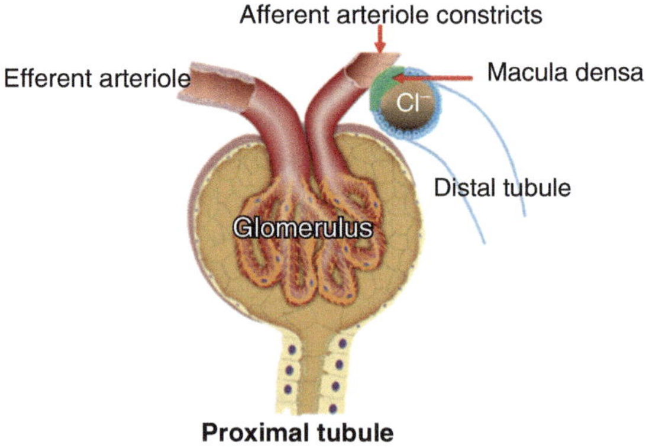

Fig. 21.1 Hyperchloremia increases chloride ions filtered through the glomeruli, leading to a high chloride concentration in the distal tubule. The macula densa cells (shaded green) sense the high chloride content and trigger vasoconstriction of the adjacent afferent arteriole causing reduced glomerular filtration

loss, greater requirement for blood products, and the higher incidence of coagulation abnormities that may ensue following resuscitation with normal saline or hydroxyethyl starch suspended in saline [6].

21.3 The Evidence

What is the current state of evidence regarding normal saline compared with balanced crystalloids in the resuscitation of critically ill patients (Table 21.1)?

Table 21.1 Randomized controlled trials that compared normal saline vs. balanced crystalloid in critically ill patients

Author/year	Study population	Location	Balanced crystalloid type	Outcomes	Comments
Young et al. (2015) [7] (SPLIT)	ICU patients who required crystalloids	4 ICUs in New Zealand	Plasmalyte 148	No difference in AKI stage injury or higher; similar requirement for RRT; similar ICU and hospital mortality	Feasibility trial, not powered for clinical endpoints
Semler et al. (2018) [8] (SMART)	ICU patients	Single center, USA. The same fluid administered if the patient was transferred to other locations	Plasma-Lyte A or lactated Ringer's solution	Major adverse kidney events, the primary outcome was higher with normal saline. No difference in hospital mortality ventilator-free, or ICU-free days	Relatively small volumes of fluid administered. Drawbacks of a composite outcome
Self et al. (2018) [9] (SALT-ED)	Patients presenting to the emergency department	Emergency department, USA	Plasma-Lyte A or lactated Ringer's solution	Hospital-free days at 30 d not different. Major adverse kidney events lower with balanced crystalloid. Hospital mortality not different	Drawbacks of a composite outcome

(continued)

Table 21.1 (continued)

Author/year	Study population	Location	Balanced crystalloid type	Outcomes	Comments
Zampieri et al. [10] (2021) (BaSICS)	ICU patients who required fluid resuscitation	75 ICUs in Brazil	Plasmalyte 148	90-day mortality the primary outcome was similar. AKI requiring RRT not different. No difference in ICU or hospital mortality. Higher 90-day mortality with normal saline in TBI	Relatively small volumes of fluid administered. Large number of patients received the non-study fluid in the first 24 h before study enrolment. The study may have been underpowered
Finfer et al. [11] (2022) (PLUS)	ICU patients	53 ICUs in Australia and New Zealand	Plasmalyte 148	90-day mortality not different. No difference in RRT, peak creatinine levels. No difference in ICU, hospital, or 28-day mortality. No difference in days alive and ICU-free, ventilator-free, or hospital-free	Study was ceased early and did not attain the planned sample size. Non-protocol fluids administered outside the ICU. Open label saline in a large number of patients in the plasmalyte arm

Abbreviations: *AKI* acute kidney injury, *RRT* renal replacement therapy, *TBI* traumatic brain injury

21.3.1 The SPLIT Trial

Young et al. compared normal saline with plasmalyte 148 in a multicentric study from four ICUs in New Zealand in a randomized controlled trial (RCT) [7]. Patients who required crystalloid fluid therapy according to the treating physician were included. If feasible, the study fluid was also administered in locations outside the ICU as required. A total of 2278 patients were enrolled; 1162 were assigned to the plasmalyte 148 group and 1116 to the normal saline group. Most patients were admitted to the ICU after elective surgical procedures, mainly cardiovascular surgery. The primary outcome was the proportion of patients who fulfilled the criteria for injury or greater according to the RIFLE classification of acute kidney injury (AKI). There was no significant difference in the incidence of AKI fulfilling the criteria for injury or higher according to the RIFLE classification between the two groups [102/1067 (9.6%) in the plasmalyte 148 group compared to 94/1025 (9.2%) in the saline group; (RR 1.04 95% CI: 0.8–1.36, $p = 0.77$)]. Among the secondary outcomes, the number of patients who suffered AKI under each category of the RIFLE score was similar between groups. The requirement for renal replacement therapy (RRT) was also similar: 3.3% with plasmalyte 148 vs. 3.4% with saline. The difference between the baseline and the highest creatinine levels was also similar between groups. ICU and hospital mortality, the length of stay in ICU and hospital, and the requirement for and duration of mechanical ventilation were also similar. The risk of AKI among subgroups of patients with sepsis, trauma, APACHE score of 25 or more, cardiac surgical patients, and patients with traumatic brain injury (TBI) remained similar between groups.

The SPLIT trial was a feasibility study and hence not powered to evaluate clinical endpoints. The largest cohort of patients was postoperative cardiac surgical with relatively few patients with other underlying causes requiring ICU admission. However, this study suggested that the use of normal saline compared to a buffered crystalloid solution may not lead to adverse clinical outcomes.

21.3.2 The SMART Trial

The SMART trial compared normal saline with a buffered crystalloid (Plasma-Lyte A or lactated Ringer's solution) as intravenous fluid among critically ill patients admitted to the ICUs of a single center (Vanderbilt University Hospital) in the USA in an RCT [8]. The choice of intravenous fluid alternated between normal saline and buffered crystalloid on a monthly basis. The trial was coordinated between ICUs, emergency department, and operation theaters that enabled the same study fluid to be administered at different locations. The trial enrolled 15,802 patients: 7942 patients received plasmalyte, while 7860 patients received normal saline. The primary outcome was the proportion of patients who met one or more criteria for a major adverse kidney event, censored at 30 days (MAKE-30), including a composite of death, RRT, or persistent renal dysfunction. A major adverse kidney event occurred in a significantly higher number of patients who received normal saline compared to those who received buffered crystalloid (15.4% vs. 14.3%; OR: 0.91, 95% CI: 0.84–0.99, $P = 0.04$). On prespecified subgroup analysis, the difference in the primary outcome was greater among patients who received larger volumes of fluid. In patients with sepsis, the 30-day mortality was lower with a buffered crystalloid compared to normal saline. The hospital mortality was not different between the two groups. The requirement for RRT and the presence of persistent renal dysfunction were also not different between groups. Furthermore, there was no difference in the ICU-free days, ventilator-free days, vasopressor-free days, and AKI stage II or higher after enrolment between the two groups. The SMART trial used either Plasma-Lyte A or lactated Ringer's solution in the balanced crystalloid arm; hence the specific impact of the particular type of fluid could not be evaluated. Other limitations include the relatively small volume of fluid administered, with a median of 1.0 L in the crystalloid group and 1.02 L in the normal saline group. Besides, it was a single-center, unblinded study. The use of a composite primary outcome may also have its own limitations.

21.3.3 The SALT-ED Trial

The SALT-ED trial also compared buffered crystalloids (Plasma-Lyte A or lactated Ringer's solution) with normal saline in a randomized controlled trial [9]. The study included consecutive patients who received crystalloids in the emergency department of the Vanderbilt University Hospital and were hospitalized outside the ICU. Patients who were admitted to the ICU were included in the SMART study. The number of hospital-free days at 30 days, the primary outcome, was not significantly different between patients who received crystalloids compared to those who received normal saline. The incidence of major adverse kidney events at 30 days was significantly lower with a buffered crystalloid compared to normal saline (4.7% vs. 5.6%; OR: 0.82, 95% CI: 0.7–0.95 $p = 0.01$). The hospital mortality was not significantly different between groups. Among patients who presented with AKI of KDIGO stage II or greater, a significantly lower incidence of a major adverse kidney event was observed with the use of a buffered crystalloid. This was again an unblinded study with the drawbacks associated with a composite outcome. Furthermore, data were not available regarding the type of fluid administered after initial care in the emergency department.

21.3.4 The BaSICS Trial

The BaSICS randomized controlled trial included patients from 75 ICUs in Brazil who required fluid expansion at least on one occasion [10]. In addition, one of the following criteria had to be met: age > 65 years, hypotension, sepsis, respiratory support with mechanical ventilation (invasive or non-invasive ventilation or high-flow nasal cannula for at least 12 h), early signs of renal dysfunction, cirrhosis, or acute liver failure. Those who were likely to require RRT within 6 h or already receiving RRT and who have high (>160 mmol/L) or low (<120 mmol/L) serum sodium levels were excluded. Patients were randomized into four arms; plasmalyte 148 or normal saline was administered, each at 333 m/h or 999 mL/h. All fluid challenges, maintenance fluid, and drug dilution were carried out with the study fluid, for up to 90 days after randomization. The overall patient care was at the discretion of the treating physician. A total of 11,052 patients were enrolled over approximately 3 years. The plasmalyte arm included 5230 patients, while 5290 patients were randomized to receive normal saline.

Patient characteristics were well balanced at baseline; 48.3% of patients were post-surgical. The primary outcome was the 90-day mortality. In the plasmalyte group, 1381/5230 (26.4%) patients had died at 90 days compared to 1439/5290 (27.2%) in the normal saline arm (hazard ratio: 0.97 95% CI: 0.9–1.05); the difference was not statistically significant. Among the secondary outcomes, the incidence of AKI requiring RRT on days 1, 2, 3, and 7 or during hospital admission was not different between groups. The composite outcome of AKI, stage II or greater by the KDIGO classification, and mortality was not different on day 3 and day 7. The total SOFA scores on days 3 and 7 were also not different between groups. The SOFA scores under individual organ systems were not different on day 3. However, the incidence of a neurological SOFA score of >2 on day 7 was significantly higher with plasmalyte (32.1%) compared to normal saline (26%). This finding suggested a worse neurological status on day 7 among patients who received plasmalyte compared to normal saline. On prespecified subgroup analysis, in patients with traumatic brain injury, the 90-day mortality was higher in the plasmalyte group compared to the normal saline group (31.3% vs. 21.1%). There was no significant difference in the 90-day mortality in subgroups of patients with AKI of KDIGO 2 or greater severity, sepsis as the underlying cause, surgical patients, and APACHE score of 25 or more. There was no difference between groups in the ICU or hospital mortality and the ICU or hospital length of stay. On post hoc analysis, the composite outcome of 90-day mortality and the requirement for RRT were not different between groups. The authors concluded that among critically ill patients who require a fluid challenge, there was no difference in the 90-day mortality with plasmalyte compared to normal saline. There was a suggestion of harm among patients with traumatic brain injury, with higher neurological SOFA on day 7 and higher 90-day mortality.

The BaSICS study echoes the findings of the SAFE study, which also revealed higher mortality among patients with traumatic brain injury who received 4% albumin compared to normal saline [11]. The study is limited by the relatively small volume of fluid infused: a median of 1.5 L on day 1 and 2.9 L in the first 3 days. Perhaps, larger volumes of fluid may lead to a difference in outcomes. A large number of patients received the non-study fluid in the first 24 h prior to study enrolment which may have confounded the results. The sample size was calculated based on 35% 90-day mortality in the normal saline arm; however, the actual mortality was lower, which could have resulted in a slightly underpowered study.

The PLUS study compared Plasmalyte 148 with normal saline as the resuscitation fluid in critically ill patients in a double-blind RCT [12]. The study included 5037 patients from 53 ICUs in Australia and New Zealand, with 2515 patients assigned to receive plasmalyte 148 and 2522 patients to receive normal saline. The patients were well matched at baseline, with a median APACHE II score of 19; 79% of patients received mechanical ventilation, and 42.3% had sepsis. The primary outcome, death within 90 days of randomization, was not significantly different between the two groups (plasmalyte 148 vs. saline: 21.8% vs. 22). Among the secondary outcomes, there was no difference in peak creatinine levels and the use of renal replacement therapy between groups. The number of days alive and ventilation-free, alive and out of ICU, and alive and out of hospital was similar. Furthermore, there was no difference between groups in the ICU mortality, hospital mortality, and mortality at day 28. On subgroup analysis, there was no difference in the 90-day mortality between plasmalyte 148 and normal saline regardless of age 65 or more vs. less, gender, presence of sepsis or acute kidney injury, APACHE score of 25 or more vs. less, and postoperative compared to nonoperative patients.

Although the original sample size was 8800 patients, the study was called off after enrolment of 5037 patients as the COVID-19 pandemic set in. The study excluded a large number (70%) of patients who were screened. The type of fluid administered was not based on the study protocol outside the ICU. Most patients (66.1%) had received normal saline within 24 h prior to randomization; besides, 63% of patients assigned to receive plasmalyte 148 received 500 mL or more of open label saline and may have confounded the results.

Hammond et al. performed a meta-analysis of 13 RCTs, including 35,884 patients that compared the effect of balanced crystalloids with normal saline in critically ill adults [13]. The relative risk of 90-day mortality in six studies with a low risk of bias was 0.96 (95% CI: 0.91–1.01). On Bayesian analysis, using vague priors, the probability of 90-day mortality with balanced salt solutions was 89.5% lower compared to saline. There was no significant difference in the relative risk for the development of AKI or use of RRT. No significant difference was observed in the number of ventilator-free days or vasopressor-free days between the two groups. In septic patients, the use of balanced crystalloids compared to saline ranged from a 14% relative reduction to 1% relative increase in the risk of death. In contrast, in brain injury, the risk of death with the use of balanced crystalloids ranged from a 60% relative increase to a 2% relative reduction. The authors concluded that there was a high probability that balanced crystalloids reduced mortality compared with saline in a heterogenous group of critically ill patients; however, the impact on mortality may be variable in subgroups of patients.

Key Points

- Normal saline has been extensively used as intravenous fluid for nearly two centuries; over the years, questions have been raised regarding possible adverse effects.
- The high chloride content compared to plasma levels has been associated with hyperchloremia and metabolic acidosis.
- Hyperchloremia has been implicated in the causation of AKI through the tubuloglomerular feedback mechanism; besides, concerns have also been raised regarding splanchnic hypoperfusion and coagulation abnormalities.
- RCTs that compared a buffered crystalloid solution with normal saline among critically ill patients have revealed conflicting results.
- The multicentric BaSICS study did not reveal any significant benefit in clinical endpoints with a buffered crystalloid compared to normal saline among a general ICU population.
- The PLUS study did not reveal significant difference in the 90-day mortality, peak creatinine levels, or the use of renal replacement therapy between saline and Plasmalyte 148 treated patients.

- A recent meta-analysis did not reveal a significant difference in the 90-day mortality with balanced crystalloids compared to saline among six RCTs with a low risk of bias. On Bayesian meta-analysis, the probability of 90-day mortality with balanced salt solutions was 89.5% lower compared to saline.
- In traumatic brain injury, there is a consistent suggestion of possible harm with the use of a buffered crystalloid from the SAFE and the BaSICS trials. Although based on subgroup analysis, it may be appropriate to prefer normal saline over a buffered crystalloid in traumatic brain injury.
- Based on the available evidence, balanced crystalloids may be the preferred resuscitation fluid in a heterogenous population of critically ill patients. However, the impact on specific subgroups of patients including those with traumatic brain injury needs further evaluation.

References

1. Awad S, Allison SP, Lobo DN. The history of 0.9% saline. Clin Nutr. 2008;27(2):179–88.
2. Lewins R. Injection of saline solutions in extraordinary quantities into the veins of malignant cholera. Lancet. 1832;18:243–4.
3. Briggs JP, Schnermann J. The tubuloglomerular feedback mechanism: functional and biochemical aspects. Annu Rev Physiol. 1987;49:251–73.
4. Rein JL, Coca SG. "I don't get no respect": the role of chloride in acute kidney injury. Am J Physiol Renal Physiol. 2019;316(3):F587–605.
5. Williams EL, Hildebrand KL, McCormick SA, Bedel MJ. The effect of intravenous lactated Ringer's solution versus 0.9% sodium chloride solution on serum osmolality in human volunteers. Anesth Analg. 1999;88(5):999–1003.
6. Martin G, Bennett-Guerrero E, Wakeling H, Mythen MG, el-Moalem H, Robertson K, et al. A prospective, randomized comparison of thromboelastographic coagulation profile in patients receiving lactated Ringer's solution, 6% hetastarch in a balanced-saline vehicle, or 6% hetastarch in saline during major surgery. J Cardiothorac Vasc Anesth. 2002;16(4):441–6.
7. Young P, Bailey M, Beasley R, Henderson S, Mackle D, McArthur C, et al. Effect of a buffered crystalloid solution vs saline on acute kidney injury among patients in the intensive care unit: the SPLIT randomized clinical trial. JAMA. 2015;314(16):1701.
8. Semler MW, Self WH, Wanderer JP, Ehrenfeld JM, Wang L, Byrne DW, et al. Balanced crystalloids versus saline in critically ill adults. N Engl J Med. 2018;378(9):829–39.
9. Self WH, Semler MW, Wanderer JP, Wang L, Byrne DW, Collins SP, et al. Balanced crystalloids versus saline in noncritically ill adults. N Engl J Med. 2018;378(9):819–28.
10. Zampieri FG, Machado FR, Biondi RS, Freitas FGR, Veiga VC, Figueiredo RC, et al. Effect of intravenous fluid treatment with a balanced solution vs 0.9% saline solution on mortality in critically ill patients: the BaSICS Randomized Clinical Trial. JAMA. 2021;326(9):1–12. https://doi.org/10.1001/jama.2021.11684.
11. Finfer S, Bellomo R, Boyce N, French J, Myburgh J, Norton R, et al. A comparison of albumin and saline for fluid resuscitation in the intensive care unit. N Engl J Med. 2004;350(22):2247–56.
12. Finfer S, Micallef S, Hammond N, Navarra L, Bellomo R, Billot L, et al. Balanced multielectrolyte solution versus saline in critically ill adults. N Engl J Med. 2022;386:815.
13. Hammond NE, Zampieri FG, Di Tanna GL, Garside T, Adigbli D, Cavalcanti AB, et al. Balanced crystalloids versus saline in critically ill adults — a systematic review with meta-analysis. NEJM Evid. 2022;1(2). https://doi.org/10.1056/EVIDoa2100010.

22 Liberal Fluid Resuscitation Vs. Early Vasopressors in Septic Shock

22.1 Introduction

Fluid resuscitation is one of the key early interventions in patients with septic shock. The Surviving Sepsis Guidelines continue to recommend an initial volume of resuscitation of 30 mL/kg, with additional boluses guided by the assessment of volume responsiveness [1]. In the landmark ProCESS, ProMisE, and ARISE trials, most patients with septic shock received approximately 5 L of fluid during the first few hours of resuscitation [2].

Septic shock is characterized by extensive vasodilatation of vascular beds accompanied by a reduction in systemic vascular resistance, leading to hypotension. Endothelial dysfunction occurs with the breakdown of the glycocalyx and leakage of fluid from the intravascular to the interstitial compartment [3]. The putative benefits of intravenous fluid administration include replenishment of the intravascular compartment that compensates for the extravasation of fluid into the interstitial space. Fluid resuscitation may also augment cardiac output and improve perfusion to the vital organs.

However, do the putative benefits of fluid resuscitation in septic patients impact clinical outcomes? Alternately, would a strategy of restricted early fluid resuscitation combined with vasopressor therapy, targeting mean arterial pressure, be more optimal?

22.2 The Evidence Behind Fluid Resuscitation

In their landmark study, Rivers et al. randomized patients presenting to the emergency department with severe sepsis or septic shock to a protocolized, early, goal-directed therapy (EGDT) or to clinician-guided resuscitation targets [4]. In the EGDT arm, crystalloid boluses of 500 mL every 30 min targeting a central venous pressure of

J. Chacko et al., *Controversies in Critical Care*,
https://doi.org/10.1007/978-981-19-9940-6_22

8–12 mm Hg and vasopressors targeting a mean arterial pressure of 65 mm Hg were administered as part of the early resuscitation strategy. Packed red cells were transfused if the $ScvO_2$ dropped below a threshold level of 70%. If the $ScvO_2$ remained persistently low despite these measures, a dobutamine infusion was commenced to augment the cardiac output. Patients randomized to the EGDT arm received significantly larger volumes of fluid in the first 6 h of resuscitation (5.0 L vs. 3.5 L). The in-hospital mortality, the primary endpoint, was significantly lower among patients in the EGDT compared to the control group (30.5 vs. 46.5%, $p = 0.009$).

Several subsequent studies seemed to corroborate the findings of this single-center study from an emergency department in the USA [5, 6]. However, it was largely unclear whether the improved clinical outcomes from EGDT resulted from a comprehensive "bundled" approach or from individual elements of the bundle. Could the favorable effects have been due to earlier recognition of sepsis, antibiotic administration, and source control? Indeed, the findings of a meta-analysis seem to suggest that the favorable effect of EGDT on mortality may arise from earlier administration of appropriate antibiotics compared to the impact of fluid resuscitation and attainment of hemodynamic goals [7].

Three RCTs evaluated the impact of EGDT on patients with septic shock after the original study by Rivers et al. The ProCESS [8], ARISE [9], and ProMISe [10] trials did not demonstrate any difference in clinical outcomes, including mortality, with EGDT compared to usual care. In these studies, the total volume of fluid administered during the initial 6 h of resuscitation was similar across all groups of patients. However, the volume of fluid administered in the first 6 h was less than both the arms of the original EGDT study.

22.3 How Does Excessive Fluid Administration Cause Harm?

Fluid-responsiveness may be highly variable in patients with septic shock. The ANDROMEDA-SHOCK trial randomized patients to a lactate-guided compared to the capillary refill-guided strategy of fluid resuscitation. In this study, only 57% of patients were fluid responsive, while fluid-responsiveness could not be determined in 18% of patients [11]. Clearly, arbitrary administration of fixed resuscitation volumes over a set period is fraught with the potential for harm from excessive fluid in patients who are not fluid responsive.

A fluid-liberal initial resuscitation strategy may lead to adverse consequences, with overfilling of the intravascular compartment and fluid leakage into the interstitial compartment due to capillary leak. Interstitial edema may lead to reduced tissue perfusion and precipitate organ dysfunction [12]. Furthermore, targeting central venous pressures may lead to a rise in the venous pressures with a drop in perfusion pressures of vital organs such as the kidneys [13] (Fig. 22.1).

Fluid resuscitation in septic shock may generate a persistent vasodilated state with reduced systemic vascular resistance and effective arterial elastance. The reduction in the systemic vascular resistance and elastance may result in increased cardiac output with no corresponding rise in blood pressure [14]. Vasodilatation resulting from fluid administration has been attributed to attenuation of baroreceptor-mediated vasoconstrictor response [14], endothelial nitric oxide release [15], and release of natriuretic peptides from increased cardiac filling pressures [16].

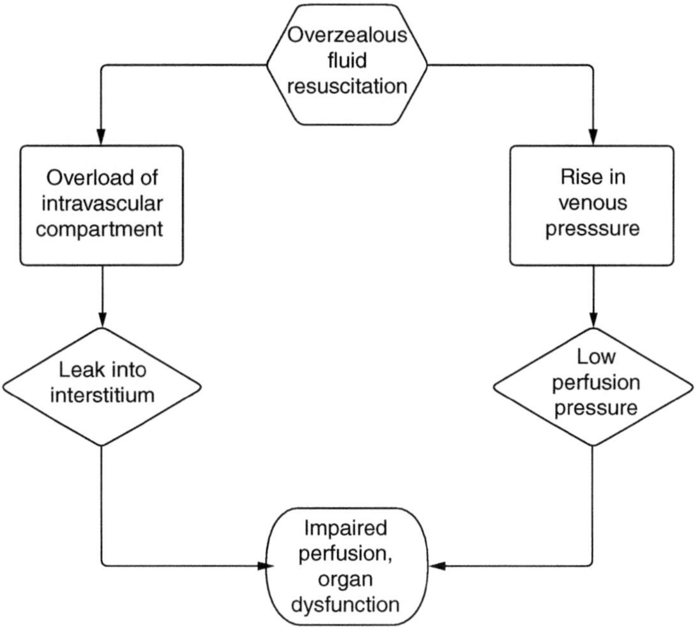

Fig. 22.1 Harmful effects of overzealous fluid resuscitation

22.4 Evidence of Possible Harm from Excess Fluid

The Fluid Expansion as Supportive Therapy (FEAST) study was carried out in children who presented with a severe febrile illness and clinical signs of impaired perfusion across multiple centers in sub-Saharan Africa. In this provocative three-armed study, initial resuscitation was performed with 20–40 mL/kg of 5% albumin or normal saline solution. This was compared with a control group that received no fluid boluses [17]. The 48 h mortality was significantly higher among children who received fluid boluses compared to those who did not (10.5% vs. 7.3%, $p = 0.003$). Shock resolution occurred more often with bolus fluids; however, improvement in blood pressures did not lead to improved survival.

In the Vasopressin in Septic Shock Trial (VAAST) trial, the mean cumulative positive fluid balance ranged from 5 to 11 L in the first week of illness among patients in septic shock [18]. The 28-day mortality was progressively higher with an increase in the cumulative fluid balance [18]. The Sepsis Occurrence in Acutely Ill Patients (SOAP) study echoed these findings with a 10% excess mortality for every liter of positive fluid balance at 72 h [19]. In the National Heart, Lung, and Blood Institute ARDS Clinical Trials Networks study, a conservative compared to a liberal strategy of fluid management was evaluated using explicit protocols for the first 7 days in 1000 patients [20]. The mean cumulative fluid balance was significantly lower in the fluid-liberal group (−136 ± 491 mL vs. 6992 ± 502 mL, $p < 0.001$). A fluid-conservative strategy was associated with a significantly lower duration of mechanical ventilation and ICU stay.

How does a liberal, goal-directed resuscitation compare with a more restrictive strategy in patient with acute pancreatitis? The WATERFALL multicenter RCT including 249 patients compared the two approaches. In the liberal group, lactated Ringer's solution was administered as an initial bolus of 20 mL/kg followed by 3 mL/kg/h. In the restrictive group, a bolus dose of 10 mL/kg was followed by 1.5 mL/kg/h. The study was terminated early as a significantly higher number of patients in the liberal resuscitation group developed fluid overload (20.5% vs. 6.3%, adjusted relative risk, 2.85; 95% CI, 1.36–5.94, $p = 0.004$). Progression to moderately severe or severe pancreatitis, the primary outcome, was not significantly different at the time of termination of the trial. The median duration of hospital stay was longer by 1 day in the liberal group (6 days, IQR: 4–8 vs. 5 days, IQR: 3–7). The WATERFALL trial adds to the body of knowledge that suggests the drawbacks associated with an aggressive resuscitative strategy in critically ill patients [21].

22.5 A Fluid-Restrictive Approach

Limitation of fluid administration with early use of vasopressors to maintain perfusion pressures and preserve organ function may be an alternative therapeutic strategy. Vasopressors decrease the venous capacitance and lead to an increase in the stressed volume in the venous circulation. An increase in the stressed volume effectively increases the venous return and cardiac output without the adverse consequences of fluid overload and tissue edema [22]. Besides, the hemodynamic effect of a fluid bolus among patients with septic shock is often transient. Repeated administration of fluid boluses may not improve the hemodynamic status even when patients appear to be fluid responsive by conventional monitoring [23].

The CLASSIC randomized controlled study was conducted across multiple centers in Scandinavia to assess the feasibility of a fluid-restrictive strategy after the initial resuscitation phase [24]. In the fluid-restrictive group, after the early resuscitation phase, further boluses were administered only in the presence of persistent signs of severe hypoperfusion. In the control group, further fluid boluses were administered if an improvement was noted in the static or dynamic hemodynamic indices. The co-primary outcomes included resuscitation volumes on day 5 and during the entire duration of ICU stay. At both time points, the resuscitation volumes were significantly lower with a restrictive strategy. The 90-day mortality, incidence of ischemic events, and acute kidney injury were similar between groups. Although the study was underpowered to evaluate patient-centered clinical outcomes, a restrictive fluid strategy was shown to be feasible in septic shock.

22.6 Early Vasopressor Administration

Is it time to reconsider the traditional fluid-liberal resuscitation strategy in light of putative harm that may arise from this approach? Should we consider the limitation of fluid resuscitation with early administration of vasopressors to maintain perfusion pressure in septic shock? The early use of vasopressors may facilitate the attainment of resuscitation targets with the administration of a lower volume of fluids.

In a retrospective observational study, the early administration of norepinephrine as the sole vasopressor was evaluated in 142 patients with septic shock. Following a limited initial fluid resuscitation, norepinephrine infusion was commenced targeting a mean arterial pressure of 75 mm Hg. The median time of commencement of norepinephrine infusion was 1.3 h after ICU admission. The target mean arterial pressure was attained in 86.3% of patients within 1 h of commencing norepinephrine infusion. The hospital mortality among the study cohort was 34.5% compared to the predicted mortality of 40.8% based on the SAPS II score. The hospital mortality was 50% compared to the predicted mortality of 74.4% among the most severely ill (SAPS score of >56) ($p = 0.07$). Although retrospective in nature, with no comparator group, this study suggested that the early administration of norepinephrine as the sole vasopressor led to the rapid achievement of target blood pressure. Besides, mortality was lower than predicted by the SAPS II score [25].

Bai et al. evaluated a retrospective cohort of 213 patients with septic shock from two surgical ICUs of a Chinese tertiary care hospital. The study was based on the hypothesis that late compared to earlier administration of norepinephrine would lead to a longer duration of hypotension leading to impaired organ perfusion. The impact of the timing of norepinephrine infusion on clinical outcomes was evaluated in patients with septic shock [26]. The 28-day mortality was significantly lower in patients who received norepinephrine within 2 h of the onset of septic shock compared with those who received it later. The authors observed an increase in mortality by 5.3% for every 1 h of delay in norepinephrine administration within the first 6 h of onset of septic shock. On univariate logistic regression analysis, the interval between the onset of septic shock and the commencement of norepinephrine infusion was an important determinant of the 28-day mortality. The odds ratio for death was 1.2 per hour of delay (1.07 to 1.35, $P = 0.002$); every 1 h delay was associated with a 20.4% increased likelihood of death. Mean arterial pressures were higher at 1, 2, 4, and 6 h, and serum lactate levels were lower at 2, 4, 6, and 8 h after the onset of septic shock among patients in the early compared to the late norepinephrine group.

In a phase II randomized, placebo-controlled trial from Thailand, norepinephrine was commenced in a dose of 0.05 mcg/kg/min within 1 h of the diagnosis of septic shock. The study patients fulfilled the definition of sepsis according to the surviving sepsis guidelines and had a mean arterial pressure of less than 65 mm Hg [27]. The norepinephrine infusion was continued for a period of 24 h, while the control group received a placebo infusion. If the mean arterial pressure remained lower than 65 mm Hg, open-label vasopressors were administered. The primary outcome was "shock control" after 6 h of diagnosis of septic shock. Shock control required a sustained mean arterial pressure of more than 65 mm Hg with evidence of adequate tissue perfusion, defined as a urine output higher than 0.5 mL/kg/h for 2 consecutive hours or a decrease by more than 10% in the serum lactate levels compared to baseline. The median time to open-label vasopressor administration was significantly lower in the early norepinephrine compared to the placebo group. The number of patients who attained shock control after 6 h of initial resuscitation was significantly higher with early administration of norepinephrine compared to placebo. In-hospital and 28-day hospital mortality were not significantly different between groups. Fewer episodes of cardiogenic pulmonary edema and arrhythmias were observed in the early norepinephrine group. This study demonstrated that the early commencement of norepinephrine results in more rapid attainment of resuscitation goals. Table 22.1 summarizes studies on the early administration of norepinephrine combined with a restrictive resuscitation strategy.

The recently published CLOVERS RCT enrolled 1563 patients at 60 centers in the US including patients with septic shock with a systolic blood pressure <100 mm Hg after ≥1000 ml of IV fluids [28]. Patients were randomized to a restrictive or a liberal fluid resuscitation strategy for a 24-hour period. In the restrictive group, fluid boluses of up to 2 L were administered, followed by early norepinephrine and a second vasopressor if necessary for MAP of <65 or sys BP <90. Rescue boluses of 500 ml were allowed based on predefined criteria. In the liberal group, patients received up to 2 L fluids at randomization followed by additional 500 ml boluses based on predefined criteria. Rescue vasopressors were administered in the liberal group for severe hypotension, persisting hyperlactatemia, fluid overload state, if >5 L of fluid had already been administered, or based on clinician judgment. Patients in the liberal group received significantly larger volumes of fluid at 6- and 24-hours post-randomization. Death before discharge at 90 days, the primary outcome, was not significantly different between the two groups. At 28 days, the number of days free of organ-support was similar in both groups. The ICU- and hospital-free days were similar at 28 days. The all-cause mortality at 90 days was also similar between both groups. The CLOVERS trial demonstrated that an early vasopressor-based resuscitation strategy is safe and effective compared with a fluid-liberal resuscitation strategy in patients with septic shock. However, the resuscitation strategy needs to be tailored to the clinical situation, especially among patients who may hypovolemic or fluid overloaded.

Key Points

- The landmark EGDT trial and the subsequent body of evidence from later trials have led to the widespread practice of fixed-volume fluid resuscitation in patients with septic shock.
- Excessive fluid administration with cumulative positive balance may lead to fluid overload, raised venous pressures, and a vasodilatory state with impairment of organ function.
- There is robust evidence that suggests adverse clinical outcomes due to overzealous fluid administration in critically ill patients.
- An alternative approach may be to adopt a fluid-restrictive resuscitation strategy combined with early use of vasopressors to maintain perfusion pressure. Preliminary evidence suggests potential improvement in clinical outcomes with a fluid-restrictive strategy.
- The optimal volume of initial fluid resuscitation, timing of commencement of vasopressor therapy, and appropriate hemodynamic targets need to be evaluated in future studies.

Table 22.1 Studies evaluating the use of early norepinephrine administration with restricted fluid resuscitation

Study/year	Design	Intervention	Control	Outcomes
Morimatsu et al. (2004) [24]	Retrospective observational	Limited fluid resuscitation, early norepinephrine (1.3 h after ICU admission)	No control group	Hospital mortality lower than predicted (by SAPS II score) with early norepinephrine. Predicted hospital mortality 40.8%; actual mortality 34.5% In the severely ill, predicted vs. actual: 74.4% vs. 50% ($p = 0.007$)
Bai et al. (2014) [25]	Retrospective observational	Norepinephrine <2 h after septic shock	Norepinephrine ≥2 h after septic shock	28-day mortality was significant with norepinephrine ≥2 h. every 1 h delay in norepinephrine administration increased mortality by 5.3% in the first 6 h
Permpikul et al. (2019) [26]	RCT	Norepinephrine within 1 h of septic shock	Placebo infusion. Open-label vasopressors for MAP <65 mm Hg	"Shock control" achieved earlier with norepinephrine. No difference in in-hospital or 28-day mortality. Less cardiogenic pulmonary edema and arrhythmias with norepinephrine
CLOVERS (2023) [28]	RCT	Fluid-restrictive: Boluses up to 2 L, including pre-randomization; norepinephrine, second vasopressor for MAP <65 or sys BP <90. Rescue boluses of 500 ml	Fluid-liberal: 2 L at randomization; (may restrict to 1 L). Additional 500 ml boluses based on pre-defined criteria	No difference between groups in mortality before discharge home by day 90

Abbreviations: *SAPS II* simplified acute physiology score II, *RCT* randomized controlled trial, *MAP* mean arterial pressure

References

1. Evans L, Rhodes A, Alhazzani W, Antonelli M, Coopersmith CM, French C, et al. Surviving sepsis campaign: international guidelines for management of sepsis and septic shock 2021. Intensive Care Med. 2021;47(11):1181–247. https://doi.org/10.1007/s00134-021-06506-y.
2. Nguyen HB, Jaehne AK, Jayaprakash N, Semler MW, Hegab S, Yataco AC, et al. Early goal-directed therapy in severe sepsis and septic shock: insights and comparisons to ProCESS, ProMISe, and ARISE. Crit Care. 2016;20(1):160.
3. Iba T, Levy JH. Derangement of the endothelial glycocalyx in sepsis. J Thromb Haemost. 2019;17(2):283–94.
4. Rivers E, Nguyen B, Havstad S, Ressler J, Muzzin A, Knoblich B, et al. Early goal-directed therapy in the treatment of severe sepsis and septic shock. N Engl J Med. 2001;345(19):1368–77. https://doi.org/10.1056/NEJMoa010307.
5. Lin SM, Huang CD, Lin HC, Liu CY, Wang CH, Kuo HP. A modified goal-directed protocol improves clinical outcomes in intensive care unit patients with septic shock: a randomized controlled trial. Shock. 2006;26(6):551–7.
6. Early Goal-Directed Therapy Collaborative Group of Zhejiang Province. The effect of early goal-directed therapy on treatment of critical patients with severe sepsis/septic shock: a multi-center, prospective, randomized, controlled study. Zhongguo Wei Zhong Bing Ji Jiu Yi Xue. 2010;22(6):331–4.
7. Xu JY, Chen QH, Liu SQ, Pan C, Xu XP, Han JB, et al. The effect of early goal-directed therapy on outcome in adult severe sepsis and septic shock patients: a meta-analysis of randomized clinical trials. Anesth Analg. 2016;123(2):371–81.
8. ProCESS Investigators, Yealy DM, Kellum JA, Huang DT, Barnato AE, Weissfeld LA, et al. A randomized trial of protocol-based care for early septic shock. N Engl J Med. 2014;370(18):1683–93.
9. ARISE Investigators, ANZICS Clinical Trials Group, Peake SL, Delaney A, Bailey M, Bellomo R, et al. Goal-directed resuscitation for patients with early septic shock. N Engl J Med. 2014;371(16):1496–506.
10. Mouncey PR, Osborn TM, Power GS, Harrison DA, Sadique MZ, Grieve RD, et al. Trial of early, goal-directed resuscitation for septic shock. N Engl J Med. 2015;372(14):1301–11.
11. Hernández G, Ospina-Tascón GA, Damiani LP, Estenssoro E, Dubin A, Hurtado J, et al. Effect of a resuscitation strategy targeting peripheral perfusion status vs serum lactate levels on 28-day mortality among patients with septic shock. JAMA. 2019;321(7):654–64.
12. Marik PE. Iatrogenic salt water drowning and the hazards of a high central venous pressure. Ann Intensive Care. 2014;4:21.
13. Legrand M, Dupuis C, Simon C, Gayat E, Mateo J, Lukaszewicz AC, et al. Association between systemic hemodynamics and septic acute kidney injury in critically ill patients: a retrospective observational study. Crit Care. 2013;17(6):R278.
14. Monge García MI, Guijo González P, Gracia Romero M, Gil Cano A, Oscier C, Rhodes A, et al. Effects of fluid administration on arterial load in septic shock patients. Intensive Care Med. 2015;41(7):1247–55.
15. Pohl U, De Wit C, Gloe T. Large arterioles in the control of blood flow: role of endothelium-dependent dilation. Acta Physiol Scand. 2000;168(4):505–10.
16. Hennig T, Mogensen C, Kirsch J, Pohl U, Gloe T. Shear stress induces the release of an endothelial elastase: role in integrin α(v)β(3)-mediated FGF-2 release. J Vasc Res. 2011;48(6):453–64.
17. Maitland K, Kiguli S, Opoka RO, Engoru C, Olupot-Olupot P, Akech SO, et al. Mortality after fluid bolus in African children with severe infection. N Engl J Med. 2011;364(26):2483–95.
18. Boyd JH, Forbes J, Nakada TA, Walley KR, Russell JA. Fluid resuscitation in septic shock: a positive fluid balance and elevated central venous pressure are associated with increased mortality. Crit Care Med. 2011;39(2):259–65.

19. Vincent JL, Sakr Y, Sprung C, Ranieri V, Reinhart K, Gerlach H, et al. Sepsis in European intensive care units: results of the SOAP study. Crit Care Med. 2006;34(2):344–53.
20. National Heart, Lung, and Blood Institute Acute Respiratory Distress Syndrome (ARDS) Clinical Trials Network, Wiedemann HP, Wheeler AP, Bernard GR, Thompson BT, Hayden D, et al. Comparison of two fluid-management strategies in acute lung injury. N Engl J Med. 2006;354(24):2564–75.
21. de-Madaria E, Buxbaum JL, Maisonneuve P, García García de Paredes A, Zapater P, Guilabert L, et al. Aggressive or moderate fluid resuscitation in acute pancreatitis. N Engl J Med. 2022;387(11):989–1000.
22. Spiegel R. Stressed vs. unstressed volume and its relevance to critical care practitioners. Clin Exp Emerg Med. 2016;3(1):52–4.
23. Nunes TSO, Ladeira RT, Bafi AT, de Azevedo LCP, Machado FR, Freitas FGR. Duration of hemodynamic effects of crystalloids in patients with circulatory shock after initial resuscitation. Ann Intensive Care. 2014;4:25. https://doi.org/10.1186/s13613-014-0025-9.
24. The CLASSIC Trial Group, The Scandinavian Critical Care Trials Group, Hjortrup PB, Haase N, Bundgaard H, Thomsen SL, et al. Restricting volumes of resuscitation fluid in adults with septic shock after initial management: the CLASSIC randomised, parallel-group, multicentre feasibility trial. Intensive Care Med. 2016;42(11):1695–705.
25. Morimatsu H, Singh K, Uchino S, Bellomo R, Hart G. Early and exclusive use of norepinephrine in septic shock. Resuscitation. 2004;62(2):249–54.
26. Bai X, Yu W, Ji W, Lin Z, Tan S, Duan K, et al. Early versus delayed administration of norepinephrine in patients with septic shock. Crit Care. 2014;18(5):532.
27. Permpikul C, Tongyoo S, Viarasilpa T, Trainarongsakul T, Chakorn T, Udompanturak S. Early use of norepinephrine in septic shock resuscitation (CENSER): a randomized trial. Am J Respir Crit Care Med. 2019;199(9):1097–105. https://doi.org/10.1164/rccm.201806-1034OC.
28. National Heart, Lung, and Blood Institute Prevention and Early Treatment of Acute Lung Injury Clinical Trials Network, Shapiro NI, Douglas IS, Brower RG, Brown SM, Exline MC, et al. Early Restrictive or Liberal Fluid Management for Sepsis-Induced Hypotension. N Engl J Med. 2023 Feb 9;388(6):499–510.

Epinephrine and Outcomes Following Cardiac Arrest

23

23.1 Introduction

Clinical outcomes from out-of-hospital cardiac arrest remain poor, with only 6.6% of patients surviving to hospital discharge according to the Cardiac Arrest Registry to Enhance Survival (CARES) report of 2020 [1]. The use of epinephrine was found to improve survival among dog models of asphyxia-induced cardiac arrest from studies conducted in the1960s [2], and guidelines continue to recommend its use [3, 4]. Epinephrine is presumed to augment myocardial perfusion through alpha-1 receptor stimulation, thereby increasing the aortic diastolic and the coronary perfusion pressures during cardiopulmonary resuscitation (CPR). However, concurrent beta-adrenergic stimulation might increase the myocardial oxygen demand and increase the propensity to arrhythmias. Besides, although epinephrine may increase the global macrocirculatory blood flow, it might compromise microcirculatory flow, particularly in the brain, which may lead to poor neurological outcomes [5, 6]. Furthermore, epinephrine-mediated alpha-1-adrenergic stimulation might trigger platelet activation and predispose to thrombogenicity [7]. The precise role of epinephrine in cardiac arrest has never been evaluated in robust clinical trials and has been the subject of debate in recent years.

23.2 Could Epinephrine Lead to Adverse Outcomes Following Out-of-Hospital Cardiac Arrest?

Several observational studies and randomized controlled trials (RCTs) have raised doubts about the purported beneficial effects of epinephrine in out-of-hospital cardiac arrest, particularly regarding long-term and neurological outcomes (Table 23.1).

J. Chacko et al., *Controversies in Critical Care*,
https://doi.org/10.1007/978-981-19-9940-6_23

Table 23.1 Main observational studies and randomized controlled trials that evaluated the efficacy of epinephrine in out-of-hospital cardiac arrest

Study/year	Country	Design	No: of patients	Main findings
Hagihara et al. (2012) [8]	Japan	Prospective observational	417,188	ROSC higher with epinephrine; 1-month survival and good neurological outcome; lower with epinephrine
Dumas et al. (2014) [9]	France	Observational	1556	Worse neurological outcomes with epinephrine; delay in epinephrine administration associated with poor outcomes
Perkins et al. (2018) [10]	UK	RCT	4015	ROSC achieved more often with epinephrine. 30-day survival, survival to hospital admission, and discharge higher with epinephrine. No difference in neurological outcomes at hospital discharge and 3 months. Severe neurological impairment higher with epinephrine
Olasveengen et al. (2012) [11]	Norway	RCT	851	Survival to hospital admission higher with epinephrine. Survival to hospital discharge, favorable neurological outcome, 1-year survival higher with no epinephrine
Jacobs et al. (2011) [12]	Australia	RCT	534	Survival to hospital admission higher with epinephrine. No difference in survival to hospital discharge. ROSC higher with epinephrine if initial rhythm non-shockable

Abbreviations: *RCT* randomized controlled trial, *ROSC* return of spontaneous circulation

23.2.1 Observational Studies

An observational study from Japan analyzed 417,188 patients who suffered out-of-hospital cardiac arrest during the period between 2005 and 2008 [8]. Return of spontaneous circulation (ROSC) was achieved in a significantly higher number of patients who received epinephrine compared to those who did not [2786/15,030 (18.5%) vs. 23,042/402,158 (5.7%), $p < 0.001$]. The attainment of ROSC remained significantly higher with epinephrine on propensity-matched analysis. In contrast, survival at 1 month was lower with epinephrine use. Besides, a good neurological outcome, defined as a cerebral performance category (CPC) score of 1–2 with independent daily living and ability to work in a sheltered environment, was lower among patients who received epinephrine. A good overall performance category (OPC) score of 1–2 (ranging from normal function up to a level of moderate disability) was also lower among patients who received epinephrine during resuscitation. These negative associations with epinephrine use remained significant on propensity-matched analysis.

In a retrospective cohort study of 1556 patients who sustained out-of-hospital cardiac arrest, epinephrine-treated patients experienced a significantly worse neurological outcome compared to those who did not receive epinephrine (17% vs. 63%; $p < 0.001$) [9]. Furthermore, a longer time interval between cardiac arrest and epinephrine administration was associated with poor outcomes. Epinephrine administration within the first 9 min of cardiac arrest resulted in more favorable outcomes.

These observational studies suggested that epinephrine may enable ROSC, but at the cost of poor long-term outcomes.

23.2.2 Randomized Controlled Trials

In light of observational studies that pointed toward worse long-term outcomes with epinephrine use in out-of-hospital cardiac arrest, the PARAMEDIC 2 RCT was conducted by the ambulance services of the National Health Services (NHS) in the UK. The trial randomized patients who suffered out-of-hospital cardiac arrest with failed initial attempts at CPR and defibrillation to receive 1 mg epinephrine or saline placebo by the intravenous or intraosseous route at 3–5 min intervals [10]. The epinephrine group included 4015 patients with 3999 patients in the placebo group. ROSC was achieved more often in patients who received epinephrine compared to placebo (36.3% vs. 11.7%). The primary outcome, survival at 30 days, was significantly higher in the epinephrine compared to the placebo group (3.2% vs. 2.4%, OR: 1.39, 95% CI: 1.06–1.82).

Among the secondary outcomes, survival to hospital admission and hospital discharge was significantly higher with epinephrine compared to placebo. However, there was no significant difference between the two groups in favorable neurological outcomes, defined as a score of 3 or less on the modified Rankin scale, at hospital discharge (2.2% vs. 1.9%) and at 3 months (2.1% vs.1.6%). Severely impaired neurological function (a score of 4 or 5 on the modified Rankin scale) was higher with the use of epinephrine (31% vs. 17.8%). This study demonstrated that although epinephrine administration in out-of-hospital may improve survival, long-term neurological outcomes may be worse compared to placebo.

An RCT from Norway including 851 patients with out-of-hospital cardiac arrest compared those who received intravenous medication according to the ACLS protocol with those in whom IV access and drug administration were delayed until 5 min after ROSC [13]. Intravenous epinephrine was administered to 330/418 (79%) patients in the IV group. Among 286 patients with a shockable rhythm (ventricular fibrillation or pulseless ventricular tachycardia), there was no difference in the attainment of ROSC, survival to ICU admission, or survival to discharge from hospital between patients who received intravenous medication compared to those who did not. Among 565 patients who presented with an initial non-shockable rhythm (asystole or pulseless electrical activity), the attainment of ROSC and survival to ICU admission were significantly higher with intravenous drug administration. However, survival to hospital discharge was low and did not differ significantly between the two groups (IV vs. no IV: 2% vs. 3%, $p = 0.65$). This study demonstrated that IV drug administration during CPR, mostly epinephrine, resulted in increased short-term survival; however, long-term outcomes including survival to hospital discharge did not differ compared with no IV drug administration.

A post hoc analysis of this RCT compared 367 patients who received epinephrine with 481 patients who did not [11]. Survival to hospital admission was significantly higher in the epinephrine group (OR: 2.5, CI 1.9–3.4). However, survival to hospital discharge and a favorable neurological outcome based on the CPC score were significantly more likely in the no-epinephrine group. The 1-year survival was also significantly higher among patients who did not receive epinephrine. On multivariate regression analysis, with VF, response time, witnessed vs. unwitnessed arrest, age, gender, and endotracheal intubation as confounders, the likelihood of survival was significantly greater among patients who did not receive epinephrine.

An RCT from Western Australia including 534 patients echoed the findings of the Norwegian study. Survival to hospital admission was significantly higher among patients randomized to receive epinephrine compared to placebo; however, there was no significant difference in the survival to hospital discharge. Attainment of ROSC was higher with epinephrine among patients who were in an initial non-shockable rhythm [12].

23.3 Evidence from Meta-Analyses

Considering the lack of conclusive evidence from RCTs, and the ethical implications associated with conducting large prospective trials, several meta-analyses have attempted to evaluate the impact of epinephrine in out-of-hospital cardiac arrest.

Lin et al., in their meta-analysis of 14 RCTs, including 12,246 patients, observed improved rates of ROSC and survival to hospital admission; however, no beneficial effect of epinephrine administration was noted on survival to hospital discharge or neurological outcomes [14]. Atiksawedparit et al. noted no improvement in the overall attainment of ROSC nor survival to hospital admission or survival to discharge [15]. Loomba et al. also found a significant increase in the attainment of ROSC with the use of epinephrine in out-of-hospital cardiac arrest, with no significant difference in survival at 1 month or survival to hospital discharge. A significant increase in the incidence of poor neurological outcomes was observed with the use of epinephrine [6]. Vargas et al. analyzed outcomes of 20,716 patients from 15 RCTs; epinephrine compared to placebo was associated with higher rates of survival to hospital admission and survival at discharge, with no significant difference in neurological outcomes. High-dose epinephrine compared to a standard dose was associated with a significantly higher likelihood of attainment of ROSC and survival to hospital admission; neurological outcomes were similar [16].

In contrast to the above studies, the meta-analysis by Ran et al. revealed possible benefit with the use of epinephrine [17]. Their meta-analysis of RCTs and observational studies included 574,392 patients from 24 studies. Epinephrine administration within 10 min of cardiac arrest was associated with an increase in the rate of ROSC, survival to hospital discharge, and favorable neurological outcomes.

The findings of these meta-analyses on the impact of epinephrine on clinical outcomes in out-of-hospital cardiac arrest have been largely conflicting, although a clear beneficial effect toward improved long-term outcomes with epinephrine has remained elusive.

23.4 Does Time to Administration Matter?

Data from earlier observational studies had suggested that earlier compared to later use of epinephrine may result in improved clinical outcomes [18–20]. The time to administration of epinephrine in out-of-hospital cardiac arrest was evaluated in a secondary analysis of the PARAMEDIC 2 RCT that compared epinephrine to placebo [21]. As expected, the likelihood of ROSC decreased in both groups over time. Although the rate of ROSC decreased over time, epinephrine administration was associated with a higher rate of ROSC compared to placebo with the passage of time. However, survival to hospital discharge and at 30 days and the neurological outcome at discharge were similar between the two groups, regardless of the timing of drug administration.

23.5 High- Vs. Standard-Dose Epinephrine

A higher compared to a standard dose of epinephrine may be hypothesized to result in higher aortic diastolic pressures and enhanced coronary perfusion with improved outcomes. In a study of patients who had suffered cardiac arrest receiving CPR, the coronary perfusion pressures were significantly higher compared to baseline only with a higher dose of 0.2 mg/kg, compared to the usual dose of 1 mg. The authors postulated that higher coronary perfusion pressures with high-dose epinephrine compared to the standard dose of 1 mg may improve the likelihood of ROSC [22].

Several RCTs have hence evaluated the impact of a higher dose ranging between 0.1 and 0.2 mg/kg compared to the standard dose of 1 mg. Attainment of ROSC was higher in some studies [23–27]; however, these studies have failed to demonstrate any effect of a higher dose on survival to hospital discharge [14–18] or survival to a favorable neurological outcome [23, 24]. The American Heart Association continues to recommend the standard dose of 1 mg epinephrine intravenously every 3–5 min [3].

Key Points

- Epinephrine is presumed to improve coronary perfusion through alpha-adrenergic stimulation; however, the beta-agonist effects may worsen neurological outcomes.
- The likelihood of ROSC may increase with epinephrine administration during CPR; however, the impact on long-term clinical outcomes, including the potential for harm, is unclear.

- As the duration of cardiac arrest becomes more prolonged, the likelihood of ROSC is higher with epinephrine administration compared to non-administration of epinephrine; nonetheless, this does not improve survival or neurological outcomes.
- Epinephrine should be administered early with an initial non-shockable rhythm; benefits are less certain with an initial shockable rhythm.
- A higher dose of epinephrine, compared to the standard dose of 1 mg every 3–5 min, is unlikely to lead to improved outcomes.

References

1. Chan PS, Girotra S, Tang Y, Al-Araji R, Nallamothu BK, McNally B. Outcomes for out-of-hospital cardiac arrest in the United States during the coronavirus disease 2019 pandemic. JAMA Cardiol. 2021;6(3):296–303.
2. Pearson JW, Redding JS. Epinephrine in cardiac resuscitation. Am Heart J. 1963;66:210–4.
3. Panchal AR, Berg KM, Hirsch KG, Kudenchuk PJ, Del Rios M, Cabañas JG, et al. 2019 American Heart Association focused update on advanced cardiovascular life support: use of advanced airways, vasopressors, and extracorporeal cardiopulmonary resuscitation during cardiac arrest: an update to the American Heart Association guidelines for cardiopulmonary resuscitation and emergency cardiovascular care. Circulation. 2019;140(24):e881–94. https://doi.org/10.1161/CIR.0000000000000732.
4. Perkins GD, Graesner JT, Semeraro F, Olasveengen T, Soar J, Lott C, et al. European resuscitation council guidelines 2021: executive summary. Resuscitation. 2021;161:1–60.
5. Link MS, Berkow LC, Kudenchuk PJ, Halperin HR, Hess EP, Moitra VK, et al. Part 7: adult advanced cardiovascular life support: 2015 American Heart Association guidelines update for cardiopulmonary resuscitation and emergency cardiovascular care. Circulation. 2015;132(18 Suppl 2):S444–64.
6. Loomba RS, Nijhawan K, Aggarwal S, Arora RR. Increased return of spontaneous circulation at the expense of neurologic outcomes: is prehospital epinephrine for out-of-hospital cardiac arrest really worth it? J Crit Care. 2015;30(6):1376–81.
7. Larsson PT, Wallén NH, Egberg N, Hjemdahl P. Alpha-adrenoceptor blockade by phentolamine inhibits adrenaline-induced platelet activation in vivo without affecting resting measurements. Clin Sci (Lond). 1992;82(4):369–76.
8. Hagihara A, Hasegawa M, Abe T, Nagata T, Wakata Y, Miyazaki S. Prehospital epinephrine use and survival among patients with out-of-hospital cardiac arrest. JAMA. 2012;307(11):1161–8.
9. Dumas F, Bougouin W, Geri G, Lamhaut L, Bougle A, Daviaud F, et al. Is epinephrine during cardiac arrest associated with worse outcomes in resuscitated patients? J Am Coll Cardiol. 2014;64(22):2360–7.
10. Perkins GD, Ji C, Deakin CD, Quinn T, Nolan JP, Scomparin C, et al. A randomized trial of epinephrine in out-of-hospital cardiac arrest. N Engl J Med. 2018;379(8):711–21.
11. Olasveengen TM, Wik L, Sunde K, Steen PA. Outcome when adrenaline (epinephrine) was actually given vs. not given - post hoc analysis of a randomized clinical trial. Resuscitation. 2012;83(3):327–32.
12. Jacobs IG, Finn JC, Jelinek GA, Oxer HF, Thompson PL. Effect of adrenaline on survival in out-of-hospital cardiac arrest: a randomised double-blind placebo-controlled trial. Resuscitation. 2011;82(9):1138–43.

13. Olasveengen TM, Sunde K, Brunborg C, Thowsen J, Steen PA, Wik L. Intravenous drug administration during out-of-hospital cardiac arrest: a randomized trial. JAMA. 2009;302(20):2222–9.
14. Lin S, Callaway CW, Shah PS, Wagner JD, Beyene J, Ziegler CP, et al. Adrenaline for out-of-hospital cardiac arrest resuscitation: a systematic review and meta-analysis of randomized controlled trials. Resuscitation. 2014;85(6):732–40.
15. Atiksawedparit P, Rattanasiri S, McEvoy M, Graham CA, Sittichanbuncha Y, Thakkinstian A. Effects of prehospital adrenaline administration on out-of-hospital cardiac arrest outcomes: a systematic review and meta-analysis. Crit Care. 2014;18(4):463.
16. Vargas M, Buonanno P, Iacovazzo C, Servillo G. Epinephrine for out of hospital cardiac arrest: a systematic review and meta-analysis of randomized controlled trials. Resuscitation. 2019;145:151–7.
17. Ran L, Liu J, Tanaka H, Hubble MW, Hiroshi T, Huang W. Early administration of adrenaline for out-of-hospital cardiac arrest: a systematic review and meta-analysis. J Am Heart Assoc. 2020;9(11):e014330.
18. Donnino MW, Salciccioli JD, Howell MD, Cocchi MN, Giberson B, Berg K, et al. Time to administration of epinephrine and outcome after in-hospital cardiac arrest with non-shockable rhythms: retrospective analysis of large in-hospital data registry. BMJ. 2014;348:g3028.
19. Andersen LW, Kurth T, Chase M, Berg KM, Cocchi MN, Callaway C, et al. Early administration of epinephrine (adrenaline) in patients with cardiac arrest with initial shockable rhythm in hospital: propensity score matched analysis. BMJ. 2016;353:i1577.
20. Okubo M, Komukai S, Callaway CW, Izawa J. Association of timing of epinephrine administration with outcomes in adults with out-of-hospital cardiac arrest. JAMA Netw Open. 2021;4(8):e2120176.
21. Perkins GD, Kenna C, Ji C, Deakin CD, Nolan JP, Quinn T, et al. The influence of time to adrenaline administration in the Paramedic 2 randomised controlled trial. Intensive Care Med. 2020;46(3):426–36.
22. Paradis NA, Martin GB, Rosenberg J, Rivers EP, Goetting MG, Appleton TJ, et al. The effect of standard- and high-dose epinephrine on coronary perfusion pressure during prolonged cardiopulmonary resuscitation. JAMA. 1991;265(9):1139–44.
23. Callaham M, Madsen CD, Barton CW, Saunders CE, Pointer J. A randomized clinical trial of high-dose epinephrine and norepinephrine vs standard-dose epinephrine in prehospital cardiac arrest. JAMA. 1992;268(19):2667–72.
24. Choux C, Gueugniaud PY, Barbieux A, Pham E, Lae C, Dubien PY, et al. Standard doses versus repeated high doses of epinephrine in cardiac arrest outside the hospital. Resuscitation. 1995;29(1):3–9.
25. Stiell IG, Hebert PC, Weitzman BN, Wells GA, Raman S, Stark RM, et al. High-dose epinephrine in adult cardiac arrest. N Engl J Med. 1992;327(15):1045–50.
26. Brown CG, Martin DR, Pepe PE, Stueven H, Cummins RO, Gonzalez E, et al. A comparison of standard-dose and high-dose epinephrine in cardiac arrest outside the hospital. The multicenter high-dose epinephrine study group. N Engl J Med. 1992;327(15):1051–5.
27. Sherman BW, Munger MA, Foulke GE, Rutherford WF, Panacek EA. High-dose versus standard-dose epinephrine treatment of cardiac arrest after failure of standard therapy. Pharmacotherapy. 1997;17(2):242–7.

Targeted Temperature Management in Out-of-Hospital Cardiac Arrest

24

24.1 Introduction

Lowering of body temperature was resorted to in ancient times for various ailments. Around 400 BCE, Hippocrates is purported to have applied snow and ice to reduce bleeding. In the early and mid-twentieth century, Temple Fay, a pioneering neurosurgeon, broadened the use of hypothermia, including its use in severe pain, reduction of tumor size, and as a neuroprotective intervention after traumatic brain injury. Wilfred Bigelow ushered in the use of hypothermia during cardiac surgery, with his pioneering animal experiments [1]. The era of deep hypothermic cardiac arrest was heralded by Barnard and Schrir, during surgery of an aneurysm involving the aortic arch and the ascending aorta [2]. Despite progress in cardiac and aortic surgery, hypothermia was cold-shouldered by clinicians due to the potential for complications until the early 1980s when Peter Safar rekindled interest as part of a cardiopulmonary-cerebral resuscitation strategy [3]. However, it was not until the twenty-first century with the publication of two landmark trials in 2002 [4, 5] that induced hypothermia opened a new resuscitative window following cardiac arrest.

Current International Liaison Committee on Resuscitation (ILCOR) guidelines advocate targeted temperature management with a target temperature of 32–36 °C for at least 24 h for all patients in coma after cardiac arrest [6]. However, the ideal temperature range and the duration of maintenance at the set level remain contentious. Although there is consensus among the intensive care community regarding the importance of targeted temperature management, practices vary around the world.

J. Chacko et al., *Controversies in Critical Care*,
https://doi.org/10.1007/978-981-19-9940-6_24

24.2 Physiologic Rationale

Therapeutic hypothermia offers cellular protection against hypoxic-ischemic encephalopathy (HIE). This is considered to be a global process that operates through mechanisms at both molecular and cellular levels. Hypothermia reduces the cerebral metabolic rate of oxygen consumption ($CMRO_2$) with a 6–10% decrease for every degree C drop in body temperature. Unlike reports from early studies, reduction in the $CMRO_2$ is not the sole mechanism of cerebral protection [7]. Ischemia-reperfusion injury results in mitochondrial dysfunction which, in turn, leads to apoptosis. Hypothermia may prevent or interrupt the apoptotic pathway at an early stage. Besides, hypothermia exerts a beneficial impact on ion pump dysfunction, with reduced calcium influx, and thereby reduces neurotoxicity [1]. The immune system is activated by the acutely injured brain. The ischemic insult triggers an inflammatory cascade with the release of interleukin-1 and tumor necrosis factor-alpha by the microglia, endothelial cells, and astrocytes [7]. Animal and clinical studies reveal that hypothermia inhibits the release of pro-inflammatory cytokines and decreases the generation of nitric oxide, a key mediator of post-ischemic brain injury [8]. Ischemia-reperfusion injury following cardiac arrest provokes a significant production of oxygen free radicals. Although hypothermia does not abolish this response, it greatly attenuates the generation of free radicals and allows their scavenging by antioxidant mechanisms [9]. Mild-moderate hypothermia may prevent blood-brain barrier disruption by reducing vascular permeability [10]. Hypothermia may also improve glucose utilization by the brain [11] and reduce seizure activity in the ischemic brain [12].

24.3 The Evidence for Targeted Temperature Management

24.3.1 The Trailblazers: The European and Australian Trials of 2002

In 2002, two pioneering trials rekindled the interest in therapeutic hypothermia following cardiac arrest. The Hypothermia after Cardiac Arrest Study Group (HACA) reported their ground-breaking trial with the use of induced hypothermia among 274 patients across 5 countries in patients who sustained out-of-hospital cardiac arrest due to ventricular fibrillation. A temperature of 32–34 °C was targeted in the hypothermia group and compared with a control group that received standard treatment, aiming for normothermia. A favorable neurological outcome, based on the cerebral-performance category scale, was significantly greater in the hypothermia group. Induced hypothermia also reduced the 6-month mortality. Bernard et al. studied 77 patients who had suffered out-of-hospital cardiac arrest with ventricular fibrillation as the initial rhythm in a quasi-randomized controlled trial. Hypothermia to 33 °C was induced within 2 h of return of spontaneous circulation (ROSC) for a total duration of 12 h; the control group was maintained normothermic. Survival with a good outcome—discharge home or to a rehabilitation facility—was higher with hypothermia. The favorable effect persisted after adjusting for differences in baseline characteristics.

24.3.2 The TTM-1 Trial

The targeted temperature management-1 (TTM-1) trial was designed to confirm the benefits of hypothermia demonstrated in the HACA and Australian trials. Besides, it was unclear whether the observed benefits were from hypothermia or control of fever alone. The trial included patients who suffered out-of-hospital cardiac arrest, regardless of the initial rhythm, and had a poor neurological response (GCS < 8). A total of 950 patients were randomized, aiming for a target temperature of 33 or 36 °C. Rapid cooling was performed using ice-cold fluids, the application of ice, and intravascular or surface cooling devices. All-cause mortality through the period of the trial, the primary outcome, occurred in 50% of patients with a target temperature of 33 °C compared to 48% maintained at 36 °C; the difference was not statistically significant. The secondary outcome, a composite of poor neurological function or death at 180 days, was also similar between the two groups (33 °C vs. 36 °C: 54% vs. 52%). Thus, the TTM-1 trial, in contrast to the 2002 landmark trials, seemed to suggest that cooling to 33 °C did not offer any additional benefit compared to maintaining a temperature of 36 °C, with the primary aim of preventing fever [13].

24.3.3 Duration of Targeted Temperature Management: 24 vs. 48 h

Although improved clinical outcomes were demonstrated with hypothermia, there was ambiguity regarding the duration of targeted temperature management. The Time-differentiated Therapeutic Hypothermia trial aimed to evaluate whether a longer duration of 48 h of hypothermia would be superior to 24 h of maintenance of a target temperature of 33 ± 1 °C. This multicentric trial included 355 patients with out-of-hospital cardiac arrest, with an initial shockable or non-shockable rhythm. The neurological outcome and mortality at 6 months were not significantly different between 24 and 48 h of targeted temperature management. The median duration of ICU stay was longer, and adverse events were higher in the 48 h group. This study demonstrated that a longer duration of 48 h compared with 24 h of targeted temperature management does not result in improved clinical outcomes [14].

24.3.4 Hypothermia in Non-shockable Rhythms: The HYPERION Trial

The efficacy of hypothermia in non-shockable rhythms remained unclear, considering the conflicting results from earlier studies [15, 16]. Against this background, the

HYPERION trial investigators conducted a multicenter randomized controlled trial (RCT) among patients who remained comatose after resuscitation from cardiac arrest following a non-shockable rhythm [17]. In the moderate hypothermia group, patients were cooled to 33 °C for 24 h. Rewarming was carried out at 0.25–0.5 °C per hour, to 36.5–37.5 °C, and maintained at that level for another 24 h. In the normothermia group, the temperature was maintained at 36.5–37.5 °C for 48 h. At 90 days, significantly more patients were alive with a favorable neurological outcome in the hypothermia group compared to the normothermia group (10.2% vs. 5.7%, $p = 0.04$). The 90-day mortality and the incidence of prespecified adverse events did not differ between the two groups. The HYPERION trial strongly suggested improved survival and neurological outcomes with a targeted temperature of 33 °C maintained for 24 h compared to normothermia.

24.3.5 The TTM-2 Trial

Although several RCTs had evaluated the use of induced hypothermia following cardiac arrest and were recommended by guidelines, the impact on clinical outcomes remained equivocal. Considering the harmful effects of fever on neurological outcomes following cardiac arrest, how would a strategy based on normothermia with early treatment of fever compare with hypothermia? The TTM-2 trial randomized 1900 patients who remained comatose after out-of-hospital cardiac arrest of cardiac or non-cardiac origin. In the hypothermia group, patients were cooled using surface or intravascular devices to a target temperature of 33 °C. The temperature was maintained at this level for 28 h after randomization, followed by gradual rewarming to 37 °C. In the normothermia group, a target temperature of 37.5 or less was aimed for. If the temperature exceeded 37.8 °C after conservative measures, cooling was commenced to a target temperature of 37.5 °C. Of the 1900 patients randomized, 1850 were included in the evaluation of all-cause mortality at 6 months, the primary outcome. There was no significant difference in the all-cause mortality at 6 months between the hypothermia and the normothermia group (50% vs. 48%; relative risk with hypothermia, 1.04; 95% CI, 0.94 to 1.14; $P = 0.37$).

Poor functional outcome at 6 months, with a modified Rankin score of 4–6, occurred in 55% of patients in both groups (relative risk with hypothermia, 1.00; 95% CI, 0.92 to 1.09). Among adverse events noted, the incidence of arrhythmia leading to hemodynamic instability was more common in the hypothermia group. The TTM-2 trial suggested no improvement in clinical outcomes including mortality and neurological outcome at 6 months with hypothermia targeting a temperature of 33 °C compared to normothermia with control of fever, maintaining the temperature at 37.5 °C or less [18]. Table 24.1 summarizes recent RCTs that evaluated the efficacy of induced hypothermia in the post-cardiac arrest setting.

Table 24.1 Recent RCTs on the efficacy of hypothermia in post-cardiac arrest patients

Study/year	Population	Group 1	Group 2	Outcomes
Nielsen et al. (TTM-1, 2013) [13]	Patients in coma after OHCA	33 °C for 28 h (total intervention period: 40 h)	36 °C for 28 h (total intervention period: 40 h)	All-cause mortality similar; secondary outcome: composite of poor neurological function or death at 180 days, similar
Kirkegaard et al. (2017) [14]	OHCA patients with any rhythm	33 ± 1 °C for 24 h	33 ± 1 °C for 48 h	Neurological outcome and mortality at 6 months similar. Median duration of ICU longer, adverse events higher in the 48 h group
Lascarrou et al. (HYPERION, 2019) [17]	OHCA with non-shockable rhythm	33 °C for 24 h	37 °C for 24 h	Significantly more patients alive with a favorable neurological outcome at 90 days with hypothermia. The 90-day mortality, adverse events similar
Dankiewicz et al. (TTM-2, 2021) [18]	Patients in coma after OHCA	33 °C for 28 h (total intervention period: 40 h)	37.5 °C for 28 h (total intervention period: 40 h)	6-month all-cause mortality, poor functional status at 6 months, similar. Arrhythmias with hemodynamic instability more common with hypothermia

Abbreviation: *OHCA* out-of-hospital cardiac arrest

24.4 Points of Contention

The TTM-1 trial aimed to address the adverse impact of fever in the control group in previous studies of hypothermia, by comparing a target temperature of 33 °C with 36 °C. This trial did not reveal superior outcomes with a target temperature of 33 °C. However, critics point to the prolonged duration of >9 h it took to establish hypothermia in the 33 °C group as a likely confounder. The mean time to attain the target temperature was >7 h in the TTM-2 trial although the investigators had aimed to achieve it by 90 min [19]. After the TTM-1 trial, many centers across the world switched to a strategy of normothermia post-cardiac arrest. In a before-after study from Melbourne, Australia, fewer patients underwent active cooling after the change of policy; the target temperature was achieved less often, and there was a higher incidence of fever after the change of strategy. Fewer patients were discharged alive and had a favorable neurological outcome after switching of target temperature from 33 to 36 °C [20].

The ANZICS database study included 16,252 patients from 140 hospitals admitted to ICU post-out-of-hospital cardiac arrest. This study revealed an increase in the mean lowest temperature of post-cardiac arrest patients during the first 24 h in ICU after the publication of the TTM-1 trial. The frequency of fever also rose during this period. A marginal trend toward increased mortality was also noted during the same period [21]. Perhaps these observational studies suggest that we should exhibit caution in abandoning the use of hypothermia in post-cardiac arrest patients.

24.5 Hypothermia in Relation to the Severity of Post-cardiac Arrest Syndrome

Do the benefits of induced hypothermia depend on the severity of the post-cardiac arrest syndrome? Nishikimi et al., in an observational study, evaluated the outcomes of 1111 patients who suffered out-of-hospital cardiac arrest and received targeted temperature management. The severity of post-cardiac arrest syndrome was classified as low, moderate, or high based on a previously validated risk assessment tool. The authors observed that TTM at 33–34 °C was associated with good neurological outcomes only in post-cardiac arrest syndrome of moderate severity [22]. Thus, large studies including patients with variable degrees of injury may not demonstrate a likely benefit in subgroups of patients who may benefit from hypothermia.

Key Points

- Peter Safar noted in the 1960s that "hypothermia should be started within 30 minutes if there is no sign of CNS recovery." The landmark trials of 2002 triggered a resurgence of enthusiasm for post-cardiac arrest hypothermia. Current international guidelines recommend targeted temperature management post-cardiac arrest to prevent hypoxic-ischemic damage to the brain.
- Hypothermia may protect the brain through several putative mechanisms including reduction of $CMRO_2$, attenuation of apoptosis, inhibition of the inflammatory response, and scavenging of free radicals.
- The 2002 trailblazers had demonstrated improved clinical outcomes in patients with a shockable rhythm; the more recent HYPERION trial suggests possible benefit with targeted temperature management in non-shockable rhythms.
- The TTM-1 and TTM-2 trials did not show additional benefit from cooling, compared to the maintenance of body temperature close to normal levels. However, the slow initiation of hypothermia in both these trials may have confounded the results.

- Observational evidence suggests that after the publication of the TTM-2 trial, temperature management has been inconsistent in many centers, with a trend toward worse outcomes with hyperthermia.
- It is plausible that the benefit related to hypothermia may be related to the severity of the post-cardiac arrest syndrome, with improved outcomes in patients with moderate severity compared to mild or high severity.
- The evidence for optimal temperature management in the post-cardiac arrest scenario remains equivocal and requires further evaluation.

References

1. Bigelow WG, Callaghan JC, Hopps JA. General hypothermia for experimental intracardiac surgery; the use of electrophrenic respirations, an artificial pacemaker for cardiac standstill and radio-frequency rewarming in general hypothermia. Ann Surg. 1950;132(3):531–9.
2. Barnard CN, Schrire V. The surgical treatment of acquired aneurysm of the throracic aorta. Thorax. 1963;18:101–15.
3. Safar P. On the future of reanimatology. Acad Emerg Med. 2000;7(1):75–89.
4. Bernard SA, Gray TW, Buist MD, Jones BM, Silvester W, Gutteridge G, et al. Treatment of comatose survivors of out-of-hospital cardiac arrest with induced hypothermia. N Engl J Med. 2002;346(8):557–63.
5. Hypothermia after Cardiac Arrest Study Group. Mild therapeutic hypothermia to improve the neurologic outcome after cardiac arrest. N Engl J Med. 2002;346(8):549–56.
6. Donnino MW, Andersen LW, Berg KM, Reynolds JC, Nolan JP, Morley PT, et al. Temperature management after cardiac arrest: an advisory statement by the advanced life support task force of the international liaison committee on resuscitation and the American Heart Association emergency cardiovascular care committee and the council on cardiopulmonary, critical care, perioperative and resuscitation. Circulation. 2015;132(25):2448–56.
7. Small DL, Morley P, Buchan AM. Biology of ischemic cerebral cell death. Prog Cardiovasc Dis. 1999;42(3):185–207.
8. Fischer S, Clauss M, Wiesnet M, Renz D, Schaper W, Karliczek GF. Hypoxia induces permeability in brain microvessel endothelial cells via VEGF and NO. Am J Phys. 1999;276(4):C812–20.
9. Globus MY, Busto R, Lin B, Schnippering H, Ginsberg MD. Detection of free radical activity during transient global ischemia and recirculation: effects of intraischemic brain temperature modulation. J Neurochem. 1995;65(3):1250–6.
10. Novack TA, Dillon MC, Jackson WT. Neurochemical mechanisms in brain injury and treatment: a review. J Clin Exp Neuropsychol. 1996;18(5):685–706.
11. Chatauret N, Zwingmann C, Rose C, Leibfritz D, Butterworth RF. Effects of hypothermia on brain glucose metabolism in acute liver failure: a H/C-nuclear magnetic resonance study. Gastroenterology. 2003;125(3):815–24.
12. Karkar KM, Garcia PA, Bateman LM, Smyth MD, Barbaro NM, Berger M. Focal cooling suppresses spontaneous epileptiform activity without changing the cortical motor threshold. Epilepsia. 2002;43(8):932–5.
13. Nielsen N, Wetterslev J, Cronberg T, Erlinge D, Gasche Y, Hassager C, et al. Targeted temperature management at 33°C versus 36°C after cardiac arrest. N Engl J Med. 2013;369(23):2197–206.
14. Kirkegaard H, Søreide E, de Haas I, Pettilä V, Taccone FS, Arus U, et al. Targeted temperature management for 48 vs 24 hours and neurologic outcome after out-of-hospital cardiac arrest: a randomized clinical trial. JAMA. 2017;318(4):341.

15. Vaahersalo J, Hiltunen P, Tiainen M, Oksanen T, Kaukonen KM, Kurola J, et al. Therapeutic hypothermia after out-of-hospital cardiac arrest in Finnish intensive care units: the FINNRESUSCI study. Intensive Care Med. 2013;39(5):826–37.
16. Chan PS, Berg RA, Tang Y, Curtis LH, Spertus JA, American Heart Association's Get With the Guidelines–Resuscitation Investigators. Association Between Therapeutic Hypothermia and Survival After In-Hospital Cardiac Arrest. JAMA. 2016;316(13):1375–82.
17. Lascarrou JB, Merdji H, Le Gouge A, Colin G, Grillet G, Girardie P, et al. Targeted temperature Management for Cardiac Arrest with nonshockable rhythm. N Engl J Med. 2019;381(24):2327–37.
18. Dankiewicz J, Cronberg T, Lilja G, Jakobsen JC, Levin H, Ullén S, et al. Hypothermia versus Normothermia after out-of-hospital cardiac arrest. N Engl J Med. 2021;384(24):2283–94.
19. Schäfer A, Bauersachs J, Akin M. Therapeutic hypothermia following cardiac arrest after the TTM2 trial - more questions raised than answered. Curr Probl Cardiol. 2021;101046. https://doi.org/10.1016/j.cpcardiol.2021.101046.
20. Bray JE, Stub D, Bloom JE, Segan L, Mitra B, Smith K, et al. Changing target temperature from 33°C to 36°C in the ICU management of out-of-hospital cardiac arrest: a before and after study. Resuscitation. 2017;113:39–43.
21. Salter R, Bailey M, Bellomo R, Eastwood G, Goodwin A, Nielsen N, et al. Changes in temperature management of cardiac arrest patients following publication of the target temperature management trial. Crit Care Med. 2018;46(11):1722–30.
22. Nishikimi M, Ogura T, Nishida K, Hayashida K, Emoto R, Matsui S, et al. Outcome related to level of targeted temperature management in postcardiac arrest syndrome of low, moderate, and high severities: a Nationwide multicenter prospective registry. Crit Care Med. 2021;49(8):e741–50.
23. Siesjö BK, Bengtsson F, Grampp W, Theander S. Calcium, excitotoxins, and neuronal death in the brain. Ann N Y Acad Sci. 1989;568:234–51.

Part III

Acute Kidney Injury and Renal Replacement Therapy

Augmented Renal Clearance: When Supranormal Renal Function May Cause Harm

25

25.1 Introduction

Augmented renal clearance (ARC) is the phenomenon of enhanced renal function in critically ill patients. ARC is characterized by a higher than predicted increase in the renal elimination of solutes. It occurs due to an increase in glomerular filtration and altered renal tubular function, usually manifesting as an increase in the creatinine clearance. ARC leads to increased clearance of drugs excreted through the kidneys resulting in suboptimal concentrations of important medications, including antibiotics, and may lead to treatment failure. This phenomenon was first described more than 40 years ago in burns patients who were observed to have higher than normal creatinine clearance, leading to a reduction in the half-life of intravenously administered tobramycin [1]. ARC has been the focus of extensive research in recent times; however, the pathophysiology is complex, and several unanswered questions remain.

25.2 Definition

ARC is defined as an increase in creatinine clearance above 130 ml/min/1.73 cm^2. It is considered clinically significant at a level of more than 150 ml/min/1.73 m^2 in female and more than 160 ml/min/1.73m^2 in male subjects [2]. ARC may occur in 20–65% of critically ill patients [3]. The duration of ARC has also been proposed as an important consideration. A substantial number of patients develop increased renal solute clearance over the first week of ICU stay, which may remain undetected [4]. In a prospective observational study from a mixed medical-surgical ICU, ARC was identified in 51.6% of patients. Therapeutic failure was defined as an impaired clinical response to the antibiotics administered with the need for alternate therapy.

J. Chacko et al., *Controversies in Critical Care*,
https://doi.org/10.1007/978-981-19-9940-6_25

Patients who had transient ARC (only for 1 day) were less likely to experience therapeutic failure (17.4%) compared to those who experienced ARC throughout the study period (33.3%) [5].

25.3 Risk Factors, Pathophysiological Mechanisms

The systemic inflammatory reaction that occurs in critically ill patients, secondary to major trauma, burns, sepsis, and following major surgery, could play an important role in triggering ARC. The release of inflammatory mediators leads to systemic vasodilatation, with a reduction in the systemic vascular resistance, leading to an increase in the cardiac output, the renal blood flow, and the glomerular filtration rate (GFR). Local release of nitric oxide and prostaglandins has also been implicated in the increase in renal blood flow [6]. Fluid resuscitation and the use of vasopressor medication may also increase the GFR, leading to ARC [7]. Another factor that may play an important role in ARC is the functional reserve of the kidney, which enables an increase in the GFR in response to critical illness (Fig. 25.1).

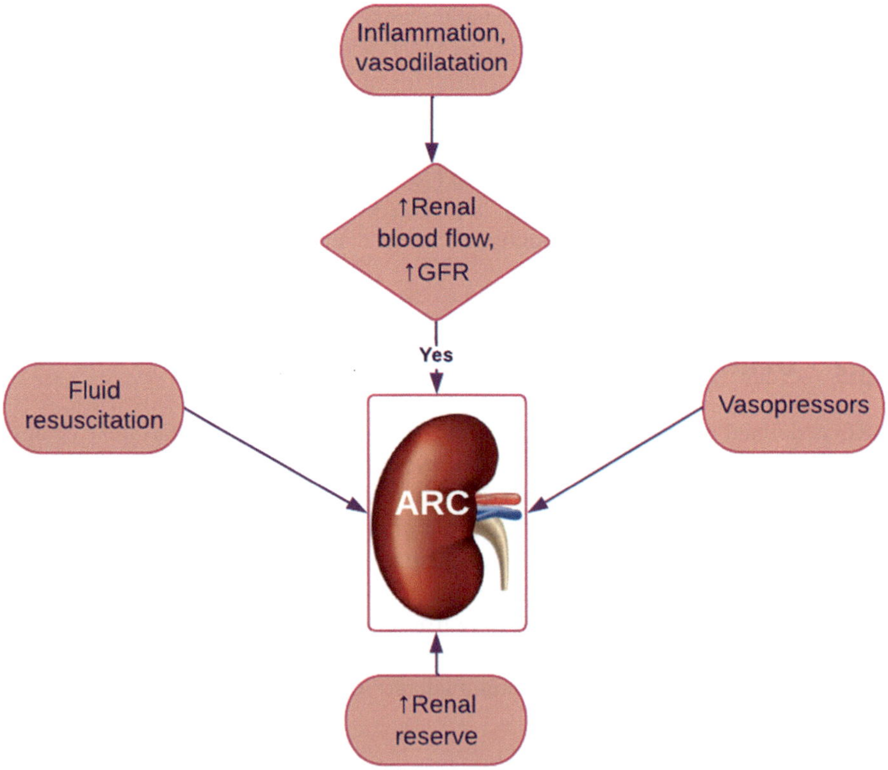

Fig. 25.1 Pathophysiological mechanisms of augmented renal clearance in critically ill patients

The functional reserve of the kidneys is higher in younger subjects, who have a greater propensity for the development of ARC [8]. ARC is frequently observed in neurocritical care, including in patients with traumatic brain injury (TBI) and subarachnoid hemorrhage; contributing factors may be the use of osmotherapy for raised intracranial pressure and vasopressors to maintain the cerebral perfusion pressure. ARC may be mediated by an increase in the atrial natriuretic peptide (ANP) levels resulting from increased sympathetic activity seen in TBI. A rise in ANP levels leads to vasodilatation of the afferent arteriole, with an increase in the renal blood flow and the GFR [9]. Younger age group (34–50 years), polytrauma, and lower severity of illness are common risk factors for ARC [3].

25.4 How Do You Diagnose ARC?

There is ongoing debate regarding the most appropriate methodology to diagnose augmented renal clearance.

The commonly used equations for the calculation of GFR, including the Cockcroft-Gault and the Modification of Diet in Renal Disease equations, are inaccurate in estimating GFR and may under- or overestimate measured values of creatinine clearance (CrCl) [10, 11]. Hence, measurement of urinary CrCl is more appropriate in the diagnosis of ARC. Although an 8–24-hour urine collection is conventionally followed, a 2-h urine collection may be adequate in most circumstances.

$$\text{CrCl} = \text{urinary creatinine } (\text{mg/dl}) \times \text{ collected urinary volume } (\text{ml}) \times 1.73 / \text{serum creatinine} \times \text{ collection time in min} \times \text{ body surface area.}$$

$$\text{Body surface area} = \text{square root of } \left[\text{height } (\text{cm}) \times \text{ weight } (\text{kg}) \ / \ 3600\right].$$

25.5 Scoring Systems to Identify Risk Factors ARC

Various scoring systems have been proposed for the early recognition of ARC. The ARC scoring system is based on age <50 years, presence of trauma, and a SOFA score ≤4 as predictive criteria [8]. It has been shown to have 100% sensitivity and 71% specificity for identifying patients with ARC, based on pharmacokinetic data after piperacillin/tazobactam administration in critically ill patients [12]. The ARCTIC scoring system, which does not include the SOFA score, has been developed to identify ARC in trauma patients and was shown to have a sensitivity of 84% and specificity of 68% in identifying ARC [13] (Table 25.1).

Table 25.1 Scoring systems for the early identification of ARC

	ARC scoring system [7]	ARCTIC scoring system [11]
Criteria	• Age 50 or less: 6 points • Trauma: 3 points • SOFA ≤4: 1 point	• S. creatinine <0.7 mg/dl: 3 points • Male gender: 2 points • Age < 56: 4 points • Age 56–75: 3 points
Risk for ARC	0–6 points: low risk 7–10 points: high risk	<6 points: low risk >6 points: high risk

25.6 What Is the Impact of ARC on Drug Clearance in Critically Ill Patients?

Enhanced renal elimination leads to a reduction in the half-life and reduced effectiveness of several antibiotics in common use among critically ill patients. ARC may lead to increased elimination of beta-lactam antibiotics, including penicillins and cephalosporins. Beta-lactams exhibit time-dependent killing, with their efficacy contingent on the duration for which the serum level of the drug is above the minimum inhibitory concentration. There may be a strong rationale for the administration of beta-lactams as a continuous infusion in patients with ARC [14]. A continuous administration may be particularly relevant as therapeutic drug level monitoring of beta-lactams is rarely carried out in clinical practice.

Therapeutic drug levels may be poorly achieved with carbapenems in the presence of ARC. Extended infusions of 2 g over 3 h after an initial loading dose of 2 g over 30 min may facilitate the attainment of appropriate serum levels of meropenem. Vancomycin is a hydrophilic drug, and 80–90% is excreted unchanged by the kidneys. Target trough levels of vancomycin are difficult to achieve with conventional dosing in the presence of ARC [15]. An initial loading dose of 25–30 mg/kg followed by 45 mg/kg/day in three divided doses or as a continuous infusion along with therapeutic drug level monitoring is recommended. Aminoglycosides and fluoroquinolones are also primarily eliminated by the kidneys and need adjustment of dosing in the presence of ARC. Apart from antibiotics, levetiracetam clearance is higher among the neurocritical care patient population. Besides, patients with ARC may have a shorter duration of action of enoxaparin. Therapeutic drug level monitoring may be an important facet of care in patients presenting with ARC. Therapeutic drug level monitoring in infected body fluids may also be an option, e.g., cerebrospinal fluid in meningitis. This may be important in situations with nonuniform antimicrobial distribution and poor correlation between levels in the plasma and infected tissues [16]. Table 25.2 summarizes recommended dosing for drugs significantly impacted by ARC [17].

Table 25.2 Suggested intravenous dosing for drugs that are significantly impacted by ARC [17]

Drug	Suggested IV dose
Meropenem	Bolus: 2 g over 30 min, followed by 2 g/8 h, administered over 3 h
Vancomycin	Loading dose: 25–30 mg/kg; maintenance: 45 mg/kg/day, as continuous infusion or divided into 3 doses. Therapeutic drug level monitoring recommended. Maintain level at 10–20 mg/l
Piperacillin/ tazobactam	4.5 g/6 h, as extended infusion over 4 h
Levofloxacin	750–1000 mg 24 hourly
Levetiracetam	1000 mg 8 hourly

25.7 ARC and the Newer Antibiotics

Ceftazidime-avibactam is a newer beta-lactam and beta-lactamase combination that is effective in gram-negative infections including strains that produce *Klebsiella pneumoniae* carbapenemase (KPC) and *Enterobacteriaceae* spp. oxacillinase (OXA-48). Ceftazidime-avibactam is predominantly excreted by the kidneys, and dose adjustment is required based on the renal function. In the REPROVE study, the ceftazidime-avibactam combination was compared with meropenem in patients with nosocomial pneumonia. In patients with ARC, the standard dose of ceftazidime 2 g and avibactam 500 mg as a 2 h infusion, administered 8 hourly, attained a target drug concentration above the minimum inhibitory concentration (fT > MIC) for 50% of the time with 95% probability [18]. Population pharmacokinetic models including five phase III trials also suggest that the dose of ceftazidime-avibactam may not require adjustments in patients with ARC [19]. No information is available on dose adjustment of the meropenem-vaborbactam combination in the presence of ARC. Imipenem-relebactam is a new carbapenem-beta-lactamase inhibitor combination. It has enhanced activity against multidrug-resistant strains of *P. aeruginosa* and other carbapenemase-producing *Klebsiella* and *Enterobacteriaceae*. The packet insert warns about insufficient drug levels if the creatinine clearance exceeds 150 ml/min; however, no recommendations are made for dose adjustment [20].

25.8 Efficacy of Combination Therapy in ARC

Combination therapy has been investigated as a possible treatment strategy to overcome ARC using the hollow fiber infection model (HFIM) [21]. HFIM is an in vitro system that enables high-density microbial cultures in an enclosed compartment [22]. Ayeman et al., using the HFIM model, demonstrated the efficacy of the meropenem-ciprofloxacin combination compared to monotherapy with maximum daily doses under ARC conditions [23]. Clinical studies are required to test the efficacy of combination compared to monotherapy among patients with ARC.

Key Points

- ARC is characterized by an enhanced rate of drug elimination by the kidneys and may result in suboptimal drug levels and treatment failure, particularly during antibiotic administration.
- ARC is commonly seen in young patients with relatively low severity of illness. It is associated with sepsis, trauma, burns, and after major surgery.
- Estimation of the glomerular filtration rate based on standard equations may be imprecise in the critical care setting and fail to identify patients with ARC. Measurement of urinary creatinine clearance is more appropriate. The ARC and the ARCTIC scoring systems enable early identification of ARC.
- Adjustment of dose to compensate for enhanced renal elimination is required with many antibiotics commonly used in the critically ill. Therapeutic drug monitoring should be carried out if feasible.
- A strategy of combination therapy with antimicrobials may be one of the options to overcome ARC and ensure antibiotic efficacy.

References

1. Loirat P, Rohan J, Baillet A, Beaufils F, David R, Chapman A. Increased glomerular filtration rate in patients with major burns and its effect on the pharmacokinetics of tobramycin. N Engl J Med. 1978;299(17):915–9.
2. Udy AA, Roberts JA, Boots RJ, Paterson DL, Lipman J. Augmented renal clearance: implications for antibacterial dosing in the critically ill. Clin Pharmacokinet. 2010;49(1):1–16.
3. Bilbao-Meseguer I, Rodríguez-Gascón A, Barrasa H, Isla A, Solinís MÁ. Augmented renal clearance in critically ill patients: a systematic review. Clin Pharmacokinet. 2018;57(9):1107–21.
4. Udy AA, Baptista JP, Lim NL, Joynt GM, Jarrett P, Wockner L, et al. Augmented renal clearance in the ICU: results of a multicenter observational study of renal function in critically ill patients with normal plasma creatinine concentrations. Crit Care Med. 2014;42(3):520–7.
5. Claus BOM, Hoste EA, Colpaert K, Robays H, Decruyenaere J, De Waele JJ. Augmented renal clearance is a common finding with worse clinical outcome in critically ill patients receiving antimicrobial therapy. J Crit Care. 2013;28(5):695–700.
6. Sharma A, Mucino MJ, Ronco C. Renal functional reserve and renal recovery after acute kidney injury. Nephron Clin Pract. 2014;127(1–4):94–100.
7. Udy AA, Jarrett P, Lassig-Smith M, Stuart J, Starr T, Dunlop R, et al. Augmented renal clearance in traumatic brain injury: a single-center observational study of atrial natriuretic peptide, cardiac output, and creatinine clearance. J Neurotrauma. 2017;34(1):137–44.
8. Udy AA, Roberts JA, Shorr AF, Boots RJ, Lipman J. Augmented renal clearance in septic and traumatized patients with normal plasma creatinine concentrations: identifying at-risk patients. Crit Care. 2013;17(1):R35.
9. Khalid F, Yang GL, McGuire JL, Robson MJ, Foreman B, Ngwenya LB, et al. Autonomic dysfunction following traumatic brain injury: translational insights. Neurosurg Focus. 2019;47(5):E8.
10. Baptista JP, Udy AA, Sousa E, Pimentel J, Wang L, Roberts JA, et al. A comparison of estimates of glomerular filtration in critically ill patients with augmented renal clearance. Crit Care. 2011;15(3):R139.

11. Grootaert V, Willems L, Debaveye Y, Meyfroidt G, Spriet I. Augmented renal clearance in the critically ill: how to assess kidney function. Ann Pharmacother. 2012;46(7–8):952–9.
12. Akers KS, Niece KL, Chung KK, Cannon JW, Cota JM, Murray CK. Modified augmented renal clearance score predicts rapid piperacillin and tazobactam clearance in critically ill surgery and trauma patients. J Trauma Acute Care Surg. 2014;77(3 Suppl 2):S163–70.
13. Barletta JF, Mangram AJ, Byrne M, Sucher JF, Hollingworth AK, Ali-Osman FR, et al. Identifying augmented renal clearance in trauma patients: validation of the augmented renal clearance in trauma intensive care scoring system. J Trauma Acute Care Surg. 2017;82(4):665–71.
14. Roberts JA, Lipman J. Optimal doripenem dosing simulations in critically ill nosocomial pneumonia patients with obesity, augmented renal clearance, and decreased bacterial susceptibility. Crit Care Med. 2013;41(2):489–95.
15. Campassi ML, Gonzalez MC, Masevicius FD, Vazquez AR, Moseinco M, Navarro NC, et al. Augmented renal clearance in critically ill patients: incidence, associated factors and effects on vancomycin treatment. Rev Bras Ter Intensiva. 2014;26(1):13–20.
16. Abdul-Aziz MH, Alffenaar JWC, Bassetti M, Bracht H, Dimopoulos G, Marriott D, et al. Antimicrobial therapeutic drug monitoring in critically ill adult patients: a position paper#. Intensive Care Med. 2020;46(6):1127–53.
17. Mahmoud S, Shen C. Augmented renal clearance in critical illness: an important consideration in drug dosing. Pharmaceutics. 2017;9(4):36.
18. Torres A, Zhong N, Pachl J, Timsit JF, Kollef M, Chen Z, et al. Ceftazidime-avibactam versus meropenem in nosocomial pneumonia, including ventilator-associated pneumonia (REPROVE): a randomised, double-blind, phase 3 non-inferiority trial. Lancet Infect Dis. 2018;18(3):285–95.
19. Li J, Lovern M, Green ML, Chiu J, Zhou D, Comisar C, et al. Ceftazidime-avibactam population pharmacokinetic modeling and pharmacodynamic target attainment across adult indications and patient subgroups. Clin Transl Sci. 2019;12(2):151–63.
20. Gorham J, Taccone FS, Hites M. Drug regimens of novel antibiotics in critically ill patients with varying renal functions: a rapid review. Antibiotics. 2022;11(5):546.
21. Yadav R, Bergen PJ, Rogers KE, Kirkpatrick CMJ, Wallis SC, Huang Y, et al. Meropenem-tobramycin combination regimens combat Carbapenem-resistant Pseudomonas aeruginosa in the hollow-fiber infection model simulating augmented renal clearance in critically ill patients. Antimicrob Agents Chemother. 2019;64(1):e01679–19.
22. Sadouki Z, McHugh TD, Aarnoutse R, Ortiz Canseco J, Darlow C, Hope W, et al. Application of the hollow fibre infection model (HFIM) in antimicrobial development: a systematic review and recommendations of reporting. J Antimicrob Chemother. 2021;76(9):2252–9.
23. Agyeman AA, Rogers KE, Tait JR, Bergen PJ, Kirkpatrick CM, Wallis SC, et al. Evaluation of Meropenem-ciprofloxacin combination dosage regimens for the pharmacokinetics of critically ill patients with augmented renal clearance. Clin Pharmacol Ther. 2021;109(4):1104–15.

Renal Replacement Therapy in Acute Kidney Injury: Is Timing All Important?

26

26.1 Introduction

Intensive care physicians often face the vexing question of when to commence renal replacement therapy (RRT) in critically ill patients with acute kidney injury (AKI). Early RRT may be employed for the correction of electrolyte and metabolic abnormalities and prevention of volume overload in patients who continue to require fluid resuscitation. However, an early strategy may entail unnecessary therapy for some patients who might recover renal function without supportive therapy. The hemodynamic instability that often accompanies RRT may perpetuate damage to the kidneys and delay recovery. The proximal convoluted tubules located at the corticomedullary junction may be particularly vulnerable to ischemic insult resulting from hemodynamic instability. This is due to a low partial pressure of oxygen of less than 40 mm Hg at the corticomedullary junction which increases the susceptibility of the tubular cells to RRT-induced damage [1]. Hence, the decision on the timing of commencement of RRT is crucial.

26.2 Renal Replacement Therapy: Benefit vs. Possible Harm

The likelihood of potential benefit compared to possibility of harmful effects must be carefully weighed prior to the commencing RRT. Particularly, in patients without imminent, life-threatening complications and those with a reasonable likelihood of recovery, RRT may impair renal function and may lead to worse clinical outcomes, including mortality [2, 3]. More than three decades ago, during the Vietnam war, Conger et al. proposed that intradialytic hypotension may potentially offset the benefits of early, aggressive RRT and impede recovery from renal failure [4]. Continuous therapies generally maintain better hemodynamic stability compared to intermittent therapies. However, hypotensive episodes do occur with continuous therapies [5]. In

J. Chacko et al., *Controversies in Critical Care*,
https://doi.org/10.1007/978-981-19-9940-6_26

the multicentric BEST trial that evaluated the period prevalence of ARF in intensive care unit, hypotension occurred in 19% of patients who underwent CRRT [6]. Vascular access-related complications and inadequate antibiotic dosing in light of insufficient pharmacokinetic information constitute potential problems related to RRT in the critically ill [7]. Besides, RRT may lead to excessive loss of electrolytes and essential nutrients [8]. Furthermore, the dialytic membrane and the extracorporeal circuit may trigger an inflammatory reaction and lead to adverse outcomes [9]. In contrast, undue delay in commencing RRT may also lead to significant clinical deterioration and adverse outcomes.

Observational studies from the past had suggested potential benefit from early commencement of RRT [10, 11]. However, RRT techniques have been refined over time; besides, overall management of critically ill patients has also progressed over the years [12]. In recent years, several randomized controlled studies (RCTs) have addressed the question of optimal timing of RRT (Table 26.1). Hence, it is appropriate to reconsider the impact of the timing of RRT in light of current evidence.

Table 26.1 RCTs evaluating the timing of RRT

Study/year	AKI stage	Early strategy	Delayed strategy	Main findings	Limitations
Zarbock et al. (ELAIN, 2016) [13]	KDIGO 2	Within 8 h of KDIGO 2	Within 12 h of KDIGO 3 or no RRT	Lower 90-day mortality with early strategy	Small sample size, mostly surgical patients, low fragility index of 3, fluid overload may have occurred in the delayed group. No difference in the 28- and 60-day mortality
Gaudry et al. (AKIKI 1, 2016) [14]	KDIGO 3	Immediately after randomization	Any of $K^+ > 6$ mmol/l, BUN >112 mg/dl, pH <7.15, acute pulmonary edema	No difference in 60-day mortality; no RRT in 49% patients in the delayed group	Advanced AKI in the study population, 50% of patients underwent IHD that may not be standard of care in many ICUs

Table 26.1 (continued)

Study/year	AKI stage	Early strategy	Delayed strategy	Main findings	Limitations
Barbar et al. (IDEAL-ICU, 2018) [15]	RIFLE—stage F	Within 12 h of stage F	After 48 h if renal recovery had not occurred by then	No difference in 90-day mortality	Study not blinded to data collectors, did not attain sample size due to early stoppage
Bagshaw et al. (STAART-AKI, 2020) [16]	KDIGO 2 or 3	Within 12 h of randomization	Any of pH <7.2, or HCO_3 < 12 mmol/l, K+ >6 mmol/l, fluid overload, persistent AKI	No difference in 90-day mortality; RRT-dependence higher at 90 d with early strategy	Decision on RRT based on clinician judgment of equipoise
Gaudry et al. (AKIKI 2, 2021) [17]	KDIGO 3 urine output <0.3 ml/kg/h or <500 ml/day for >72 h, or BUN level between 112–140 mg/dl	Within 12 h of fulfilling criteria	BUN ≥140 mg/dl, urgent need for RRT while waiting	No difference in RRT-free days at 28 day; HR for 60-day mortality higher with delayed strategy	Underpowered to detect difference in RRT-free days. Threshold BUN level to commence RRT is questionable

Abbreviations: *KDIGO* Kidney Disease Improving Global Outcomes score, *BUN* blood urea nitrogen, *AKI* acute kidney injury, *IHD* intermittent hemodialysis, *RIFLE* Risk, Injury, Failure, Loss of function, End-stage renal disease score, *RRT* renal replacement therapy, *HR* hazard ratio

26.3 Early vs. Late: The Evidence

26.3.1 The ELAIN Trial

The ELAIN trial randomized 231 postoperative patients with AKI from a single center in Germany. Among these, 108 (47%) were postoperative cardiac surgical patients [13]. The early group were randomized to receive RRT within 8 h of the diagnosis of KDIGO stage 2 AKI; patients in the late group were randomized to receive RRT within 12 h of KDIGO stage 3. Patients had to meet at least one of the following conditions: severe sepsis, catecholamine infusion, refractory fluid overload, and onset or worsening of non-renal organ dysfunction. In the early group, all

112 patients who were randomized received RRT compared to 108/119 patients in the late group. The primary outcome, the 90-day mortality, was significantly lower in the early group. According to predefined criteria, approximately 75% of all patients had evidence of fluid overload. This finding raises the question whether RRT may have been delayed in some patients with evidence of fluid overload who were randomized to the late group. It is plausible that delay in RRT may have contributed to worse outcomes in this subgroup of patients who were randomized to the late group. Besides, the study revealed a low fragility index of only three patients for 90-day mortality, the primary outcome. This meant that the difference in the 90-day mortality between the two groups would have been non-significant if three more patients had suffered 90-day mortality in the early group. Furthermore, it is difficult to explain a mortality benefit at 90 days, while no difference was observed in the 28- and 60-day mortality.

26.3.2 The AKIKI Trial

In the AKIKI 1 trial, patients with AKI, KDIGO stage 3 were randomized to receive early or late RRT [14]. In the early group, patients were scheduled to undergo RRT immediately after randomization. In the late group, RRT was carried out only if any of the following criteria were present: $K^+ > 6.0$ mmol/l (>5.5 mmol/l after corrective measures), BUN >112 mg/dl, pH < 7.15, and acute pulmonary edema due to fluid overload. In the early group, 305/311 (98.1%) actually received RRT, compared to 157/308 (51%) patients who were randomized to the late group. Mortality at 60 days, the primary outcome, was not significantly different between the two groups. Thus, although nearly half of all patients who were randomized to the late arm did not require RRT, no adverse clinical outcomes were observed.

26.3.3 The IDEAL-ICU Trial

In a multicentric French study, the IDEAL-ICU investigators randomized patients in early-stage septic shock who were in the failure stage (stage F) of the RIFLE classification [15]. The early group underwent RRT within 12 h of reaching stage F, while the late group received RRT after 48 h if recovery of renal function had not occurred during this period. The study was stopped for futility after the second interim analysis. At the time of cessation of the trial, no difference was observed in the 90-day mortality, the primary outcome, between the early and late groups (58% vs. 54%, $p = 0.38$). Among patients randomized to the late group, 38% did not receive RRT.

26.3.4 The STARRT-AKI Trial

The STARRT-AKI trial was a multicentric RCT including critically ill patients from168 sites across 15 countries [16]. Patients who were in KDIGO stage 2 or 3 AKI were randomized if the treating physician considered that there was sufficient equipoise in the choice between an accelerated and a standard strategy. RRT was commenced within 12 h of randomization in the accelerated strategy group. In the standard strategy group, RRT was commenced in the presence of metabolic acidosis (pH <7.2, or $HCO_3 < 12$ mmol/l), hyperkalemia ($K^+ > 6$ mmol/l), fluid overload with hypoxemia, or persistent AKI lasting >72 h after randomization. There was no difference in the 90-day mortality, the primary outcome, between the accelerated and the standard strategy of RRT (43.9% vs. 43.7%; RR: 1, [95% CI 0.93–1.09], $P = 0.92$). At 90 days, RRT-dependence was significantly higher in the accelerated compared to the standard strategy group (10.4% vs. 6%), RR 1.74 [95% CI 1.24–2.43]). Besides, there was a higher incidence of adverse events, including hypotension and hypophosphatemia, in the accelerated strategy group. The composite outcome of all-cause mortality and RRT-dependence at 90 days was not different between the two groups. The ICU, 28-day, and hospital mortality were not significantly different between the two groups. The number of RRT-free days at 90 days was similar between groups. The number of ventilation- and vasopressor-free days at 28 days also did not differ significantly different between the two groups. This study demonstrated no improvement in the 90-day survival with an accelerated strategy of RRT; besides, the accelerated strategy significantly increased RRT-dependence at 90 days.

26.3.5 The AKIKI 2 Trial

Two delayed strategies of RRT were compared in the AKIKI 2 trial among critically ill patients who were mechanically ventilated or on a catecholamine infusion with KDIGO stage 3 of AKI [17]. The study patients were oliguric or anuric (urine output <0.3 ml/kg/h or <500 ml/day for >72 h) or had a blood urea nitrogen level of 112–140 mg/dl. In the delayed group, RRT was carried out within 12 h of meeting the above criteria. In the "more delayed" group, RRT was postponed until the blood urea nitrogen concentration level reached 140 mg/dl or an urgent requirement for RRT arose in the meantime. The primary outcome was the number of RRT-free days until day 28; no significant difference was noted between the delayed and the more-delayed strategies (12 vs. 10 days; $P = 0.93$). The more delayed strategy was one of the risk factors associated with 60-day mortality on multivariable analysis. Other risk factors identified for 60-day mortality included a higher SAPS III score and the requirement for mechanical ventilation. RRT-dependence at 60 days and potential complications of acute kidney injury or RRT were similar between groups.

26.4 Summary

Apart from the ELAIN trial, recently published RCTs support a delayed strategy of RRT in critically ill patients with AKI in the absence of life-threatening complications. These studies reinforce the perspective that initiation of RRT should not depend solely on the stage of AKI. It may be more appropriate to decide on commencement of RRT based on presence of complications, including fluid overload or metabolic abnormalities. Furthermore, a strategy of watchful waiting may enable optimization of clinical status and thus enhance the possibility of renal recovery. In contrast, RRT-related hemodynamic instability could lead to worsening or perpetuation of renal injury and adversely impact recovery.

Other key factors while considering the requirement for RRT are the trajectory of the underlying disease process and the presence of non-renal organ dysfunction. In a patient with clinical resolution of non-renal organ dysfunction, a waiting strategy would probably be more appropriate. However, in the presence of a continued hypermetabolic state or continued requirement for fluid resuscitation, early RRT may be more appropriate. The metabolic and fluid demands far exceed renal capacity in such situations, necessitating prompt supportive therapy. The "frusemide test" has been used to identify patients who may require renal replacement therapy in a previous study [18]. Intravenous frusemide is administered in a dose of 1.0 mg/kg to frusemide-naïve patients and 1.5 mg/kg to those already on frusemide. A urine output of less than 200 ml in 2 h following frusemide administration was highly predictive of patients who required RRT.

Key Points

- Observational studies from the past had suggested that an early-RRT strategy may lead to more favorable clinical outcomes in critically ill patients with AKI.
- However, more recent RCTs support a delayed strategy in the absence of life-threatening complications of AKI.
- Besides complications directly related to therapy, hemodynamic perturbations associated with RRT may adversely impact the recovery from AKI.
- The trajectory of the underlying illness and the metabolic state are also crucial factors to consider in the timing of RRT.
- A dogmatic approach with fastidious reliance on physiological or biochemical parameters is unlikely to be helpful in deciding upon the optimal timing of RRT.
- A holistic, individualized approach based on the clinical situation, physiological, and biochemical parameters is more reasonable compared to a "one-size-fits-all" approach.

References

1. Gaudry S, Quenot J-P, Hertig A, Barbar SD, Hajage D, Ricard J-D, et al. Timing of renal replacement therapy for severe acute kidney injury in critically ill patients. Am J Respir Crit Care Med. 2019;199(9):1066–75. https://doi.org/10.1164/rccm.201810-1906CP.
2. Clec'h C, Gonzalez F, Lautrette A, Nguile-Makao M, Garrouste-Orgeas M, Jamali S, et al. Multiple-center evaluation of mortality associated with acute kidney injury in critically ill patients: a competing risks analysis. Crit Care. 2011;15(3):R128.
3. Elseviers MM, Lins RL, Van der Niepen P, Hoste E, Malbrain ML, Damas P, et al. Renal replacement therapy is an independent risk factor for mortality in critically ill patients with acute kidney injury. Crit Care. 2010;14(6):R221.
4. Conger JD. Does hemodialysis delay recovery from acute renal failure? Semin Dial. 1990;3(3):146–8.
5. Shawwa K, Kompotiatis P, Jentzer JC, Wiley BM, Williams AW, Dillon JJ, et al. Hypotension within one-hour from starting CRRT is associated with in-hospital mortality. J Crit Care. 2019;54:7–13.
6. Uchino S, Kellum JA, Bellomo R, Doig GS, Morimatsu H, Morgera S, et al. Acute renal failure in critically ill patients: a multinational, multicenter study. JAMA. 2005;294(7):813–8.
7. Fissell WH. Antimicrobial dosing in acute renal replacement. Adv Chronic Kidney Dis. 2013;20(1):85–93.
8. Finkel KW, Podoll AS. Complications of continuous renal replacement therapy. Semin Dial. 2009;22(2):155–9.
9. Gutierrez A, Alvestrand A, Wahren J, Bergström J. Effect of in vivo contact between blood and dialysis membranes on protein catabolism in humans. Kidney Int. 1990;38(3):487–94.
10. Gettings LG, Reynolds HN, Scalea T. Outcome in post-traumatic acute renal failure when continuous renal replacement therapy is applied early vs. late. Intensive Care Med. 1999;25(8):805–13. https://doi.org/10.1007/s001340050956.
11. Demirkiliç U, Kuralay E, Yenicesu M, Cağlar K, Oz BS, Cingöz F, Günay C, Yildirim V, Ceylan S, Arslan M, Vural A, Tatar H. Timing of replacement therapy for acute renal failure after cardiac surgery. J Card Surg. 2004;19(1):17–20. https://doi.org/10.1111/j.0886-0440.2004.04004.x.
12. Bagshaw SM, Uchino S, Bellomo R, Morimatsu H, Morgera S, Schetz M, et al. Timing of renal replacement therapy and clinical outcomes in critically ill patients with severe acute kidney injury. J Crit Care. 2009;24(1):129–40.
13. Zarbock A, Kellum JA, Schmidt C, Van Aken H, Wempe C, Pavenstädt H, et al. Effect of early vs delayed initiation of renal replacement therapy on mortality in critically ill patients with acute kidney injury: the ELAIN randomized clinical trial. JAMA. 2016;315(20):2190.
14. Gaudry S, Hajage D, Schortgen F, Martin-Lefevre L, Pons B, Boulet E, et al. Initiation strategies for renal-replacement therapy in the intensive care unit. N Engl J Med. 2016;375(2):122–33.
15. Barbar SD, Clere-Jehl R, Bourredjem A, Hernu R, Montini F, Bruyère R, et al. Timing of renal-replacement therapy in patients with acute kidney injury and sepsis. N Engl J Med. 2018;379(15):1431–42.
16. STARRT-AKI Investigators, Canadian Critical Care Trials Group, Australian and New Zealand Intensive Care Society Clinical Trials Group, United Kingdom Critical Care Research Group, Canadian Nephrology Trials Network, Irish Critical Care Trials Group, Bagshaw SM, Wald R, Adhikari NKJ, et al. Timing of initiation of renal-replacement therapy in acute kidney injury. N Engl J Med. 2020;383(3):240–51. https://doi.org/10.1056/NEJMoa2000741; Erratum in: N Engl J Med. 2020 Jul 15.
17. Gaudry S, Hajage D, Martin-Lefevre L, et al. Comparison of two delayed strategies for renal replacement therapy initiation for severe acute kidney injury (AKIKI 2): a multicentre, open-label, randomised, controlled trial. Lancet. 2021;397(10281):1293–300. https://doi.org/10.1016/S0140-6736(21)00350-0.
18. Lumlertgul N, Peerapornratana S, Trakarnvanich T, Pongsittisak W, Surasit K, Chuasuwan A, et al. Early versus standard initiation of renal replacement therapy in furosemide stress test non-responsive acute kidney injury patients (the FST trial). Crit Care. 2018;22(1):101.

Optimizing the Dose of Renal Replacement Therapy

27

Critically ill patients with acute kidney injury (AKI) often require renal replacement therapy. Compared to conventional, intermittent hemodialysis, continuous renal replacement therapy (CRRT) enables precise control of the volume status with gradual and steady correction of acid-base and electrolyte abnormalities, in contrast to the fluctuating character of intermittent therapies [1]. The ideal approach to renal replacement therapy, however, remains unclear. Continuous therapies may be optimal in critically ill patients, especially in the presence of hemodynamic instability. Although CRRT may be preferred in most critically ill patients, optimization of the dose has been the subject of debate.

27.1 Calculation of CRRT Dose

The total effluent rate represents the CRRT dose and correlates with the solute clearance during therapy. The effluent rate, or dose, depends on the modality of CRRT and is expressed as mL/kg/h. Calculation of the dose of CRRT with various modalities is as follows. Volumes are expressed in mL/kg/h. Figure 27.1 depicts various modalities of CRRT.

- Continuous veno-venous hemofiltration (CVVH): Total replacement fluid (pre- and post-dilution) + fluid removed
- Continuous veno-venous hemodialysis (CVVHD): Dialysate fluid + fluid removed
- Continuous veno-venous hemodiafiltration (CVVHDF): Total replacement fluid (pre and post-dilution) + dialysate + fluid removed

There is no consensus on whether the actual or ideal body weight should be used to calculate the dose; however, it may be preferable to use the actual body weight as it more closely correlates with changes in volume distribution occurring from fluid overload [2].

J. Chacko et al., *Controversies in Critical Care*,
https://doi.org/10.1007/978-981-19-9940-6_27

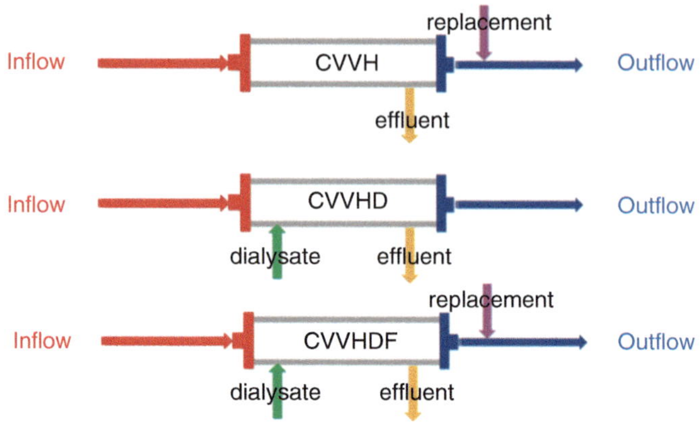

Fig. 27.1 The different modalities of CRRT. Red arrow, inflow to the filter; blue arrow, outflow from the filter; purple arrow, replacement fluid; yellow arrow, effluent fluid; green arrow, dialysate fluid

27.2 Evidence for Dosing

In their seminal paper from more than two decades ago, Ronco et al. had suggested a dose of 35 mL/kg/h with post-dilution CVVH [3]. They based this recommendation on lower mortality at 15 days after cessation of CVVH, compared with a dose of 25 mL/kg/h. A still higher dose of 45 mL/kg/h of this three-arm trial did not result in a further improvement in mortality compared to 35 mL/kg/h. In a subsequent study, CVVH using a dose of 1–2.5 L/h of replacement fluid was compared to CVVDHF with an additional dialysate dose of 1–1.5 L/h in a prospective randomized controlled trial (RCT). The high- and low-dose arms of this trial received 42 mL/kg/h and 25 mL/kg/h, respectively. The 28-day and 3-month survival were significantly higher in the CVVHDF arm at a higher total dose [4]. In contrast to these early studies, most recent trials do not support high-dose CRRT.

The VA/NIH Acute Renal Failure Trial Network study compared high- with low-intensity renal replacement therapy in patients with AKI and at least one other organ failure or sepsis [5]. Hemodynamically stable patients with a cardiovascular SOFA score of 2 or less underwent intermittent hemodialysis, while hemodynamically unstable patients with a score of 3 or 4 underwent CRRT. In the high-intensity arm, CVVHDF was carried out at 35 mL/kg/h; intermittent therapy was performed six times a week in the sustained, low-efficiency dialysis mode. In the low-intensity arm, CVVHDF was carried out at 20 mL/kg/h; sustained, low-efficiency dialysis was performed three times a week. A total of 1124 patients were randomized; 563 patients were included in the high-intensity arm and 561 patients in the low-intensity arm. All-cause mortality at 60 days, the primary endpoint, was 53.6% in the high-intensity and 51.5% in the low-intensity group; the difference was not statistically significant (OR: 1.09; 95% confidence interval: 0.86–1.40; $P = 0.47$). Among the secondary outcomes, renal recovery at 28 days, RRT-free days until day 28, and hospital and ICU-free days until day 60 were also similar between the two groups. The progress of non-renal organ failure, according to organ-specific SOFA scores, was also similar. A higher incidence of hypokalemia and hypophosphatemia was noted in the high-intensity group.

Patients with AKI deemed to require renal replacement therapy by the treating clinician, and fulfilled pre-defined inclusion criteria were randomized to undergo high- or low-intensity CRRT in the RENAL trial [6]. CRRT was performed in the CVVHDF mode, with replacement fluid administered post-filter. In the high-intensity arm, an effluent flow of 40 mL/kg/h was targeted, compared to 25 mL/kg/h in the low-intensity arm. Among 1508 patients enrolled, 747 received high-intensity therapy, and 761 low-intensity therapy. Mortality at 60 days was nearly identical, at 44.7% in each group. RRT-dependence at 28 and 90 days was similar between the two groups. Among other key clinical outcomes, the duration of ICU and hospital stay, duration of mechanical ventilation, and the incidence of non-renal organ failure were also similar between the two groups of patients. The incidence of hypophosphatemia was significantly more in the high-intensity group. Compared to the VA/NIH Acute Renal Failure Trial Network study, the RENAL trial used CRRT as the sole modality of therapy, according to local practice guidelines. Table 27.1 summarizes landmark RCTs that evaluated the dose of RRT in critically ill patients with AKI.

Table 27.1 RCTs comparing high vs. low dose of RRT

Study/year	Population	High-dose	Low-dose	Outcomes
Ronco et al. (2000) [3]	ICU patients with acute renal failure	45 mL/kg/h	Two low doses—35 and 20 mL/kg/h	Survival similar with 35 and 45 mL/kg/h; significantly lower with 25 mL/kg/h
Saudan et al. (2006) [4]	Critically ill patients with acute renal failure	CVVHDF with 1–2.5 L/h replacement fluid +1–1.5 L/h dialysate	CVVH with 1–2.5 L/h replacement fluid	28-day and 3-month survival significantly higher in the high-dose arm
Palevsky et al. (2008) [5]	Critically ill patients with AKI, failure of at least one non-renal organ or sepsis	CVVHDF at 35 mL/kg/h or SLED 6 times/week	CVVHDF at 20 mL/kg/h or SLED thrice weekly	No difference in all-cause mortality at 60 days, renal recovery at 28 days, ICU and hospital-free days at 60 days. Similar progression of non-renal organ failure
Bellomo et al. (RENAL 2009) [6]	Critically ill patients with AKI	CVVHDF at 25 mL/kg/h	CVVHDF at 40 mL/kg/h	60-day mortality, RRT-dependence at 28 and 90 days, duration of hospital and ICU stay, duration of mechanical ventilation, non-renal organ failure similar

CVVH continuous veno-venous hemofiltration, *CVVHDF* continuous veno-venous hemodiafiltration, *SLED* sustained, low-efficiency dialysis

27.3 Meta-Analysis Comparing Doses

The evidence from RCTs is supported by meta-analysis that compared low- vs. high-intensity RRT in critically ill patients. A 2016 Cochrane review included five RCTs. No significant difference was observed between high- and low-intensity RRT in the mortality risk at 30 days or later. The number of patients who were RRT-free was also similar among patients who underwent different levels of intensity of RRT. As observed previously, hypophosphatemia was more common with higher-intensity therapy [7].

Wang et al. analyzed individual patient data in a meta-analysis of seven RCTs, including 3682 patients. The 28-day mortality was similar with standard compared to higher-intensity RRT. However, RRT-dependence at 28 days was greater with high-intensity therapy. Besides, cessation of RRT was significantly more delayed in the high-intensity compared to the standard intensity group. This meta-analysis also suggested no difference in mortality with high-intensity compared to standard dose CRRT; besides, renal recovery appeared to be delayed with high-intensity therapy [8]. The meta-analysis by Jun et al. compared standard dose RRT at 20–25 mL/kg/h or equivalent with high-intensity therapy of 35–48 mL/kg/h or equivalent. Higher intensity therapy did not improve survival or renal recovery in patients with AKI [9].

27.4 Prescribed Vs. Delivered Dose

Interruptions to therapy often occur during CRRT. Therapy may have to be temporarily halted for procedures that require transfer out of the ICU, filter clotting, or catheter malfunction, with delays in recommencement. Hence, the delivered dose may be considerably lower than the prescribed dose. The delivered dose should be evaluated at regular intervals to assess the efficacy of CRRT and may be calculated using the equation below [10].

$$\begin{aligned}&\text{Delivered dose of CRRT} = \text{Total effluent volume } (V) \times \\&\quad \text{Urea nitrogen level in the effluent fluid}(U)/ \\&\quad \text{Urea nitrogen level in the arterial limb of the circuit}(P)\end{aligned}$$

In a retrospective study by Venkataraman et al., the mean duration of CRRT was only around 16 h/day. Although the mean prescribed dose was 24.46 ± 6.73 mL/kg/h, the actual delivered dose was much lower at 16.55 ± 5.41 mL/kg/h [11]. Similarly, among patients who were prescribed a CRRT dose of >35 mL/kg/h, only 22% received the target dose [12]. In the VA/NIH Acute Renal Failure Trial Network study, 89% of the prescribed dose was delivered in the high-intensity arm compared to 95% in the low-intensity arm [5]. The RENAL study achieved 84% of the prescribed dose in the high-intensity compared to 88% in the low-intensity arm [6]. These studies suggest that a considerable gap may exist between the prescribed and delivered dose in patients who are on CRRT. Hence, appropriate adjustments in the prescribed dose need to be undertaken. The KDIGO recommends the prescription of a dose range between 25–30 mL/kg/h aiming to deliver a dose of 20–25 mL/kg/h, to compensate for possible interruptions to therapy. They also suggest frequent assessment and dose adjustment [13].

27.5 High-Volume Hemofiltration (HVHF)

Sepsis is characterized by a dysregulated host response to infection, leading to high circulating levels of cytokines as part of the inflammatory response. The use of HVHF may enable convective clearance of middle molecules including endotoxin, cytokines, and oxygen free radicals that may potentially improve clinical outcomes in sepsis. Techniques aimed at cytokine removal may offer putative benefits by halting the inflammatory cascade and preventing cytokine accumulation, thereby mitigating organ dysfunction [14]. HVHF is conventionally defined as a dose of >35 mL/kg/h, although most studies have used a dose of >50 mL/kg/h [15].

The HEROICS study evaluated the effect of HVHF at 80 mL/kg/h compared to standard care in patients with severe shock 3–24 h post-cardiac surgery [16]. The authors hypothesized that convective removal of toxins and pro-inflammatory mediators and correction of metabolic acidosis may improve clinical outcomes. However, no reduction was observed in the 30-day mortality compared to standard care involving delayed CVVHDF only for conventional indications in AKI.

In a study of septic patients, Zhang et al. compared HVHF at a dose of 50 mL/kg/h with "extra" HVHF at a dose of 85 mL/kg/h. The mortality at 28, 60, and 90 days was comparable between the two groups; besides, the renal outcomes among survivors at 90 days did not differ [17].

The multicenter IVOIRE study compared high vs. conventional volume hemofiltration therapy among patients with septic shock and AKI. In this RCT, HVHF was performed at 70 mL/kg/h compared to standard therapy with 35 mL/kg/h for 96 h [18]. Although the study was ceased prematurely, no reduction was noted in the 28-day mortality in patients who underwent CVVHDF. Besides, there was no apparent improvement in the hemodynamic status or organ dysfunction. Excessive removal of antibiotics was noted during therapy, which could have offset possible beneficial effects. Meta-analyses of RCTs do not support the use of HVHF in patients with sepsis, with no difference observed in mortality or organ dysfunction [19–21].

Key Points

- CRRT is preferred over intermittent therapies in critically ill patients with AKI; it enables precise control of the volume status with gradual and steady correction of acid-base and electrolyte abnormalities.
- The optimal dose of CRRT has been the focus of intense research; early studies had suggested improved clinical outcomes with a dose of ≥35 mL/kg/h.

- More recent RCTs suggest that high-dose therapy does not lead to improved clinical outcomes; besides, it may lead to adverse outcomes including hypophosphatemia, hyperkalemia, and excessive removal of antibiotics.
- The efficacy of CRRT depends on uninterrupted therapy; however, interruptions in therapy are common in critically ill patients who frequently undergo procedures that require transfer out of the ICU. Filter clotting may occur with the delayed recommencement of therapy. Hence, the delivered dose may be considerably lower than the prescribed dose. Consequently, periodic evaluation of the delivered dose is a crucial component of care.
- Based on the available evidence, a prescribed dose of 25–30 mL/kg/h may be appropriate, targeting a delivered dose of 20–25 mL/kg/h.
- High-volume hemofiltration (>50 mL/kg/h) has been investigated for possible benefits from convective removal of endotoxin, cytokines, and oxygen free radicals; however, there is no evidence to support improvement in clinical outcomes.

References

1. Ronco C, Ricci Z. Renal replacement therapies: physiological review. Intensive Care Med. 2008;34(12):2139–46.
2. Vásquez Jiménez E, Anumudu SJ, Neyra JA. Dose of continuous renal replacement therapy in critically ill patients: a bona fide quality indicator. Nephron. 2021;145(2):91–8.
3. Ronco C, Bellomo R, Homel P, Brendolan A, Dan M, Piccinni P, et al. Effects of different doses in continuous veno-venous haemofiltration on outcomes of acute renal failure: a prospective randomised trial. Lancet. 2000;356(9223):26–30.
4. Saudan P, Niederberger M, De Seigneux S, Romand J, Pugin J, Perneger T, et al. Adding a dialysis dose to continuous hemofiltration increases survival in patients with acute renal failure. Kidney Int. 2006;70(7):1312–7.
5. Palevsky PM, Zhang JH, O'Connor TZ, Chertow GM, Crowley ST, et al. For the VA/NIH acute renal failure trial network. Intensity of renal support in critically ill patients with acute kidney injury. N Engl J Med. 2008;359(1):7–20.
6. Bellomo R, Cass A, Cole L, Finfer S, Gallagher M, et al. For the RENAL replacement therapy study investigators. Intensity of continuous renal-replacement therapy in critically ill patients. N Engl J Med. 2009;361(17):1627–38.
7. Fayad AI, Buamscha DG, Ciapponi A. Intensity of continuous renal replacement therapy for acute kidney injury. Cochrane Database Syst Rev. 2016;10:CD010613.
8. Wang Y, Gallagher M, Li Q, Lo S, Cass A, Finfer S, et al. Renal replacement therapy intensity for acute kidney injury and recovery to dialysis independence: a systematic review and individual patient data meta-analysis. Nephrol Dial Transplant. 2018;33(6):1017–24.
9. Jun M, Heerspink HJL, Ninomiya T, Gallagher M, Bellomo R, Myburgh J, et al. Intensities of renal replacement therapy in acute kidney injury: a systematic review and meta-analysis. Clin J Am Soc Nephrol. 2010;5(6):956–63.
10. Macedo E, Claure-Del Granado R, Mehta RL. Effluent volume and dialysis dose in CRRT: time for reappraisal. Nat Rev Nephrol. 2011;8(1):57–60.
11. Venkataraman R, Kellum JA, Palevsky P. Dosing patterns for continuous renal replacement therapy at a large academic medical center in the United States. J Crit Care. 2002;17(4):246–50.

12. Vesconi S, Cruz DN, Fumagalli R, Kindgen-Milles D, Monti G, Marinho A, et al. Delivered dose of renal replacement therapy and mortality in critically ill patients with acute kidney injury. Crit Care. 2009;13(2):R57.
13. Kellum JA, Lameire N, Aspelin P, Barsoum RS, Burdmann EA, Goldstein SL, et al. Kidney disease: improving global outcomes (KDIGO) acute kidney injury work group. KDIGO clinical practice guideline for acute kidney injury. Kidney Int Suppl. 2012;2(1):1–138.
14. Ronco C, Ricci Z, Bellomo R. Importance of increased ultrafiltration volume and impact on mortality: sepsis and cytokine story and the role of continuous veno-venous haemofiltration. Curr Opin Nephrol Hypertens. 2001;10(6):755–61.
15. Joannes-Boyau O, Dewitte A, Honoré PM. High-volume hemofiltration in the intensive care unit. In: Ronco C, Bellomo R, Kellum JA, editors. Critical care nephrology. 2nd ed. Philadelphia, PA: Elsevier; 2019. p. 1034–1037.e2. https://linkinghub.elsevier.com/retrieve/pii/B9780323449427001710.
16. Combes A, Bréchot N, Amour J, Cozic N, Lebreton G, Guidon C, et al. Early high-volume hemofiltration versus standard care for post-cardiac surgery shock. The HEROICS study. Am J Respir Crit Care Med. 2015;192(10):1179–90.
17. Zhang P, Yang Y, Lv R, Zhang Y, Xie W, Chen J. Effect of the intensity of continuous renal replacement therapy in patients with sepsis and acute kidney injury: a single-center randomized clinical trial. Nephrol Dial Transplant. 2012;27(3):967–73.
18. Joannes-Boyau O, Honoré PM, Perez P, Bagshaw SM, Grand H, Canivet JL, et al. High-volume versus standard-volume haemofiltration for septic shock patients with acute kidney injury (IVOIRE study): a multicentre randomized controlled trial. Intensive Care Med. 2013;39(9):1535–46.
19. Lehner GF, Wiedermann CJ, Joannidis M. High-volume hemofiltration in critically ill patients: a systematic review and meta-analysis. Minerva Anestesiol. 2014;80(5):595–609.
20. Clark E, Molnar AO, Joannes-Boyau O, Honoré PM, Sikora L, Bagshaw SM. High-volume hemofiltration for septic acute kidney injury: a systematic review and meta-analysis. Crit Care. 2014;18(1):R7.
21. Borthwick EM, Hill CJ, Rabindranath KS, Maxwell AP, McAuley DF, Blackwood B. High-volume haemofiltration for sepsis in adults. Cochrane Database Syst Rev. 2017;1:CD008075.

Renal Replacement Therapy in the Critically Ill: Continuous Vs. Prolonged Intermittent Therapies

28

28.1 Introduction

The incidence of acute kidney injury (AKI) in critically ill patients varies between 15 and 38% depending on the diagnostic criteria employed [1]. Renal replacement therapy (RRT) is often required for patients with severe AKI. Overall, 5–10% of ICU patients may develop AKI; the incidence may be as high as 20% in patients at risk [2]. AKI is an independent predictor of mortality [3]; 50–70% of patients who undergo RRT do not survive [4].

28.2 How Do Continuous Vs. Prolonged Intermittent Therapies Differ?

In critically ill patients with acute kidney injury who are hemodynamically unstable, continuous renal replacement therapy (CRRT), introduced in 1977 by Kramer et al. [5], is preferred by most clinicians. CRRT enables slow, gradual solute clearance and fluid removal and offers the potential for greater hemodynamic stability compared to the intermittent modalities of renal replacement therapy [6]. The slower, gradual removal of osmotically active particles that accumulate in renal failure results in less pronounced fluid shifts between the intra- and extracellular fluid compartments. Such fluid shifts are particularly deleterious in patients with cerebral edema; a rapid reduction of urea levels and serum osmolality by conventional dialytic techniques may lead to worsening of cerebral edema [7].

Prolonged, intermittent renal replacement therapies (PIRRT) constitute a hybrid modality of RRT carried out over an extended duration in patients who are at risk of hemodynamic instability with conventional, intermittent modalities of RRT. PIRRT may be performed for a variable duration, ranging from 6 to 18 h, most often on a daily basis during the acute phase of illness. PIRRT is also variably described as

J. Chacko et al., *Controversies in Critical Care*,
https://doi.org/10.1007/978-981-19-9940-6_28

Table 28.1 Comparison between prolonged intermittent (PIRRT) and continuous renal replacement therapies (CRRT)

	PIRRT	CRRT
Equipment	Dedicated machines	Conventional dialysis machines
Ease of performance	Less complex	Requires special training
Duration, frequency	Performed daily for 6–18 h per session	Continuous
Clearance	More rapid	Slower clearance over a longer duration
Hemodynamic stability	Usually maintained	May be superior in patients who are unstable
Fluid shift	More likely	Relatively less, lower risk of cerebral edema
Anticoagulation	Lower requirement; may be possible to perform anticoagulation-free treatment	Usually requires some degree of anticoagulation
Patient mobility/ treatment flexibility	Able to mobilize, transfer out of ICU may be scheduled during RRT-free periods	Interruption of therapy required for transfer out of ICU
Expense	Less expensive	More expensive

RRT renal replacement therapy

sustained low-efficiency dialysis (SLED), extended daily dialysis (EDD), or slow, continuous dialysis (SCD). PIRRT may be carried out using conventional dialysis machines and saves on the expense associated with replacement fluids required for CRRT. Thus, PIRRT represents a hybrid therapy by combining the features of CRRT and intermittent therapies with greater flexibility and cost-effectiveness [8]. The other potential advantages of PIRRT include its less labor-intensive nature, a reduced requirement for anticoagulation, and easier availability of expertise. The salient differences between PIRRT and CRRT are summarized in Table 28.1. There is ongoing debate regarding the efficacy of hybrid therapies and their impact on clinical outcomes compared with CRRT among critically ill patients.

28.3 Urea Clearance and Correction of Acidosis with PIRRT

In an early RCT, Kielstein et al. compared the efficacy and hemodynamic tolerance of SLED with CVVH in 39 mechanically ventilated patients with oliguric AKI [9]. The CVVH effluent rate was set at 30 mL/kg/h for a minimum duration of 24 h, while SLED was carried out for 12 h using a single-pass, batch dialysis system. Single-pass machines generate dialysate online using water purified by reverse osmosis; they use a closed reservoir filled with a large volume (75 L) of dialysate. Fresh dialysate is drawn from the top portion of the reservoir, while the return fluid is reintroduced to the bottom portion of the container without mixing [10].

The blood flow rate was set at 200 mL/min in both groups of patients. Both treatment modalities resulted in similar hemodynamic tolerance. The urea clearance was comparable between the two groups of patients; however, correction of acidosis was achieved more rapidly with SLED compared to CVVH. Furthermore, the heparin dose was lower in the SLED group. This study demonstrated that SLED resulted in similar efficacy and hemodynamic tolerance compared to CVVH.

28.4 Hemodynamic Stability During PIRRT

Hypotensive episodes are generally no more frequent with PIRRT compared to continuous therapies [11, 12]. Intra-dialytic hypotension may require an increase in the dose of vasopressor support, especially in patients in shock. Intractable hypotension may occasionally occur; however, these patients may remain unstable even when switched to the CRRT mode [13].

28.5 Electrolyte Abnormalities

Hypokalemia and hypophosphatemia are relatively common complications associated with PIRRT [14] and often require intravenous correction. Regional citrate anticoagulation use may lead to hypernatremia and metabolic alkalosis [15].

28.6 Outcomes of CRRT Vs. PIRRT: Clinical Studies

During the past few years, the efficacy of PIRRT as a viable alternative to CRRT in critically ill patients with AKI has been the focus of clinical research (Table 28.2).

The RESCUE randomized controlled trial (RCT) aimed to evaluate clinical outcomes and cost of care with SLED using a single-pass batch dialysis system among patients with AKI in a surgical ICU [16]. SLED was carried out with a blood flow rate of 100–120 mL/min over a 12-h duration. In the CRRT arm, continuous venovenous hemofiltration (CVVH) was performed at an effluent rate of 35 mL/kg/h with replacement fluid administered pre-filter. The blood flow was set at 100–120 mL/min, and the therapy was scheduled for a 24-h period. The study enrolled 232 patients; 115 underwent SLED, while 117 received CVVH. Pre- and post-treatment blood pressures and vasopressor doses were not different between the two groups. The 90-day mortality, the primary outcome, was similar between the SLED and CVVH groups (49.6% vs. 55.6%, $p = 0.434$). There was no significant difference in the hospital and ICU mortality; the duration of mechanical ventilation and ICU stay was lower in the SLED group. The nursing time dedicated to RRT was significantly lower with SLED therapy, leading to a lower cost of care in this group of patients.

Table 28.2 Controlled studies that compare continuous vs. prolonged intermittent renal replacement therapies

Study/year	Population	Intervention	Control	Outcomes
Schwenger et al. (RESCUE 2012) [16]	AKI patients in a surgical ICU	SLED with blood flow 100–120 mL/min for 12 h	CVVH with effluent rate of 35 mL/kg/h, pre-filter replacement fluid, for 24 h	90-day, hospital, and ICU mortality similar. Duration of ventilation, ICU stay, less with SLED. Blood pressure, vasopressor dose, not different between the two groups. Cost of care less with SLED
Kitchlu et al. (2015) [17]	AKI patients from 4 ICUs in a single center	SLED with blood flow 200 mL/min, dialysate 350 mL/min, minimum 6 h	CVVHD or CVVHDF. Blood flow, 100–200 mL/min; effluent rate, 20–35 mL/kg/h	30-day all-cause mortality similar. RRT dependence at 30 day, early clinical worsening, 48-h mortality similar
Mishra et al. (2017) [18]	Patients with septic shock and AKI	SLED with blood flow 200 mL/min, dialysate 250 mL/min	CVVHDF with effluent rate 30 mL/kg/h	Vasopressor dose similar; efficacy of treatment, assessed by equivalent urea clearance was greater with CRRT. Cost of therapy less with SLED
Abe et al. (2011) [22]	Critically ill patients with AKI	SLED-*f* using dialysate flow 300–500 mL/min, replacement fluid >14 L/session. Each session of 6–8 h	CVVHDF with effluent rate 25 mL/kg/h	30-day survival similar. Renal recovery significantly greater with SELD-*f*
Sun et al. (2014) [23]	Patients with septic shock and AKI	EDHF for 8–12 h/day	CVVH for >72 h	Rate of renal recovery greater, time to recovery shorter with CVVH. 60-day all-cause mortality similar

AKI acute kidney injury, *SLED* sustained, low efficiency dialysis, *CVVH* continuous veno-venous hemofiltration, *CVVHDF* continuous veno-venous hemodiafiltration, *RRT* renal replacement therapy, *CRRT* continuous renal replacement therapy, *SLED-f* sustained low-efficiency daily diafiltration, *EDHF* extended daily hemofiltration

A retrospective cohort study by Kitchlu et al. evaluated patients with AKI who underwent RRT from four ICUs in a single center in Canada [17]. CRRT was performed in the CVVH or continuous veno-venous hemodiafiltration (CVVHDF) mode. The blood flow was set at 100–200 mL/min and effluent rates at 20–35 mL/kg/h. SLED was carried out with a blood flow of 200 mL/min and dialysate flow of 350 mL/min, for a minimum duration of 6 h. The frequency of SLED sessions was based on clinician judgment. The all-cause mortality at 30 days was not significantly different between the SLEDD and CRRT groups (54% vs. 61%). After adjustment for likely confounders, mortality remained similar between the two groups (OR: 1.07, 95% CI: 0.56–2.03). RRT dependence at 30 days and early clinical worsening denoted by an increase in the SOFA score or mortality within 48 h of commencement of RRT were similar between the two groups.

Mishra et al. conducted a pilot RCT comparing the efficacy and hemodynamic stability of SLED compared to CVVHDF [18]. SLED was performed with a blood flow rate of 200 mL/min and dialysate flow of 250 mL/min. An effluent dose of 30 mL/kg/h was used with CVVHDHF. Hemodynamic stability, assessed using the relative dose of vasopressors, was similar between the two groups. The efficacy of treatment, evaluated using equivalent urea clearance, was greater with CRRT compared to SLED. The cost of therapy was significantly lower with SLED compared to CRRT.

28.6.1 Sustained Low-Efficiency Daily Diafiltration (SLED-f)

High flux membranes with greater permeability are employed in CRRT, allowing convective clearance, compared with standard intermittent therapies that rely on diffusive clearance alone. PIRRT may be modified to allow convective clearance using such high-flux membranes. This technique, termed SLED-*f*, overcomes the disadvantage of relying on largely diffusive clearance associated with conventional SLED [19]. Convective clearance using more porous membranes allows clearance of large- and middle-sized molecules including inflammatory mediators in septic patients [20]. Newer machines allow cost-efficient, online generation of replacement fluid [21].

Abe et al. compared CCVHDF with SLED-*f* in 50 critically ill patients with AKI [22]. The CVVHDF effluent rate was 25 mL/kg/h; in the SLED-*f* group, the dialysate flow was set at 300–500 mL/min, and the replacement fluid was administered at >14 L/session. Each SLED-*f* session was between 6 and 8 h. The 30-day survival was similar in both the groups (CVVHDF 76% vs. SLED-*f* 88%). However, renal recovery, based on creatinine clearance, urine output, and spontaneous reduction in the creatinine level, was significantly higher among patients who received SLED-*f* compared to CVVHDF. Besides, the hospital length of stay was also significantly lower in the SLED-*f* group. This study suggested that compared to CVVHDF, prolonged, intermittent therapy with SLED-*f* may result in a higher rate of renal recovery.

A retrospective analysis compared CVVH performed for >72 h with extended daily hemofiltration (EDHF) of 8–12 h daily in patients with septic shock and AKI [23]. A polyacrylonitrile membrane with a bicarbonate-based replacement fluid was used with both modalities. The study included 75 patients who underwent CVVH and 80 who received extended daily hemofiltration. The renal recovery at 60 days was significantly higher, and the time to renal recovery shorter with CVVH compared to extended daily hemofiltration. However, the 60-day all-cause mortality was similar between the CVVH and EDHF groups (CVVH: 44.62%, EDHF 46.25, $p = 0.844$).

28.7 Meta-analysis: CRRT Vs. PIRRT

Several recent meta-analyses have evaluated outcomes with PIRRT compared to CRRT in AKI among critically ill patients. Zhang et al. included 17 studies—7 RCTs and 10 observational studies in their analysis [24]. This meta-analysis comprised of a total of 1208 patients, including 533 from RCTs and 675 from observational studies. There was no mortality difference on a pooled analysis of RCTs that compared SLED with CRRT. Analysis of observational studies revealed marginally lower mortality with CRRT compared to SLED (RR, 0.86; 95% CI, 0.74–1.00; $p = 0.05$). The likelihood of recovery of renal function was similar in both groups (RR 1.14; 95% CI, 0.90–1.46; $p = 0.3$). No significant difference was observed in the volume of fluid removed, the duration of ICU stay, and the biochemical efficacy of the treatment modality, assessed by the serum urea, creatinine, and phosphate levels.

Al Dalbhi et al. analyzed 11 studies of 1160 patients, including 6 RCTs and 5 prospective cohort studies [25]. No statistically significant difference was observed between SLED and CRRT regarding the mortality rate, rate of renal recovery, or dialysis dependence. The rate of fluid removal and length of ICU stay also did not differ significantly between the two groups of patients.

In a network meta-analysis, Ye et al. compared four modalities of RRT, including CRRT, conventional intermittent hemodialysis, SLED, and peritoneal dialysis in critically ill patients with AKI. Network meta-analysis allows the comparison of three or more different types of interventions in a single analysis [26]. The authors observed a possible increase in mortality with CRRT compared to SLED with a low level of certainty (relative risk, 1.06; 95% CI, 0.85–1.33). SLED was associated with the highest rate of renal recovery and the least duration of hospital stay and mechanical ventilation (low certainty).

Key Points

- PIRRT provides gradual removal of fluid and solutes compared to conventional intermittent hemodialysis. It allows greater flexibility to allow for procedures that require the transfer of patients out of ICU for procedures and imaging. Mobilization and rehabilitation are also better facilitated with intermittent compared to continuous therapies.
- Conventional dialysis machines may be used to perform PIRRT. Machines with single-pass batch systems enable online production of ultrapure dialysate, offering ease and convenience of therapy.
- The duration of PIRRT needs individualization and is usually between 6 and 18 h. The duration of therapy may be adjusted to allow scheduled procedures that require transfer out of the ICU.
- Observational studies and RCTs provide strong evidence that PIRRT leads to efficient clearance of solutes and allows adequate fluid removal compared to CRRT. Hemodynamic stability is also maintained in most patients with shock who require vasopressors.
- SLED-*f* uses high flux membranes with greater permeability allowing convective clearance in addition to diffusive clearance alone. Convective clearance enables the clearance of medium and large molecules, including inflammatory mediators.
- Clinical outcomes including mortality and duration of ICU and hospital stay are comparable between PIRRT and CRRT across broad patient cohorts. The cost of care is significantly less with PIRRT modalities.

References

1. Koeze J, Keus F, Dieperink W, van der Horst ICC, Zijlstra JG, van Meurs M. Incidence, timing and outcome of AKI in critically ill patients varies with the definition used and the addition of urine output criteria. BMC Nephrol. 2017;18(1):70.
2. Gupta S, Coca SG, Chan L, Melamed ML, Brenner SK, Hayek SS, et al. AKI treated with renal replacement therapy in critically ill patients with COVID-19. J Am Soc Nephrol. 2021;32(1):161–76.
3. Bagshaw SM, Mortis G, Doig CJ, Godinez-Luna T, Fick GH, Laupland KB. One-year mortality in critically ill patients by severity of kidney dysfunction: a population-based assessment. Am J Kidney Dis. 2006;48(3):402–9.
4. Brown JR, Rezaee ME, Marshall EJ, Matheny ME. Hospital mortality in the United States following acute kidney injury. Biomed Res Int. 2016;2016:4278579.
5. Kramer P, Wigger W, Rieger J, Matthaei D, Scheler F. Arteriovenous haemofiltration: a new and simple method for treatment of over-hydrated patients resistant to diuretics. Klin Wochenschr. 1977;55(22):1121–2.

6. Gasparović V, Filipović-Grcić I, Merkler M, Pisl Z. Continuous renal replacement therapy (CRRT) or intermittent hemodialysis (IHD)—what is the procedure of choice in critically ill patients? Ren Fail. 2003;25(5):855–62.
7. Silver SM, Sterns RH, Halperin ML. Brain swelling after dialysis: old urea or new osmoles? Am J Kidney Dis. 1996;28(1):1–13.
8. Berbece AN, Richardson RMA. Sustained low-efficiency dialysis in the ICU: cost, anticoagulation, and solute removal. Kidney Int. 2006;70(5):963–8.
9. Kielstein JT, Kretschmer U, Ernst T, Hafer C, Bahr MJ, Haller H, et al. Efficacy and cardiovascular tolerability of extended dialysis in critically ill patients: a randomized controlled study. Am J Kidney Dis. 2004;43(2):342–9.
10. Dhondt AW, Vanholder RC, De Smet RV, Claus SA, Waterloos MA, Glorieux GL, et al. Studies on dialysate mixing in the genius® single-pass batch system for hemodialysis therapy. Kidney Int. 2003;63(4):1540–7.
11. Fieghen HE, Friedrich JO, Burns KE, Nisenbaum R, Adhikari NK, Hladunewich MA, et al. The hemodynamic tolerability and feasibility of sustained low efficiency dialysis in the management of critically ill patients with acute kidney injury. BMC Nephrol. 2010;11:32.
12. Kron J, Kron S, Wenkel R, Schuhmacher HU, Thieme U, Leimbach T, et al. Extended daily on-line high-volume haemodiafiltration in septic multiple organ failure: a well-tolerated and feasible procedure. Nephrol Dial Transplant. 2012;27(1):146–52.
13. Kumar VA, Yeun JY, Depner TA, Don BR. Extended daily dialysis vs. continuous hemodialysis for ICU patients with acute renal failure: a two-year single center report. Int J Artif Organs. 2004;27(5):371–9.
14. Ballarin Albino B, Balbi AL, Ponce D. Dialysis complications in AKI patients treated with extended daily dialysis: is the duration of therapy important? Biomed Res Int. 2014;2014:e153626.
15. Morgera S, Scholle C, Melzer C, Slowinski T, Liefeld L, Baumann G, et al. A simple, safe and effective citrate anticoagulation protocol for the genius dialysis system in acute renal failure. Nephron Clin Pract. 2004;98(1):c35–40.
16. Schwenger V, Weigand MA, Hoffmann O, Dikow R, Kihm LP, Seckinger J, et al. Sustained low efficiency dialysis using a single-pass batch system in acute kidney injury—a randomized interventional trial: the REnal replacement therapy study in intensive care unit PatiEnts. Crit Care. 2012;16(4):R140.
17. Kitchlu A, Adhikari N, Burns KEA, Friedrich JO, Garg AX, Klein D, et al. Outcomes of sustained low efficiency dialysis versus continuous renal replacement therapy in critically ill adults with acute kidney injury: a cohort study. BMC Nephrol. 2015;16(1):127.
18. Mishra SB, Azim A, Prasad N, Singh RK, Poddar B, Gurjar M, et al. A pilot randomized controlled trial of comparison between extended daily hemodialysis and continuous veno-venous hemodialysis in patients of acute kidney injury with septic shock. Indian J Crit Care Med. 2017;21(5):262–7.
19. Marshall MR, Ma T, Galler D, Rankin APN, Williams AB. Sustained low-efficiency daily diafiltration (SLEDD-f) for critically ill patients requiring renal replacement therapy: towards an adequate therapy. Nephrol Dial Transplant. 2004;19(4):877–84.
20. Schetz M. Non-renal indications for continuous renal replacement therapy. Kidney Int Suppl. 1999;72:S88–94.
21. 5008 & 5008S—Fresenius Medical Care [Internet]. https://www.freseniusmedicalcare.asia/en/healthcare-professionals/hemodialysis/machines/5008-5008s. Accessed 25 Apr 2022.
22. Abe M, Maruyama N, Matsumoto S, Okada K, Fujita T, Matsumoto K, et al. Comparison of sustained hemodiafiltration with acetate-free dialysate and continuous venovenous hemodiafiltration for the treatment of critically ill patients with acute kidney injury. Int J Nephrol. 2011;2011:1–8.

23. Sun Z, Ye H, Shen X, Chao H, Wu X, Yang J. Continuous venovenous hemofiltration versus extended daily hemofiltration in patients with septic acute kidney injury: a retrospective cohort study. Crit Care. 2014;18(2):R70.
24. Zhang L, Yang J, Eastwood GM, Zhu G, Tanaka A, Bellomo R. Extended daily dialysis versus continuous renal replacement therapy for acute kidney injury: a meta-analysis. Am J Kidney Dis. 2015;66(2):322–30.
25. Dalbhi SA, Alorf R, Alotaibi M, Altheaby A, Alghamdi Y, Ghazal H, et al. Sustained low efficiency dialysis is non-inferior to continuous renal replacement therapy in critically ill patients with acute kidney injury: a comparative meta-analysis. Medicine. 2021;100(51):e28118.
26. Ye Z, Wang Y, Ge L, Guyatt GH, Collister D, Alhazzani W, et al. Comparing renal replacement therapy modalities in critically ill patients with acute kidney injury: a systematic review and network meta-analysis. Crit Care Explor. 2021;3(5):e0399.

Part IV

Neurocritical Care

Does Intracranial Pressure Monitoring Help in Severe Traumatic Brain Injury? 29

29.1 Introduction

One of the key principles that guide the management of traumatic brain injury (TBI) is based on the doctrine established by Alexander Munro and George Kellie in the early nineteenth century [1]. According to this principle, the volume of the intracranial contents is fixed and comprises of the brain parenchyma (83%), intracranial blood volume (6%), and the cerebrospinal fluid volume (11%) [2]. If the intracranial volume increases, compensation occurs to a limited extent by shift of the cerebrospinal fluid out of the intracranial compartment. However, compensatory mechanisms fail once a threshold intracranial volume is reached; any further rise in the intracranial volume results in a steep rise in the intracranial pressure (ICP) (Fig. 29.1). As the ICP continues to rise, the brain parenchyma is compressed, leading to a fall in the cerebral perfusion pressure according to the equation:

$$CPP = \text{Mean arterial pressure}(\text{MAP}) - ICP.$$

If the ICP continues to rise relentlessly, cerebral blood flow is compromised with secondary injury culminating in severe ischemia to the brain.

J. Chacko et al., *Controversies in Critical Care*,
https://doi.org/10.1007/978-981-19-9940-6_29

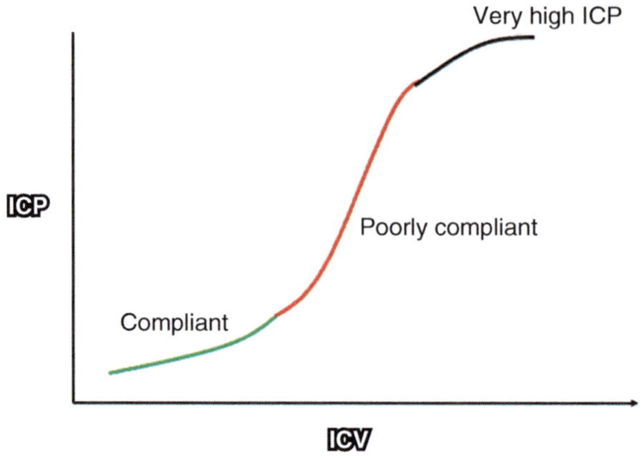

Fig. 29.1 The intracranial pressure-volume compliance curve. The initial segment of the curve (green) represents high baseline compliance and adequate compensatory reserve. As the intracranial volume rises, the compliance decreases and overwhelms the compensatory reserve (red). Further rise in ICP (black) leads to collapse of the cerebral microvasculature. *ICP* intracranial pressure, *ICV* intracranial volume

29.2 Early Studies on ICP Monitoring

In one of the early reports, Lundberg et al. carried out continuous ICP monitoring through an intraventricular catheter connected to a strain gauge transducer in 30 patients with TBI. They hypothesized that continuous ICP monitoring offers a more rational approach to guide interventions in TBI [3]. In a larger cohort study performed a decade later, Miller et al., in their series of 160 patients with severe TBI, observed that raised ICP above a threshold level of 20 mmHg was associated with poor outcomes in patients with underlying mass lesions and diffuse brain injury. They proposed that ICP measurement needs to be considered as part of the management protocol for severe TBI [4]. The only discriminatory factor was the level of intracranial pressure (ICP). All the patients with ICP greater than 30 mmHg deteriorated and required surgical intervention, but only one patient whose ICP was less than 20 mmHg experienced deterioration. In another landmark study of 26 patients with intracranial hematoma, clinical features were unhelpful in predicting the requirement for surgical intervention. However, all patients with an ICP level greater than 30 mmHg required surgical intervention. Surgical intervention was required in 50% of patients with ICP between 20 and 30 mmHg. Thus, a threshold ICP level greater than 20 mmHg was closely associated with neurological deterioration [5].

29.3 Pros and Cons of ICP Monitoring

Continuous ICP monitoring enables therapeutic interventions based on the CPP. Patients with severe TBI require controlled ventilation with administration of sedatives and muscle relaxants for control of ICP. In this situation, neurological assessment is often impracticable; besides, periodic interruption of sedation for evaluation of neurological status may be detrimental in patients with raised ICP. The ICP level is a reliable guide to identify neurological deterioration that may require imaging or surgical intervention [6]. Insertion of an intraparenchymal catheter is relatively easy and safe, especially if the ventricles are dilated [7]. Training of staff improves familiarity and skill with ICP monitoring, thus improving the overall level of care.

Paradoxically, aggressive interventions directed toward ICP control may lead to potential harm. Injudicious use of use of osmotherapy, particularly in the elderly with compromised cardiovascular and renal function, may be injurious [8]. Decompressive craniectomy in patients with TBI and refractory intracranial hypertension has been associated with poor functional outcomes [9]. ICP monitoring is recommended by the guidelines of the Brain Trauma Foundation. However, in the Trauma Quality Improvement Program database study that included 13,188 patients with isolated severe TBI, ICP monitoring was performed in only 11.5% of patients who met the eligibility criteria. This finding may suggest an ambivalent approach to ICP monitoring in TBI among neurosurgeons [10].

29.4 What Is the Evidence for the Usefulness of ICP Monitoring?

ICP monitoring is generally resorted to for titration of interventions including osmotherapy, optimization of sedation, and ventilator management. A high ICP may also trigger the requirement for surgical intervention including decompressive craniectomy. The impact of ICP monitoring on clinical outcomes is largely based on observational studies (Table 29.1).

Table 29.1 Main studies evaluating the efficacy of ICP monitoring in TBI

Study/year	Design	ICP monitoring	Control	Outcomes
Alali et al. (2013) [11]	Observational			ICP-guided management associated with lower in-hospital mortality on adjusted analysis. Centers that perform ICP monitoring frequently had lower mortality
Dawes et al. (2015) [12]	Observational			In-hospital mortality lower with ICP-guided management on unadjusted and propensity-matched analysis

(continued)

Table 29.1 (continued)

Study/year	Design	ICP monitoring	Control	Outcomes
Robba et al. (2021) [13]	Prospective cohort study			6-month mortality lower with ICP monitoring. More favorable neurological outcome and lower mortality with ICP monitoring in patients with at least one non-reactive pupil. Therapeutic intensity higher with ICP-guided management
Cremer et al. (2005) [14]	Retrospective cohort study involving two level 1 trauma centers	Target ICP <20 mmHg, CPP >70 mmHg	MAP target of 90 mmHg, clinical, and CT-guided therapeutic interventions	Similar functional outcomes after 12 months. Lower median duration of ventilator support with clinical and CT-based management
Shafi et al. (2008) [15]	Database analysis			After adjusting for confounders including admission GCS, age, blood pressure, head AIS, and ISS, ICP monitoring associated with 45% reduction in survival
Aiolfi et al. (2017) [10]	Database analysis			ICP monitoring not independently protective against mortality. ICP monitoring associated with higher overall and infectious complications and less functional independence
Chestnut et al. (2012) [16]	Randomized controlled trial	Intraparenchymal monitor with ICP target of <20 mmHg	Management based on clinical examination and imaging according to standard of care protocol	No significant difference in the composite primary outcome including duration of survival, level and duration of impaired consciousness, functional status at 3 and 6 months, and neuropsychological state at 6 months. 6-month mortality and median duration of ICU stay similar. More prolonged cerebral protective interventions with clinical imaging-based management

ICP intracranial pressure, *MAP* mean arterial pressure, *GCS* Glasgow coma scale, *AIS* abbreviated injury score, *ISS* injury severity score

The impact of ICP monitoring on severe TBI was evaluated in 10,628 adults with severe TBI from centers that participated in the American College of Surgeons Trauma Quality Improvement Program (TQIP). After adjustment for possible confounders, ICP-guided management was associated with significantly lower in-hospital mortality. Besides, centers that employed ICP monitoring more frequently revealed a lower mortality [11]. In a 2-year observational study, 844 patients with severe TBI were evaluated from 14 trauma centers in the USA. ICP monitoring was performed in 46% of patients who met eligibility criteria. Propensity score matching was performed to adjust for confounders. The in-hospital mortality was significantly lower among patients who received ICP-guided management on both unadjusted and propensity-matched analysis [12].

Robba et al. conducted a prospective cohort study including 146 ICUs across 42 countries [13]. They aimed to evaluate contemporary ICU monitoring practices and therapeutic interventions. Besides, long-term patient outcomes were compared between patients who underwent ICP monitoring and those who did not. This study included 4776 patients with TBI or intracranial hemorrhage. A substantial variability was noted in the use of ICP monitoring across centers. The 6-month mortality was significantly lower among patients who underwent ICP monitoring compared to those who did not. ICP monitoring was also associated with a more favorable neurological outcome and lower mortality among patients with at least one non-reactive pupil. The therapeutic intensity level was significantly higher among patients who underwent ICP-guided management. Furthermore, an increase in the therapeutic intensity level by 1 point was associated with a significant reduction in mortality.

Findings from other studies have revealed conflicting results. A two-center Dutch study compared a center that employed therapeutic interventions guided by clinical features and computed tomography (CT) findings with another center that carried out interventions targeting an ICP of less than 20 mmHg and CPP of more than 70 mmHg. Functional outcomes were assessed after 12 months using the Glasgow outcome score. On adjusted analysis, no differences were observed in functional outcomes between the two centers. A significantly lower median duration of ventilator support was noted among patients who underwent clinical features and CT-based management [14]. In another large US National Trauma Databank (NTDB) study, patients with TBI who underwent ICP monitoring were compared to those who did not. The study included patients with blunt TBI with a GCS of 8 or less, an abnormal brain CT scan, and ICU stay of 3 days or more. On multivariate analysis, after adjusting for confounders, ICP monitoring was associated with a 45% reduction in survival [15].

The Trauma Quality Improvement Program (TQIP) database study evaluated compliance with the BTF guidelines for ICP monitoring and the impact of ICP monitoring on clinical outcomes. Patients with isolated TBI with a GCS of less than 9 and a score of 3 or more on the head Abbreviated Injury Scale (AIS) were included. This study included 13,188 patients. ICP monitoring was carried out only in 11.5% of eligible patients. There was no difference in overall mortality among patients who underwent ICP monitoring. Besides, ICP monitoring was independent predictor of the overall incidence of complications, especially infectious complications. Functional independence was also significantly lower in patients who underwent ICP monitoring. Among the subgroup of patients with the most severe injuries according to the AIS, ICP monitoring remained an independent predictor of mortality [10].

Chestnut et al. conducted a randomized controlled trial among patients with severe TBI comparing the impact of ICP-based management with clinical assessment and imaging-based management. The study included 324 patients across 6 centers in Bolivia and Ecuador. The authors evaluated a composite primary outcome including the duration of survival, the level and duration of impaired consciousness, the functional status at 3 and 6 months, and the neuropsychological state at 6 months. No significant difference was observed between the two groups in the composite primary outcome. Furthermore, the 6-month mortality and the median duration of ICU stay were also similar between groups. Cerebral protective therapies were carried out for a longer duration among patients who underwent clinical assessment and imaging-based management. This study demonstrated that ICP-guided management was not superior to clinical assessment and image-based management of severe TBI [16]. However, the study needs to be interpreted against the background of clinical settings in which ICP monitoring may not have been the standard of care.

Key Points

- The potential beneficial effect of ICP monitoring-based care in severe TBI remains unclear; observational studies have shown conflicting results.
- The only large-sized randomized controlled trial that evaluated the potential benefit of ICP monitoring did not demonstrate any improvement in clinical outcomes compared to management based on clinical examination and CT imaging. However, the generalizability of this study in centers that routinely follow ICP monitoring-based care is uncertain.
- Timely clinical assessment is often impracticable among patients with severe TBI who are mechanically ventilated, sedated, and administered neuromuscular blocking agents as part of neuroprotective care. Continuous ICP monitoring enables early identification of neurological deterioration and may facilitate appropriate therapeutic intervention.
- The skill and familiarity with continuous ICP monitoring among caregivers may be an important factor that determines effective therapeutic intervention that may impact clinical outcomes. However, continued equipoise needs to be maintained on this still unresolved aspect of neurocritical care until more robust evidence is available.

References

1. Mokri B. The Monro-Kellie hypothesis: applications in CSF volume depletion. Neurology. 2001;56(12):1746–8.
2. Smith M. Monitoring intracranial pressure in traumatic brain injury. Anesth Analg. 2008;106(1):240–8.
3. Lundberg N, Troupp H, Lorin H. Continuous recording of the ventricular-fluid pressure in patients with severe acute traumatic brain injury. J Neurosurg. 1965;22(6):581–90.
4. Miller JD, Becker DP, Ward JD, Sullivan HG, Adams WE, Rosner MJ. Significance of intracranial hypertension in severe head injury. J Neurosurg. 1977;47(4):503–16.
5. Gallbraith S, Teasdale G. Predicting the need for operation in the patient with an occult traumatic intracranial hematoma. J Neurosurg. 1981;55(1):75–81.
6. Huijben JA, Wiegers EJA, Lingsma HF, Citerio G, Maas AIR, Menon DK, et al. Changing care pathways and between-center practice variations in intensive care for traumatic brain injury across Europe: a CENTER-TBI analysis. Intensive Care Med. 2020;46(5):995–1004.
7. Hawthorne C, Piper I. Monitoring of intracranial pressure in patients with traumatic brain injury. Front Neurol. 2014;5:121.
8. Grände PO, Romner B. Osmotherapy in brain edema: a questionable therapy. J Neurosurg Anesthesiol. 2012;24(4):407–12.
9. Cooper DJ, Rosenfeld JV, Murray L, Arabi YM, Davies AR, D'Urso P, et al. Decompressive craniectomy in diffuse traumatic brain injury. N Engl J Med. 2011;364(16):1493–502.
10. Aiolfi A, Benjamin E, Khor D, Inaba K, Lam L, Demetriades D. Brain trauma foundation guidelines for intracranial pressure monitoring: compliance and effect on outcome. World J Surg. 2017;41(6):1543–9.
11. Alali AS, Fowler RA, Mainprize TG, Scales DC, Kiss A, de Mestral C, et al. Intracranial pressure monitoring in severe traumatic brain injury: results from the American College of Surgeons trauma quality improvement program. J Neurotrauma. 2013;30(20):1737–46.
12. Dawes AJ, Sacks GD, Cryer HG, Gruen JP, Preston C, Gorospe D, et al. Intracranial pressure monitoring and inpatient mortality in severe traumatic brain injury: a propensity score-matched analysis. J Trauma Acute Care Surg. 2015;78(3):492–501; discussion 501-502.
13. Robba C, Graziano F, Rebora P, Elli F, Giussani C, Oddo M, et al. Intracranial pressure monitoring in patients with acute brain injury in the intensive care unit (SYNAPSE-ICU): an international, prospective observational cohort study. Lancet Neurol. 2021;20(7):548–58.
14. Cremer OL, van Dijk GW, van Wensen E, Brekelmans GJF, Moons KGM, Leenen LPH, et al. Effect of intracranial pressure monitoring and targeted intensive care on functional outcome after severe head injury. Crit Care Med. 2005;33(10):2207–13.
15. Shafi S, Diaz-Arrastia R, Madden C, Gentilello L. Intracranial pressure monitoring in brain-injured patients is associated with worsening of survival. J Trauma. 2008;64(2):335–40.
16. Chesnut RM, Temkin N, Carney N, Dikmen S, Rondina C, Videtta W, et al. A trial of intracranial-pressure monitoring in traumatic brain injury. N Engl J Med. 2012;367(26):2471–81.

Therapeutic Hypothermia in Traumatic Brain Injury

30

30.1 Introduction

Traumatic brain injury (TBI) often leads to severe neurological disability or death [1]. Mitigation of secondary brain injury is one of the key interventions in improving clinical outcomes following severe TBI. Induced hypothermia has been the focus of interest in alleviating the impact of ischemic-related injury to the brain due to stroke, raised intracranial pressure (ICP), and in the post-cardiac arrest setting [2]. Therapeutic hypothermia may attenuate the impact of secondary brain injury following TBI by reducing the adverse outcomes arising from the activation of inflammatory and biochemical cascades [3].

30.2 Hypothermia: Mechanisms

Hypothermia reduces the formation of oxygen free radicals and inhibits excitatory amino acid release in TBI. Besides, it may reduce the large influx of calcium into the cells and inhibit the release of inflammatory mediators following ischemic injury. Astrocytes, microglia, and the endothelial cells of the brain release inflammatory mediators with an hour after injury with the levels remaining high for several days [4].

Therapeutic hypothermia reduces the cerebral metabolic rate and oxygen consumption by approximately 6–10% for each degree Celsius. It may also prevent spreading cortical depolarization and exert a mitochondrial protective effect. These actions may delay apoptosis of neurons and glial cells. The onset of apoptosis occurs relatively late after injury and continues for 48–72 h which offers an opportunity for mitigatory interventions including hypothermia [3]. Hypothermia may also suppress iNOS expression resulting in improved neurological outcomes.

J. Chacko et al., *Controversies in Critical Care*,
https://doi.org/10.1007/978-981-19-9940-6_30

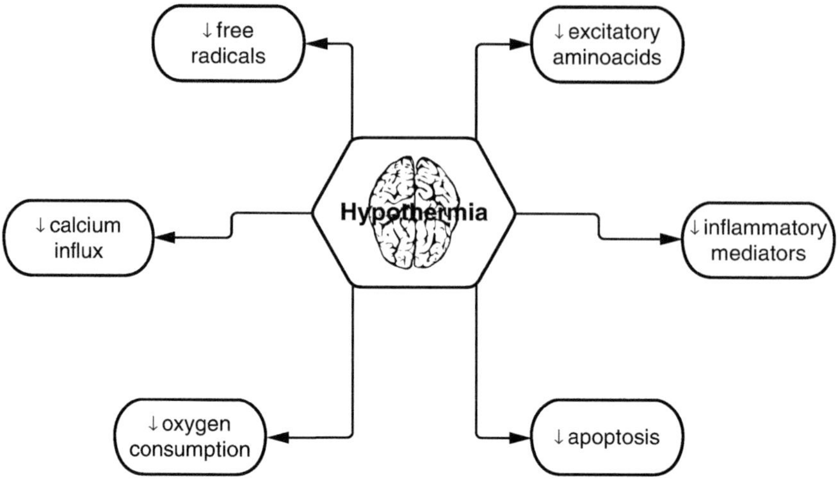

Fig. 30.1 Potential mechanisms of hypothermia-mediated neuroprotection

Furthermore, it may exert a protective effect on the blood-brain barrier, thus reducing cerebral edema and rise in the ICP. Figure 30.1 depicts the putative mechanisms of benefit with induced hypothermia in TBI.

30.3 Adverse Effects of Cooling

Induced hypothermia may cause coagulopathy and bleeding, immunosuppression, arrhythmias, and predispose to infections. A drop in the body temperature is accompanied by a decrease in the secretion of insulin and leads to insulin resistance. Thus, hyperglycemia may occur during the period of hypothermia. However, during the rewarming phase, insulin sensitivity recovers, with a profound fall in blood glucose levels. Hence, blood glucose levels should be monitored frequently during hypothermia and rewarming [5].

30.4 Methods of Cooling

The commonly employed methods for induced hypothermia include the following:

- IV saline at 4 °C during induction
- Endovascular cooling devices: central venous heat exchange catheter—enables quick cooling and maintains temperature effectively, with more precise rewarming
- Surface cooling: circulating cold water blankets, pads, or cold air blower blankets, with an automatic feedback system
- Intranasal cooling: rhinochill—for selective brain cooling

30.5 The Evidence

30.5.1 Early Studies of Hypothermia in TBI

Early studies suggested improved outcomes with the use of induced hypothermia in severe TBI.

Marion et al. (1997), in a randomized controlled trial (RCT), compared moderate hypothermia with normothermia in 82 patients with severe TBI, defined as GCS of 3–7 [6]. The patients randomized to hypothermia were cooled to 33 °C within 10 h of injury. The temperature was maintained at 32–33 °C for 24 h, followed by rewarming. Glasgow outcome scores were evaluated at 3, 6, and 12 months. At 12 months more patients who underwent hypothermia had a good neurological outcome according to the Glasgow outcome score (62% vs. 38%). No improvement in outcomes was observed among patients with GCS of 3 or 4 on admission. However, among patients with a GCS of 5–7, hypothermia resulted in significantly improved outcomes at 3 and 6 months.

In the study by Jiang et al., the effect of mild hypothermia (33–35 °C) was evaluated in 87 patients with TBI, defined as a GCS of 8 or less [7]. Cooling was carried out within a mean duration of 15 h after injury and maintained at 33–35 °C for 3–14 days. Rewarming was commenced once the ICP returned to normal levels. In the normothermia group, the temperature was maintained between 37 and 38 °C. The 1-year mortality was significantly lower with hypothermia (25.58 vs. 46.51%). Favorable neurological outcomes were also greater with hypothermia. Besides, mild hypothermia resulted in significantly reduced ICP and less hyperglycemia. The incidence of complications was similar between the two groups.

Zhi et al. randomized 396 patients with severe TBI to hypothermia (198 patients) or control (198 patients). Hypothermia was induced within 24 h of injury [8]. Rewarming was carried out within 1–7 days (average 62.4 ± 27.6 h), once rectal temperature reached 32–35 °C. Mild hypothermia resulted in lower ICP, blood glucose, and lactate levels with improved cerebral blood flow. Hypothermia was also associated with reduced mortality and improved neurological outcomes.

The NABIS: H (The National Acute Brain Injury Study: Hypothermia) RCTs evaluated the efficacy of hypothermia induced at variable intervals after severe TBI in improving neurological outcomes.

30.5.2 Clifton et al. (NABIS: H, 2001)

The study included 392 patients with severe TBI and coma (GCS of 3–8 after resuscitation) from 11 centers in the USA [9]. Patients were randomly assigned to undergo hypothermia (33 °C), initiated within 6 h after injury and maintained for 48 h. The control group was maintained at normothermia. The outcomes were poor; 57% of patients in each group suffered severe disability, were in a vegetative state, or died. Mortality was also similar; 28% of patients died in the hypothermia group compared with 27% in the normothermia group, the difference being non-significant

($P = 0.79$). The authors concluded that hypothermia induced within 8 h of injury does not improve outcomes in patients with severe TBI.

30.5.3 Clifton et al. (NABIS: H II, 2011)

The National Acute Brain Injury Study: Hypothermia II (NABIS: H II) was designed to evaluate the early induction of hypothermia on outcomes [10]. The study included patients from six centers in the USA and Canada. In this randomized, multicenter clinical trial, patients with severe TBI were enrolled within 2.5 h of injury. Patients were randomized to induced hypothermia to 35 °C until their trauma assessment was complete or maintained normothermic. The mean time to attain 35 °C is 2.6 h (SD 1.2) after injury and 4.4 h to reach 33 °C. Outcomes were poor (severe disability, vegetative state, or death) in 31 of 52 patients in the hypothermia group and 25 of 56 in the normothermia group (relative risk [RR] 1.08, 95% CI 0.76–1·53; $p = 0·67$). The mortality was also similar between groups. This trial failed to show any beneficial effect of early induction of hypothermia in TBI.

30.5.4 Maekawa et al. (B-HYPO, 2015)

In this Japanese study, patients with severe TBI were randomly assigned in a 2:1 ratio to therapeutic hypothermia (32–34 °C, $n = 98$) or control of fever (35.5–37 °C, $n = 50$) [11]. The incidence of poor neurological outcomes was similar between the hypothermia and the control groups (53 vs. 48%). The authors concluded that tight hemodynamic management and slow rewarming, combined with prolonged therapeutic hypothermia (32–34 °C), did not improve the neurological outcomes or reduce the risk of death compared with temperature control (35.5–37 °C) alone.

30.5.5 Andrews et al. (EUROTHERM, 2015)

The EUROTHERM study randomized patients with raised intracranial pressure of >20 mmHg despite level 1 interventions, including sedation and mechanical ventilation, to hypothermia (32–35 °C) or standard care alone [12]. Level 2 interventions including osmotherapy were carried out in the control group to reduce ICP. In the hypothermia group, level 2 interventions were carried out only if hypothermia failed to reduce the ICP. The study was stopped due to safety concerns after enrolling 387 patients. Level 3 interventions were required to control intracranial pressure in 54% of the patients in the control group and in 44% of the patients in the hypothermia group. Assessment of neurological outcomes by the GOS-E score revealed worse outcomes in the hypothermia group compared to the control group. Favorable outcomes were lower with hypothermia compared to controls (26 vs. 37%) The authors concluded that among patients with ICP >20 mmHg TBI, therapeutic hypothermia did not improve clinical outcomes.

30.5.6 Cooper et al. (POLAR, 2018)

The POLAR study evaluated the effect of early, prophylactic hypothermia after severe TBI [13]. The study randomized 266 patients to prophylactic hypothermia group and 245 to normothermic management. Prophylactic hypothermia involved the early induction of hypothermia (33 °C–35 °C) for at least 72 h and up to 7 days if the ICP remained high, followed by gradual rewarming. Hypothermia was induced at a median of 1.8 h (IQR, 1.0–2.7 h) with slow rewarming (median, 22.5 h [IQR, 16–27 h]). The temperature was maintained at 37 °C in the control group. The temperature was maintained within normal range for up to 7 days in both groups. All other care was at the discretion of the treating physician. Favorable neurological outcomes (Glasgow Outcome Scale Extended score, 5–8) at 6 months were not significantly different between groups: 48.8% in the hypothermia group vs. 49.1% in the normothermia group. The incidence of pneumonia and intracranial bleed was not different between groups. Early, prophylactic hypothermia did not improve clinical outcomes at 6 months compared to normothermia in this study.

30.6 Meta-analyses

Against the background of conflicting evidence from RCTs, several meta-analyses have been carried out to evaluate the impact of therapeutic hypothermia on clinical outcomes in TBI. Early systematic reviews and meta-analyses revealed marginal benefits regarding mortality and neurologic outcomes, with a higher risk for pneumonia with therapeutic hypothermia [14, 15]. Wu et al. included 6 RCTs including 1207 patients, in whom hypothermia was induced within 6 h after injury. No significant difference was observed in mortality or favorable neurological outcomes. Besides, complications were significantly higher with hypothermia in three included studies [16]. A Cochrane review found heterogeneity in design and characteristics of trial subjects. Visual assessment of outcomes revealed a high degree of inconsistency among studies. The direction of effect was dissimilar and hence data were not pooled for meta-analysis. The authors concluded that there is a lack of high-quality evidence that therapeutic hypothermia is beneficial in TBI [17].

Key Points

- Prevention of secondary brain injury is the cornerstone of improving clinical outcomes following severe TBI.
- Following TBI, several deleterious phenomena occur, including the release of oxygen free radicals, excitatory amino acids, and calcium influx into the cells. A profound pro-inflammatory response occurs, with neuronal death due to apoptosis. Induced hypothermia may potentially alleviate these injurious effects.

- Induced, therapeutic hypothermia has been extensively evaluated for improved outcomes following TBI based on its neuroprotective effects, the potential to reduce ICP, and possible prevention of secondary brain injury.
- Early RCTs revealed the potential for improved neurological outcomes; however, large multicentric RCTs have consistently failed to establish beneficial effects from therapeutic hypothermia in severe TBI. Targeted temperature management for severe traumatic brain injury remains the mainstay treatment and avoiding hyperthermia is more beneficial than inducing hypothermia.
- Considering the lack of robust evidence, therapeutic hypothermia in TBI should be confined to clinical trials.

References

1. Maas AIR, Menon DK, Adelson PD, Andelic N, Bell MJ, Belli A, et al. Traumatic brain injury: integrated approaches to improve prevention, clinical care, and research. Lancet Neurol. 2017;16(12):987–1048.
2. Sun YJ, Zhang ZY, Fan B, Li GY. Neuroprotection by therapeutic hypothermia. Front Neurosci. 2019;13:586.
3. Polderman KH. Mechanisms of action, physiological effects, and complications of hypothermia. Crit Care Med. 2009;37(7 Suppl):S186–202.
4. Schmidt OI, Heyde CE, Ertel W, Stahel PF. Closed head injury—an inflammatory disease? Brain Res Brain Res Rev. 2005;48(2):388–99.
5. Polderman KH, Herold I. Therapeutic hypothermia and controlled normothermia in the intensive care unit: practical considerations, side effects, and cooling methods. Crit Care Med. 2009;37(3):1101–20.
6. Marion DW, Penrod LE, Kelsey SF, Obrist WD, Kochanek PM, Palmer AM, et al. Treatment of traumatic brain injury with moderate hypothermia. N Engl J Med. 1997;336(8):540–6.
7. Jiang J, Yu M, Zhu C. Effect of long-term mild hypothermia therapy in patients with severe traumatic brain injury: 1-year follow-up review of 87 cases. J Neurosurg. 2000;93(4):546–9.
8. Zhi D, Zhang S, Lin X. Study on therapeutic mechanism and clinical effect of mild hypothermia in patients with severe head injury. Surg Neurol. 2003;59(5):381–5.
9. Clifton GL, Miller ER, Choi SC, Levin HS, McCauley S, Smith KR, et al. Lack of effect of induction of hypothermia after acute brain injury. N Engl J Med. 2001;344(8):556–63.
10. Clifton GL, Valadka A, Zygun D, Coffey CS, Drever P, Fourwinds S, et al. Very early hypothermia induction in patients with severe brain injury (the national acute brain injury study: hypothermia II): a randomised trial. Lancet Neurol. 2011;10(2):131–9.
11. Maekawa T, Yamashita S, Nagao S, Hayashi N, Ohashi Y, Brain-Hypothermia Study Group. Prolonged mild therapeutic hypothermia versus fever control with tight hemodynamic monitoring and slow rewarming in patients with severe traumatic brain injury: a randomized controlled trial. J Neurotrauma. 2015;32(7):422–9.
12. Andrews PJD, Sinclair HL, Rodriguez A, Harris BA, Battison CG, Rhodes JKJ, et al. Hypothermia for intracranial hypertension after traumatic brain injury. N Engl J Med. 2015;373(25):2403–12.
13. Cooper DJ, Nichol AD, Bailey M, Bernard S, Cameron PA, Pili-Floury S, et al. Effect of early sustained prophylactic hypothermia on neurologic outcomes among patients with severe traumatic brain injury: the POLAR randomized clinical trial. JAMA. 2018;320(21):2211–20.

14. Georgiou AP, Manara AR. Role of therapeutic hypothermia in improving outcome after traumatic brain injury: a systematic review. Br J Anaesth. 2013;110(3):357–67.
15. Harris OA, Colford JM, Good MC, Matz PG. The role of hypothermia in the management of severe brain injury: a meta-analysis. Arch Neurol. 2002;59(7):1077–83.
16. Wu X, Tao Y, Marsons L, Dee P, Yu D, Guan Y, et al. The effectiveness of early prophylactic hypothermia in adult patients with traumatic brain injury: a systematic review and meta-analysis. Aust Crit Care. 2021;34(1):83–91.
17. Lewis SR, Evans DJ, Butler AR, Schofield-Robinson OJ, Alderson P. Hypothermia for traumatic brain injury. Cochrane Database Syst Rev. 2017;9:CD001048.

Decompressive Craniectomy in Traumatic Brain Injury

31

31.1 Introduction

Among patients hospitalized with severe traumatic brain injury (TBI), 60% die or survive with severe disability. TBI is a significant contributor to community morbidity and mortality, particularly among the young. The main goal in the intensive care management of TBI is to minimize secondary brain injury, including maintaining optimal cerebral perfusion and cerebral blood flow. In the context of severe brain edema, the brain swelling leads to elevated intracranial pressure (ICP) and compromised cerebral blood flow. Intracranial hypertension is independently associated with worse neurological outcomes.

Decompressive craniectomy involves removing a sufficiently large segment of the skull to relieve the ICP in patients with severe intracranial hypertension despite first- and second-tier medical therapies. From a previous era of therapeutic nihilism, decompressive craniectomy is now used in many neurotrauma centers as a third-tier treatment after optimizing medical therapy. While there is no doubt that decompressive craniectomy improves ICP [1], it remains controversial *whether* it improves clinical outcomes, and there is a significant risk of creating profoundly disabled survivors.

31.2 Pathophysiology

One of the consequences of diffuse TBI is cerebral edema. When cerebral edema peaks, raised ICP may limit blood flow and thus cause a mismatch between cerebral oxygen demand and supply. First-tier therapies are directed at reducing metabolic demand with deep sedation and neuromuscular blockade, tight control of oxygen and carbon dioxide levels, maintenance of cerebral perfusion pressure, treatment of seizures, avoidance of fever, and optimization of blood flow by reducing impedance

J. Chacko et al., *Controversies in Critical Care*,
https://doi.org/10.1007/978-981-19-9940-6_31

to venous return. Second-tier therapies reduce cerebral volume by drainage of cerebrospinal fluid (CSF) or medically with osmotic agents such as mannitol and hypertonic saline. Some centers use agents such as barbiturates to decrease the cerebral metabolic requirement for oxygen.

When these measures are insufficient to control ICP, decompressive craniectomy has sometimes been used. Early case series [1] and anecdotes reported good outcomes, but with a high likelihood of reporting bias. Decompressive surgery is resource intensive and limited to major neurocritical care centers with comprehensive neurosurgical services. Following decompressive craniectomy, patients will need significant rehabilitation, long-term follow-up, and ultimately cranioplasty to either replace the bone flap if it has been saved and stored or a titanium or acrylic cranioplasty. Possible longer-term complications include infection, seizures, the development of hygroma, and paradoxical herniation.

Additionally, the general term "decompressive craniectomy" (DC) encompasses a number of procedures, and this makes interpretation of the literature more complex. This includes variations in anatomical segment (bifrontal or temporoparietal), surgical technique (including combined durotomy and duroplasty), extent of decompression, and the presence of underlying mass lesion or other indication for craniotomy.

31.3 Evidence

An early randomized trial in 27 children in a single center suggested strongly positive outcomes [2]. Two larger prospective, randomized trials of decompressive craniectomy in TBI (DECRA and RescueICP) have been reported in the last decade.

DECRA (Decompressive Craniectomy in Diffuse Traumatic Brain Injury) [3] was a multicenter randomized controlled trial of 155 patients with severe non-penetrating TBI [defined as Glasgow Coma Score (GCS) 3–8 or Marshall class 3 on CT scan] in an adult population aged between 15 and 59 years. Patients were excluded if moribund, with fixed dilated pupils, or with mass lesions requiring operative intervention. The primary inclusion criteria included a spontaneous (not stimulated) increase in ICP >20 mmHg for >15 min (continuous or intermittent within a 1 h period), despite optimum first-tier interventions (sedation, optimized $PaCO_2$, use of mannitol/hypertonic saline, neuromuscular blockade, and external ventricular drainage), within the first 72 h of injury. Patients were randomized to decompressive craniectomy (a large bifrontotemporoparietal craniectomy with bilateral cruciate durotomy) combined with best standard care (consistent with Brain Trauma Foundation guidelines and including mild hypothermia to 35 °C in tier 2) vs. best standard care alone. Rescue decompression at 72 h or beyond was allowed in the control group.

The primary outcome was a composite unfavorable outcome [composite of death, vegetative state, or severe disability—a score of 1–4 on the extended Glasgow Outcome Score (GOS-E)] at 6 months after injury]. There was no difference in mortality between groups, but functional outcomes were worse in the surgical group (median GOS-E 3 vs. 4, OR 1.83, 95% CI 1.05–3.24, $P = 0.03$), despite significantly less time with ICP above treatment threshold, fewer interventions for ICP, and fewer days in the ICU.

A subsequent 12-month follow-up of survivors confirmed this finding [4]. There were more survivors who were vegetative or severely disabled in the surgical group and no improvement in favorable functional outcomes.

RescueICP [5] was a multicenter randomized controlled trial of 408 patients, with slightly broader inclusion criteria. Patients were recruited if aged 10–65 years with an abnormal CT brain and an ICP monitor in situ with raised ICP (>25 mmHg) for 1–12 h despite tier 1 and two measures (included mannitol/hypertonic saline, hypothermia >34 °C, and ventriculostomy but not barbiturates). Postoperative patients could be included if they had not undergone a craniectomy. Patients were randomized to surgery (large unilateral frontotemporoparietal or bifrontal craniectomy at the surgeon's discretion) within 6 h.

Of randomization vs. best medical therapy (continue tiers 1 and 2, with barbiturates as required). The primary outcome was extended GOS-E at 6 months. Unlike DECRA there was lower mortality in the surgical group but higher rates of survival with vegetative state and severe disability (lower and upper) in surgical group compared to medical group. A substantial proportion of the medical group (37.2%) went on to have a delayed DC.

31.4 Controversies

Despite these largely negative trials of decompressive craniectomy, the practice continues. Supporters of RescueICP look at the distinction between "upper" and "lower" severe outcomes on the extended Glasgow Outcome Score. "Upper severe" is defined as "largely independent around their homes but needing assistance with traveling or shopping," whereas patients who are in the category of "lower severe disability" live in a supervised facility (care facility) or, if at home, need assistance most of the time. Conventionally the extended GOS-E is dichotomized as "unfavorable" [1–4] and "favorable" [5–8], but if the dichotomy is moved to only include death, vegetative, and "lower severe" [1–3] as unfavorable outcomes (in a prespecified secondary analysis), then the trial can be viewed as showing benefit for decompression. This requires a very clear understanding of the degree of disability described as "upper severe" and whether this would be acceptable to the patient or family.

DECRA has been criticized for the inclusion criterion of unstimulated ICP > 20 mmHg for 15 min (compared to >25 mmHg in RescueICP), questioning whether patients were recruited too early. Both trials examined early DC; these trials were conducted before the Eurotherm 3235 and POLAR trials [6, 7] and included mild therapeutic hypothermia as a tier 2 strategy. There were also differences in the exact operation performed.

It is clear that decompressive craniectomy helps reduce the ICP. Hence, the question arises as to why it does not result in improved outcomes? Other approaches to management which do not focus on ICP may be equally effective [8]. One possible explanation for harm after decompression is the axonal stretching that occurs as the brain swells outside the confines of the skull that may lead to worsening in contrast to prevention of the secondary brain injury. Decompression of a relatively smaller segment of the cranium may be a problem, as the brain can become ischemic as it bulges around the edges of the bone defect; however, too large a decompression may also be harmful.

The international Brain Trauma Foundation guidelines were updated in 2020 to incorporate these results [9]. The term "secondary DC" is used to distinguish from primary decompression at the time of evacuation of a hemorrhage or mass lesion. They present four level IIA recommendations:

1. Secondary DC performed for *late* refractory ICP elevation is recommended to improve mortality and favorable outcomes.
2. Secondary DC performed for *early* refractory ICP elevation is <u>not</u> recommended to improve mortality and favorable outcomes.
3. A large frontotemporoparietal DC (not less than 12 × 15 cm or 15 cm in diameter) is recommended over a small frontotemporoparietal DC for reduced mortality and improved neurological outcomes in patients with severe TBI.
4. Secondary DC performed as a treatment for either early or late refractory ICP elevation is suggested to reduce ICP and duration of intensive care, though the relationship between these effects and favorable outcomes is uncertain.

Key Points

- The role of decompressive craniectomy after severe TBI remains uncertain.
- While DC certainly reduces ICP, it may not improve or may even worsen functional outcomes.
- DC should be performed in carefully selected patients and only after an honest discussion with family about possible poor functional outcomes.
- A small pediatric study demonstrated benefit; it is likely that DC will be more effective in younger patients.
- There is no role for *early* DC but a possible role after maximizing other therapies for intracranial hypertension in patients who have no other adverse features that suggest a poor prognosis.

References

1. Whitfield PC, Patel H, Hutchinson PJA, et al. Bifrontal decompressive craniectomy in the management of posttraumatic intracranial hypertension. Br J Neurosurg. 2001;15:500–7.
2. Taylor A, Butt W, Rosenfeld J, et al. A randomized trial of very early decompressive craniectomy in children with traumatic brain injury and sustained intracranial hypertension. Childs Nerv Syst. 2001;17:154–62.
3. Cooper DJ, Rosenfeld JV, Murray L, et al. Decompressive craniectomy in diffuse traumatic brain injury. N Engl J Med. 2011;364:1493–502.
4. Cooper DJ, Rosenfeld JV, Murray L, et al. Patient outcomes at twelve months after early decompressive craniectomy for diffuse traumatic brain injury in the randomized DECRA clinical trial. J Neurotrauma. 2020;37:810–6.
5. Hutchinson PJ, Kolias AG, Tomofeev IS, et al. Trial of decompressive craniectomy for traumatic intracranial hypertension. N Engl J Med. 2016;375:1119–30.
6. Andrews PJD, Sinclair HL, Rodriguez A, et al. Hypothermia for intracranial hypertension after traumatic brain injury. N Engl J Med. 2015;373:2403–12.
7. Cooper DJ, Nichol AD, Bailey M, et al. Effect of early sustained prophylactic hypothermia on neurologic outcomes among patients with severe traumatic brain injury. JAMA. 2018;320:2211–20.
8. Chesnut RM, Temkin N, Carney N, et al. A trial of intracranial-pressure monitoring in traumatic brain injury. N Engl J Med. 2012;367:2471–81.
9. Hawryluk GWJ, Rubiano AM, Totten AM, et al. Guidelines for the management of severe traumatic brain injury: 2020 update of the decompressive craniectomy recommendations. Neurosurgery. 2020;87:427–34.

32 Optimization of Osmotherapy in Cerebral Edema

32.1 Introduction

Cerebral edema occurs due to pathological swelling of brain tissue following varied types of neurological injury. Excessive fluid accumulates in the intra- and extracellular compartments of the brain. Cerebral edema may occur due to a disrupted blood-brain barrier (BBB), inflammatory, or vascular phenomena or due to alteration in the cellular metabolism. The early recognition and management of cerebral edema are the key toward improving clinical outcomes in acute neurological injury.

Urea was the first hyperosmolar agent to be employed in the treatment of cerebral edema [1]. Hyperosmolar agents reduce cerebral edema, lower the intracranial pressure (ICP), and thereby improve cerebral blood flow and oxygen delivery. In current clinical practice, hyperosmolar agents are the cornerstone in the management of raised ICP due to cerebral edema among critically ill patients. Mannitol and hypertonic saline are the most common hyperosmolar agents used in the treatment of cerebral edema. Despite several decades of use and extensive research, the choice of the ideal hyperosmolar agent remains elusive and shrouded in controversy.

32.2 Basic Pharmacology and Mechanism of Action

The intravenous administration of hyperosmotic fluids results in an osmotic gradient across the BBB. The permeability of a solute across the BBB depends on its reflection coefficient. Permeability is measured on a scale of 0–1, with 0 representing complete permeability and 1 representing total impermeability. Thus, a higher reflection coefficient indicates lower permeability across the BBB. Sodium has a

J. Chacko et al., *Controversies in Critical Care*,
https://doi.org/10.1007/978-981-19-9940-6_32

reflection coefficient of 1.0, indicating complete impermeability, while mannitol comes close with a reflection coefficient of 0.9 [2].

According to the Monro-Kellie doctrine, the volume of the intracranial compartment remains constant. Any potential rise in the intracranial volume leads to a rise in the intracranial pressure unless there is displacement of intracranial contents out of the skull. Hyperosmotic fluids lead to the transfer of parenchymal fluid across the BBB into the intravascular compartment, resulting in a reduction in the ICP.

Besides their osmotic effect, hyperosmolar fluids improve the rheological properties of the blood. Intracellular water shifts to the extracellular compartment due to the osmotic effect. Through this mechanism, water escapes from the erythrocytes into the plasma. The dehydrating effect of the erythrocytes leads to dilution of the plasma, thereby reducing viscosity. Reduced viscosity leads to improved cerebral blood flow (CBF) and oxygen delivery. Besides, reflex vasoconstriction results in a decrease in the cerebral blood volume and the ICP [3, 4]. Hyperosmolar fluids may also exert a neuroprotective effect by reducing oxidative stress and inflammation [5]. Figure 32.1 summarizes the mechanisms of action of osmotic agents.

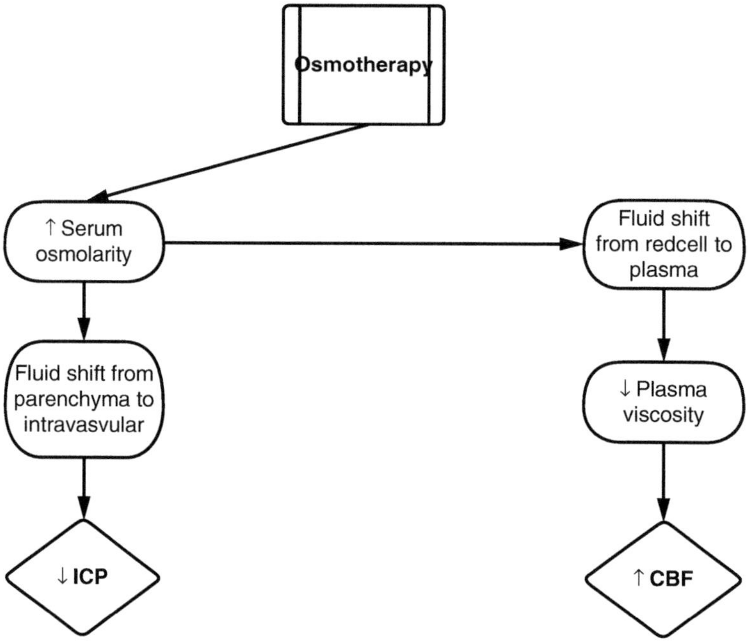

Fig. 32.1 The mechanism of action of osmotherapy

32.2.1 Mannitol

Mannitol is usually administered as a 20% solution and has an osmolality of 1098 mOsmol/L. The onset of action is within 10–20 min, with a duration of action of around 6 h. Conventionally, a dose of 0.5–1.5 g/kg is administered over 5–15 min and repeated 6–8 hourly as appropriate. Mannitol may be administered through the peripheral or central venous route.

The mannitol level in the plasma may be estimated from the plasma osmolar gap (normally ±10 mOsm/L).

$$\text{Calculated osmolarity} = 2\,\text{Na}^{+}\left(\text{mmol}/\text{L}\right) + \text{BUN}\left(\text{mg}/\text{dL}\right)/2.8 + \text{glucose}\left(\text{mg}/\text{dL}\right)/18$$

$$\text{Osmolar gap} = \text{measured osmolality} - \text{calculated osmolarity}$$

The osmolar gap should be maintained at <20 mOsmol/L during mannitol therapy [6]. An osmolar gap greater than 60–75 mOsm/kg with mannitol therapy leads to an increased likelihood of acute kidney injury.

32.2.2 Hypertonic Saline

The osmolality of hypertonic saline varies from 1026 mOsmol/L in a 3% solution to 8008 mOsmol/L in a 23.4% solution. A typical bolus dose is 150–250 mL of a 3% solution or 30 mL of a 23.4% solution. A continuous infusion may be administered targeting a Na^{+} level between 145 and 155 mmol/L. Although central venous administration is preferred for higher concentrations, 3% saline may be safely administered through a peripheral IV line [7]. The onset of action of hypertonic saline is more rapid compared to mannitol, and the effect lasts for up to 12 h [8]. The serum Na^{+} levels must be measured 4–6 hourly during therapy with hypertonic saline.

The Na^{+} content of hypertonic saline varies from 513 mmol/L in a 3% solution to 4004 mmol/L in a 23.4% solution. Hyperchloremia with a narrow strong ion difference in the plasma may occur with hypertonic saline therapy leading to metabolic acidosis. The hyperosmolar state may lead to central pontine myelinolysis, although the actual incidence of this complication with hypertonic saline therapy is unknown. Acute kidney injury, seizures, coagulopathies, and local adverse effects including thrombophlebitis may occur [9].

Let us consider the evidence for the relative efficacy of hypertonic saline compared with mannitol in various clinical situations that lead to cerebral edema and raised ICP.

32.3 Traumatic Brain Injury

A case-controlled study of prospectively collected data compared the effect of hypertonic saline with 20% mannitol in patients with severe TBI [10]. Patients who received HTS were matched in 1:1 and 1:2 ratios with those who received mannitol. Matching was based on factors known to increase the 2-week mortality, including age, GCS, pupillary reaction, hypotension, abnormalities on the CT scan, and the requirement for craniotomy. The primary outcome evaluated was the combination of a high ICP of >25 mmHg and a low cerebral perfusion pressure (CPP) of <60 mmHg. The authors identified 25 matched pairs for 1:1 comparison and 24 matched pairs for 1:2 comparison. The total number of days with high ICP and low CPP was significantly lower with hypertonic saline compared to 20% mannitol (0.6 ± 0.8 vs. 2.4 ± 2.3 day, $p < 0.01$). The percentage of days with high ICP and low CPP was also lower with hypertonic saline compared to mannitol ($8.8 \pm 10.6\%$ vs. $28.1 \pm 26.9\%$, $p < 0.01$). The duration of time with a high ICP and low CPP was longer with 20% mannitol compared to hypertonic saline (30.56 ± 31.89 h vs. 11.12 ± 14.11 h, $p = 0.01$). This case-controlled study showed that the composite adverse outcome of high ICP and low CPP was significantly lower among patients who received hypertonic saline compared with 20% mannitol.

Schwimmbeck et al. performed a meta-analysis of 12 randomized controlled trials (RCTs) including 464 patients that compared the effect of hypertonic saline with mannitol in patients with TBI [11]. The concentration of the hypertonic saline varied between 3 and 23.4% as intermittent boluses or a continuous infusion. Six studies including 318 patients reported on mortality at the end of the study period. A non-significant trend toward lower mortality was noted with hypertonic saline compared with mannitol (RR: 0.69, 95% CI: 0.45, 1.04; $P = 0.08$). Favorable neurological outcomes did not differ significantly between the two groups. The ICP levels were comparable between 30 and 60 min of commencement of treatment; however, they were significantly lower between 90 and 120 min with hypertonic saline compared to mannitol. The cerebral perfusion pressure was also significantly higher at 30–60 min and 90–120 min with hypertonic saline compared to mannitol. This meta-analysis suggested better ICP control and improved cerebral perfusion pressures with hypertonic saline compared to mannitol in TBI, although clinical outcomes including mortality were comparable between the two groups.

Riha et al. studied patients with intracerebral hemorrhage who developed moderate hyperchloremia (chloride ≥115 mmol/L) infusion of 3% saline [12]. They included 219 patients in an unmatched cohort; propensity matching was performed in 100 patients. The in-hospital mortality was significantly higher among patients who developed chloride levels of ≥115 mmol/L in the propensity-matched cohort (34% vs. 14%; $p = 0.02$). Chloride level of ≥115 mmol/L was an independent predictor of in-hospital mortality on multivariable logistic regression analysis (OR: 4.4 [95% CI, 1.4–13.5]; $p = 0.01$).

32.4 Acute Ischemic Stroke

The potential benefits of hyperosmolar therapy with either hypertonic saline or mannitol in ischemic stroke remain unclear. Hyperosmolar therapy may worsen the lateral parenchymal shift in large ischemic strokes by increasing the ICP gradient between the normal and edematous brain parenchyma resulting from the debulking effect of normal tissue [13]. There are few RCTs that evaluate the clinical efficacy of hyperosmolar therapy in patients with ischemic stroke. Evidence from two older RCTs suggests no improvement in neurological outcomes among patients with hemispheric stroke or intracerebral hemorrhage with the use of mannitol [14, 15].

Osmotic agents may, paradoxically, increase CBF and cerebral blood volume (CBV). The effect of mannitol and hypertonic saline (23.4%) on the CBF and cerebral blood volume (CBV) was studied in patients with ischemic stroke with >2 mm midline shift on imaging [16]. At normal blood pressures, hypertonic saline and mannitol had a minimal effect on the CBF; however, at high blood pressures, they resulted in a significant increase in the CBF. The findings of this study argue against the hypothesis that osmotic agents reduce ICP through a fall in the CBV due to vasoconstriction.

Does a continuous infusion of 3% saline targeting sodium levels between 145 and 155 mmol/L result in improved clinical outcomes? In one study, a reduction in ICP was observed in TBI and postoperative edema; however, there was no significant effect in patients with ischemic stroke [17]. A significant reduction in the number of episodes of ICP crisis was noted in patients with cerebral ischemia [17].

32.5 Intracerebral Hemorrhage

There is a paucity of studies that compare the effect of hypertonic saline with mannitol in intracerebral hemorrhage. Wagner et al. evaluated patients with intracerebral hemorrhage of more than 30 mL who were treated with 3% saline within 72 h, targeting a serum sodium level of 145–155 mmol/L. They compared these patients with historical controls from a database with similar hematoma volume. The authors observed a significantly lower absolute edema volume, lower incidence of ICP crisis, and lower in-hospital mortality with 3% saline infusion compared to the control group [18]. However, other studies have demonstrated conflicting findings [17].

Sun et al., in their meta-analysis, evaluated the effect of hyperosmolar therapy with mannitol in patients with hypertensive intracerebral hemorrhage and compared it with a non-mannitol group. The meta-analysis included 34 studies consisting of 3627 patients. In this meta-analysis, mannitol use was associated with an increase in the hematoma size, worsening of cerebral edema, and higher mortality [19].

Considering the implication of possible harm with mannitol use, hypertonic saline may be preferred in patients with intracerebral hemorrhage, although the level of evidence is weak [20].

32.6 Subarachnoid Hemorrhage

There is no robust evidence to guide the choice of the hyperosmolar agent in subarachnoid hemorrhage. Most treatment protocols are based on ICP lowering therapy in TBI. However, there are physiological differences between the characteristics of ICP rise in TBI compared with SAH. The mechanical shear and stress that arise from TBI do not exist in SAH. In SAH, the unique problems include hydrocephalus and delayed cerebral ischemia due to vasospasm. Two RCTs have examined the effect of hypertonic saline on ICP in SAH. In one study, the mean ICP reduction with hypertonic saline treatment was 9.9% compared to baseline [21]. In another study, hypertonic saline was compared to normal saline; hypertonic saline resulted in a reduction of ICP by 3 mmHg compared to baseline levels [22].

Pasarikovski et al. performed a systematic review to evaluate the level of ICP reduction in response to hypertonic saline and its impact on clinical outcomes in patients with SAH [23]. They also evaluated the efficacy of hypertonic saline compared to mannitol in reducing ICP. Five studies were included in this systematic review with a total of 175 patients. The strength of hypertonic saline varied between 3 and 23.4%. Hypertonic saline use reduced the mean ICP by 8.9 mmHg compared to baseline levels or to placebo and was as effective as mannitol in reducing ICP following subarachnoid hemorrhage.

The ideal strength, dose, and efficacy of bolus compared to infusion of hypertonic saline in ICP reduction in SAH remain unclear.

Key Points

- Hyperosmolar agents reduce cerebral edema through a shift of fluid from the brain parenchyma across the BBB into the intravascular compartment. Besides, they improve blood flow by reducing plasma viscosity and attenuation of the inflammatory response and oxidative stress.
- Mannitol and hypertonic saline are the agents commonly used in patients with cerebral edema and raised intracranial pressure.
- Current evidence supports the use of mannitol and hypertonic saline in reducing the ICP in patients with TBI. ICP control and cerebral perfusion pressures are better maintained with hypertonic saline compared to mannitol in patients with TBI. However, clinical outcomes appear to be similar with both agents.
- In ischemic stroke, although both mannitol and hypertonic saline may reduce edema, there is scant evidence for improved neurological outcomes.
- Hypertonic saline may be preferred over mannitol in patients with intracerebral hemorrhage; mannitol use has been shown to increase hematoma size, worsening of cerebral edema, and higher mortality.
- Hypertonic saline may be preferred in patients with subarachnoid hemorrhage and cerebral edema; however, there is no consensus on the concentration, dose, and relative efficacy of intermittent boluses compared to a continuous infusion.

References

1. Javid M, Settlage P. Effect of urea on cerebrospinal fluid pressure in human subjects; preliminary report. JAMA. 1956;160(11):943–9.
2. Boone MD, Oren-Grinberg A, Robinson TM, Chen CC, Kasper EM. Mannitol or hypertonic saline in the setting of traumatic brain injury: what have we learned? Surg Neurol Int. 2015;6:177.
3. Hartwell RC, Sutton LN. Mannitol, intracranial pressure, and vasogenic edema. Neurosurgery. 1993;32(3):444–50; discussion 450.
4. Machi T, Kassell NF, Scheld MW, Lehmann GA. Effect of mannitol on the permeability of cultured endothelial cells. Fukuoka Igaku Zasshi. 1996;87(8):178–83.
5. Rosner MJ, Coley I. Cerebral perfusion pressure: a hemodynamic mechanism of mannitol and the postmannitol hemogram. Neurosurgery. 1987;21(2):147–56.
6. García-Morales EJ, Cariappa R, Parvin CA, Scott MG, Diringer MN. Osmole gap in neurologic-neurosurgical intensive care unit: its normal value, calculation, and relationship with mannitol serum concentrations. Crit Care Med. 2004;32(4):986–91.
7. Perez CA, Figueroa SA. Complication rates of 3% hypertonic saline infusion through peripheral intravenous access. J Neurosci Nurs. 2017;49(3):191–5.
8. Alnemari AM, Krafcik BM, Mansour TR, Gaudin D. A comparison of pharmacologic therapeutic agents used for the reduction of intracranial pressure after traumatic brain injury. World Neurosurg. 2017;106:509–28.
9. Froelich M, Ni Q, Wess C, Ougorets I, Härtl R. Continuous hypertonic saline therapy and the occurrence of complications in neurocritically ill patients. Crit Care Med. 2009;37(4):1433–41.
10. Mangat HS, Wu X, Gerber LM, Schwarz JT, Fakhar M, Murthy SB, et al. Hypertonic saline is superior to mannitol for the combined effect on intracranial pressure and cerebral perfusion pressure burdens in patients with severe traumatic brain injury. Neurosurgery. 2019;86(2):221–30.
11. Schwimmbeck F, Voellger B, Chappell D, Eberhart L. Hypertonic saline versus mannitol for traumatic brain injury: a systematic review and meta-analysis with trial sequential analysis. J Neurosurg Anesthesiol. 2021;33(1):10–20.
12. Riha HM, Erdman MJ, Vandigo JE, Kimmons LA, Goyal N, Davidson KE, et al. Impact of moderate hyperchloremia on clinical outcomes in intracerebral hemorrhage patients treated with continuous infusion hypertonic saline: a pilot study. Crit Care Med. 2017;45(9):e947–53.
13. Kotek T, Zlotnik A, Rozet I. Chapter 6—hyperosmolar therapy. In: Prabhakar H, editor. Essentials of evidence-based practice of neuroanesthesia and neurocritical care [internet]. Cambridge, MA: Academic Press; 2022. p. 53–65. https://www.sciencedirect.com/science/article/pii/B9780128217764000068.
14. Misra UK, Kalita J, Ranjan P, Mandal SK. Mannitol in intracerebral hemorrhage: a randomized controlled study. J Neurol Sci. 2005;234(1–2):41–5.
15. Santambrogio S, Martinotti R, Sardella F, Porro F, Randazzo A. Is there a real treatment for stroke? Clinical and statistical comparison of different treatments in 300 patients. Stroke. 1978;9(2):130–2.
16. Diringer MN, Scalfani MT, Zazulia AR, Videen TO, Dhar R. Cerebral hemodynamic and metabolic effects of equi-osmolar doses mannitol and 23.4% saline in patients with edema following large ischemic stroke. Neurocrit Care. 2011;14(1):11–7.
17. Qureshi AI, Suarez JI, Bhardwaj A, Mirski M, Schnitzer MS, Hanley DF, et al. Use of hypertonic (3%) saline/acetate infusion in the treatment of cerebral edema: effect on intracranial pressure and lateral displacement of the brain. Crit Care Med. 1998;26(3):440–6.
18. Wagner I, Hauer EM, Staykov D, Volbers B, Dörfler A, Schwab S, et al. Effects of continuous hypertonic saline infusion on perihemorrhagic edema evolution. Stroke. 2011;42(6):1540–5.
19. Sun S, Li Y, Zhang H, Wang X, She L, Yan Z, et al. The effect of mannitol in the early stage of supratentorial hypertensive intracerebral hemorrhage: a systematic review and meta-analysis. World Neurosurg. 2018;S1878-8750(18):32818–3.

20. Cook AM, Morgan Jones G, Hawryluk GWJ, Mailloux P, McLaughlin D, Papangelou A, et al. Guidelines for the acute treatment of cerebral edema in neurocritical care patients. Neurocrit Care. 2020;32(3):647–66.
21. Huang XC, Yang LL. Comparison clinical efficacy of 3% hypertonic saline solution with 20% mannitol in treatment of intracranial hypertension in patients with aneurysmal subarachnoid hemorrhage. Zhejiang Da Xue Xue Bao Yi Xue Ban. 2015;44(4):389–95.
22. Bentsen G, Breivik H, Lundar T, Stubhaug A. Hypertonic saline (7.2%) in 6% hydroxyethyl starch reduces intracranial pressure and improves hemodynamics in a placebo-controlled study involving stable patients with subarachnoid hemorrhage. Crit Care Med. 2006;34(12):2912–7.
23. Pasarikovski CR, Alotaibi NM, Al-Mufti F, Macdonald RL. Hypertonic saline for increased intracranial pressure after aneurysmal subarachnoid hemorrhage: a systematic review. World Neurosurg. 2017;105:1–6.

How Much Sedation in Critically Ill Patients on Mechanical Ventilation? 33

33.1 Introduction

Sedative agents are commonly administered to patients who undergo mechanical ventilation in the ICU. The late Thomas Petty, who described ARDS, summed up his ICU of 1998—"what I see these days are paralyzed, sedated patients, lying without motion, appearing to be dead, except for the monitors that tell me otherwise" [1]. Alleviation of anxiety and stress and ventilator synchrony are considered to be important reasons for the administration of sedatives. However, the newer-generation ventilators synchronize better with spontaneous respiratory efforts and may be more comfortable to patients. The duration of action of conventional sedative drugs, including opioids and benzodiazepines, may be prolonged in the critically ill with organ dysfunction and may lead to a longer duration of ventilation, besides increasing the risk of delirium and cognitive impairment [2]. Furthermore, observational studies have revealed that early, deep sedation may be an independent predictor of mortality [3, 4]. On the other hand, lack of adequate sedation incurs the risk of accidental device removal [5] and may complicate the nursing care of patients who undergo mechanical ventilation [6].

There are several subgroups of critically ill patients in whom an adequate level of sedation is a crucial component of care. These include patients who require mechanical ventilation for severe hypoxia, those with raised intracranial pressure, refractory seizures, and sedation use in combination with neuromuscular blocking drugs. However, in most other clinical situations, a deep level of sedation may be unnecessary among critically ill patients on mechanical ventilation.

J. Chacko et al., *Controversies in Critical Care*,
https://doi.org/10.1007/978-981-19-9940-6_33

33.2 Importance of Monitoring the Level of Sedation

In an ideal world, the level of sedation must ensure a calm, cooperative patient who can comply with therapeutic interventions and enable mobilization as required. However, in the real world, titration of sedative agents to an ideal level may often remain elusive. Several scales have been proposed to guide the titration of sedation by the bedside. The commonly used tools include the Richmond Agitation and Sedation Scale (RASS) [7] and Riker Sedation-Agitation Scale (SAS) [8]. The RASS score ranges from −5 (unresponsive) to +4 (combative); a score of −2 (light sedation; briefly awakens and makes eye contact to voice) to −3 (any movement, but no eye contact to voice) is generally considered appropriate. The Riker scale ranges from 1 (unarousable) to 7 (dangerously agitated); a score of 4 (calm and easy to arouse, obeys commands) is the ideal target to aim for. Although these are useful tools to employ by the bedside, the subjective nature of assessment is a disadvantage. There is no general consensus on the frequency of monitoring; fluctuating levels of sedation may be difficult to monitor if the assessment is infrequent. Besides, assessment is not possible in the presence of neuromuscular blockade.

33.3 Evidence Supporting the Level of Sedation

Several controlled trials have evaluated the impact of the level of sedation among critically ill patients on mechanical ventilation (Table 33.1). These studies have compared different levels of sedation or a strategy of sedation compared with no sedation. The basic approach has revolved around seeking the most optimal methodology to titrate sedative agents to ensure patient comfort and safety without compromising clinical outcomes.

33.3.1 Daily Interruption of Sedation

Kress et al., in a seminal study, evaluated the impact of daily interruption of sedative infusions on the duration of mechanical ventilation and the length of stay in the ICU and in hospital [9]. The sedative agents used included infusions of propofol and midazolam, combined with morphine for analgesia. In the intervention group (68 patients), all sedative infusions were stopped daily until patients were awake or became uncomfortable or agitated necessitating the resumption of sedation. In the control group (60 patients), the requirement for sedation and dosage adjustment was left to physician judgment. Apart from sedation interruption and titration, all other decision-making was carried out as deemed appropriate by the treating clinician.

The median duration of mechanical ventilation was significantly lower with a daily interruption strategy compared to the control arm (4.9 vs. 7.3 days, $p = 0.004$). Patients who underwent daily interruption of sedation had a significantly shorter

Table 33.1 Landmark clinical trials that assessed the impact of sedation in mechanically ventilated patients

Study/year	Population	Intervention	Control	Outcomes
Kress et al. (2000) [9]	Sedated, mechanically ventilated patients	Sedative drugs were interrupted daily until the patients were awake	Sedative drugs were ceased at the discretion of clinicians	Reduced duration of mechanical ventilation and ICU stay with daily sedation interruption. Less diagnostic evaluation for neurological impairment less with interruption. Accidental device removal similar
Mehta et al. (SLEAP, 2012) [10]	Critically ill, mechanically ventilated patients	Patients on continuous opioid and benzodiazepine infusions underwent protocolized sedation with daily interruption	Protocolized sedation alone	Time to extubation, duration of ICU and hospital stay similar. Device removal and incidence of delirium were similar. Nursing workload higher with sedation interruption
Girard et al. (2008) [11]	Mechanically ventilated patients	Daily awakening trial combined with a daily spontaneous breathing trial	Daily awakening trial combined with usual sedation practice	More ventilation-free days in 28 days, shorter ICU and hospital stay with daily awakening and spontaneous breathing (intervention) arm. Self-extubations more common in the intervention arm; reintubation rates similar
Strøm et al. (2010) [12]	Critically ill, mechanically ventilated patients	No sedation. Morphine analgesia	Propofol or midazolam for Ramsay score of 3–4, with daily awakening. Morphine analgesia	Shorter duration of mechanical ventilation until day 28; duration of ICU and hospital stay shorter with no sedation. Accidental extubations, VAP rates, and neurological imaging similar

(continued)

Table 33.1 (continued)

Study/year	Population	Intervention	Control	Outcomes
Olsen et al. (NONSEDA, 2020) [13]	ICU patients expected to require mechanical ventilation for >24 h	No sedation	Light sedation to a level wherein the patient could be aroused	90-day mortality, ventilation-free days, duration of ICU stay, delirium or coma-free days, and peak RIFLE score similar. However, the intended difference between levels of sedation between the two groups was not achieved

VAP ventilator-associated pneumonia, *RIFLE* risk, injury, failure, loss of function, and end-stage renal disease classification of acute kidney injury

ICU stay (6.4 vs. 9.9 days, $p = 0.02$). Besides, diagnostic testing for the evaluation of neurological impairment was less frequent among patients who underwent daily interruption of sedation compared to the control group. Accidental removal of devices was uncommon and similar in both groups of patients.

The multicentric SLEAP trial conducted by the Canadian Critical Care Trials Group across 16 centers in Canada and the USA came up with contrasting findings [10]. In this study, among patients receiving continuous infusion of sedative agents, protocolized sedation combined with daily interruption did not improve clinical outcomes compared with protocolized sedation alone. However, among patients who underwent daily interruption, a higher dose of benzodiazepines and opioids was administered; besides, the requirement for bolus sedation was also greater to achieve sedation targets in this group. Furthermore, this study also used a high dose of benzodiazepines, compared to other studies that evaluated daily interruption, which could explain the conflicting findings.

33.3.2 Daily Interruption Combined with a Spontaneous Breathing Trial

Girard et al. compared a strategy of a daily awakening trial combined with a spontaneous breathing trial with usual sedation practice and spontaneous breathing trial in mechanically ventilated patients [11]. In this multicentric RCT, 335 patients were included in the final analysis, with 167 in the intervention and 168 in the control group. Patients in the intervention arm experienced more ventilation-free days during the 28-day study period (14.7 days vs. 11.6 days $p = 0.02$); the duration of ICU and hospital stay was also significantly shorter. Self-extubations were more common in the intervention arm, but this did not lead to a higher rate of reintubation compared to the control arm.

33.3.3 Sedation vs. No Sedation

A single-center study from Denmark compared a strategy of no sedation with daily interruption of sedation until the patient was awake [12]. In the sedation arm, propofol or midazolam was infused aiming for a target Ramsay score of 3–4. Patients in both groups were administered bolus morphine, 2.5–5.0 mg for pain relief. Seventy patients were included in each group. A strategy of no sedation resulted in a shorter duration of mechanical ventilation from intubation until day 28, with a mean difference of 4.2 days between the two groups. The duration of stay in the ICU and in hospital was also significantly shorter in the no sedation group. The incidence of accidental extubations, ventilator-associated pneumonia, and investigation with neurological imaging were not different between the two groups.

The NONSEDA trial was conducted across eight centers in Denmark, Norway, and Sweden as a more detailed evaluation of the aforementioned trial. The study included patients who were intubated within 24 h prior to screening and were expected to receive mechanical ventilation for longer than 24 h [13]. Randomization was carried out in a 1:1 ratio to a plan of no sedation or light sedation with daily cessation. In the no sedation group, bolus morphine could be administered as deemed appropriate. In the light sedation group, a target score of −2 (wakes up briefly with eye contact to voice) to −3 (any movement, but no eye contact to voice) was targeted. A total of 710 patients were enrolled; 354 were assigned to the no sedation group and 356 to the light sedation group. The RASS scores in the no sedation compared to the light sedation group were −2.3 vs. −1.3 on day 1 and −1.8 vs. −0.8 on day 7.

The all-cause mortality at 90 days, the primary outcome, was not significantly different between the two groups (no sedation vs. light sedation: 42.4% vs. 37%, $p = 0.65$). Among the secondary outcomes, there was no significant difference in the number of mechanical ventilation-free days and the duration of ICU stay until 28 days after randomization. The number of delirium or coma-free days within 28 days was 1 day less in the no sedation group. A major thromboembolic event within 90 days occurred in ten patients in the sedation group compared to one patient in the no sedation group. The peak RIFLE score was not significantly different between the two groups. Although this RCT did not reveal a significant difference in important clinical outcomes, this may have been because the intended difference in the level of sedation between groups was not attained.

33.4 Does Sedation Use Lead to Hemodynamic Instability and Organ Dysfunction?

The use of sedative agents might lead to hemodynamic instability, an increase in the dose of vasopressor agents, and a higher incidence of renal dysfunction. In a post hoc analysis of their original study, Strom et al. evaluated the impact of sedative agents on the hemodynamic status, the requirement for vasopressors and additional intravenous fluid, and the incidence of acute kidney injury (AKI) [14]. No significant difference was observed in the dose of vasopressors between patients randomized to a strategy of no sedation compared with those who received targeted sedation. The cumulative fluid balance was higher in the sedation group, but the difference was not significant. Sedation use was associated with a higher frequency of AKI by the RIFLE criteria. However, the number of patients who required continuous renal replacement therapy was similar between groups.

33.5 The Impact of Sedation During the Early Phase of Mechanical Ventilation

The required depth of sedation varies depending on the stage of illness. Sedation requirements are usually higher during the first few days, followed by a reduced level depending on the trajectory of illness. Most studies have compared the level of sedation in critically ill patients after the initial 24–48 h of mechanical ventilation. It is plausible that the depth of sedation in the early phase of critical illness may be an important predictor of clinical outcomes. In a prospective observational study, early, deep sedation was found to delay extubation and an independent predictor of mortality [15]. These findings were corroborated in a secondary analysis of a prospective cohort study [4]. Deeper levels of sedation in the first 48 h of mechanical ventilation were associated with a longer duration of ventilatory support and a higher rate of tracheostomies. The correlation between deep sedation and adverse outcomes persisted on multivariate analysis.

Key Points

- Mechanically ventilated patients in the ICU occasionally require a deep level of sedation; however, the majority may be managed with light or no sedation. It is important to ensure that even when a no sedation strategy is followed, adequate pain relief is provided.
- Excessive sedation in mechanically ventilated patients has been shown to prolong the duration of ventilation, ICU, and hospital stay. On the other hand, inadequate sedation may lead to ventilator dyssynchrony, patient discomfort, accidental device removal, and an increase in the nursing workload. Hence, a balance has to be struck to avoid excessive sedation while ensuring patient comfort and safety.
- The currently available sedation scales rely mostly on subjective assessment and may not be ideal with rapid, wide fluctuations in patient behavior.
- The practice of a protocolized strategy with predefined target levels of sedation is likely to improve clinical outcomes including reduced duration of ventilation and a shorter ICU and hospital stay.
- Daily interruption of sedation may be a reasonable strategy in patients who are improving from the underlying illness with a likelihood of liberation from mechanical ventilation. The basic concept revolves around cessation of sedation, re-evaluation, and re-titration to a minimum level if appropriate.

- A spontaneous breathing trial is often combined with a sedation interruption strategy in patients who have recovered sufficiently from the underlying illness and are ready for liberation from mechanical ventilation.
- A strategy of no sedation may be appropriate among patients who are cooperative and compliant with therapeutic interventions, provided caregivers are experienced with this approach.

References

1. Petty TL. Suspended life or extending death? Chest. 1998;114(2):360–1.
2. Girard TD, Jackson JC, Pandharipande PP, Pun BT, Thompson JL, Shintani AK, et al. Delirium as a predictor of long-term cognitive impairment in survivors of critical illness. Crit Care Med. 2010;38(7):1513–20.
3. Balzer F, Weiß B, Kumpf O, Treskatsch S, Spies C, Wernecke KD, et al. Early deep sedation is associated with decreased in-hospital and two-year follow-up survival. Crit Care. 2015;19:197.
4. Tanaka LMS, Azevedo LCP, Park M, Schettino G, Nassar AP, Réa-Neto A, et al. Early sedation and clinical outcomes of mechanically ventilated patients: a prospective multicenter cohort study. Crit Care. 2014;18(4):R156.
5. Tanios MA, de Wit M, Epstein SK, Devlin JW. Perceived barriers to the use of sedation protocols and daily sedation interruption: a multidisciplinary survey. J Crit Care. 2009;24(1):66–73.
6. Kydonaki K, Hanley J, Huby G, Antonelli J, Walsh TS. Challenges and barriers to optimising sedation in intensive care: a qualitative study in eight Scottish intensive care units. BMJ Open. 2019;9(5):e024549.
7. Sessler CN, Gosnell MS, Grap MJ, Brophy GM, O'Neal PV, Keane KA, et al. The Richmond agitation-sedation scale: validity and reliability in adult intensive care unit patients. Am J Respir Crit Care Med. 2002;166(10):1338–44.
8. Riker RR, Picard JT, Fraser GL. Prospective evaluation of the sedation-agitation scale for adult critically ill patients. Crit Care Med. 1999;27(7):1325–9.
9. Kress JP. Daily interruption of sedative infusions in critically ill patients undergoing mechanical ventilation. N Engl J Med. 2000;342(20):1471–7.
10. Mehta S, Burry L, Cook D, Fergusson D, Steinberg M, Granton J, et al. Daily sedation interruption in mechanically ventilated critically ill patients cared for with a sedation protocol: a randomized controlled trial. JAMA. 2012;308(19):1985–92.
11. Girard TD, Kress JP, Fuchs BD, Thomason JWW, Schweickert WD, Pun BT, et al. Efficacy and safety of a paired sedation and ventilator weaning protocol for mechanically ventilated patients in intensive care (awakening and breathing controlled trial): a randomised controlled trial. Lancet. 2008;371(9607):126–34.
12. Strøm T, Martinussen T, Toft P. A protocol of no sedation for critically ill patients receiving mechanical ventilation: a randomised trial. Lancet. 2010;375:475.
13. Olsen HT, Nedergaard HK, Strøm T, Oxlund J, Wian KA, Ytrebø LM, et al. Nonsedation or light sedation in critically ill, mechanically ventilated patients. N Engl J Med. 2020;382(12):1103–11.
14. Strøm T, Johansen RR, Prahl JO, Toft P. Sedation and renal impairment in critically ill patients: a post hoc analysis of a randomized trial. Crit Care. 2011;15(3):R119.
15. Shehabi Y, Bellomo R, Reade MC, Bailey M, Bass F, Howe B, et al. Early intensive care sedation predicts long-term mortality in ventilated critically ill patients. Am J Respir Crit Care Med. 2012;186(8):724–31.

Delirium in the Intensive Care Unit: Are We Paying Enough Attention?

34

34.1 Introduction

Delirium is an acute dysfunctional state of the brain, typically seen among critically ill patients. The characteristic clinical feature of delirium is a disturbance in attention that evolves rapidly, associated with cognitive impairment and unrelated to the underlying disease process. Impaired memory and disorientation, with impediment of speech and perception, are also common features. Critical illness-associated delirium adds to the disease burden and often leads to deleterious outcomes. Although a relatively common manifestation of multiorgan dysfunction in the critically ill, it is generally unmonitored, unnoticed, and an often-neglected aspect of care [1]. Cognitive dysfunction may also be accepted by clinicians as the inevitable effect of sedative medication [2].

34.2 Delirium and Clinical Outcomes

The incidence of delirium ranges between 20 and 80% and is related to the severity of the underlying illness [3]. Among hospitalized patients, delirium is an independent predictor of mortality. Furthermore, it increases the duration of hospital stay, with a higher likelihood of rehospitalization, long-term cognitive impairment, and adds to the cost of care [4].

A prospective cohort study of 275 mechanically ventilated patients evaluated the impact of delirium on clinical outcomes [5]. Fifty-one patients (18.5%) remained comatose and died in hospital. Among the 224 survivors, 183 (81.7%) experienced delirium during their ICU stay. The 6-month mortality was significantly higher among patients who developed delirium compared to those who did not (34% vs. 15%, $P = 0.03$). Delirium was also associated with a significantly longer duration of

J. Chacko et al., *Controversies in Critical Care*,
https://doi.org/10.1007/978-981-19-9940-6_34

hospital stay and was an independent predictor of 6-month mortality on adjusted analysis. The incidence of cognitive impairment was higher at hospital discharge in patients who experienced delirium.

34.3 Delirium Assessment Tools

Screening for delirium and early identification are the key to timely and effective management. The Prevention and Management of Pain, Agitation/Sedation, Delirium, Immobility, and Sleep Disruption (PADIS) guidelines of the Society of Critical Care Medicine (SCCM) recommend delirium assessment in every nursing shift and more often as necessary using a reliable tool [6]. The Confusion Assessment Method for the ICU (CAM-ICU) evaluates patients in four domains, including acute change or fluctuation of mental status, inattention, altered conscious level, and disorganized thinking [3]. Fluctuation of mental status and inattention along with either altered conscious level or disorganized thinking is considered to indicate delirium (Fig. 34.1). The CAM-ICU assessment is rapid and relatively easy to

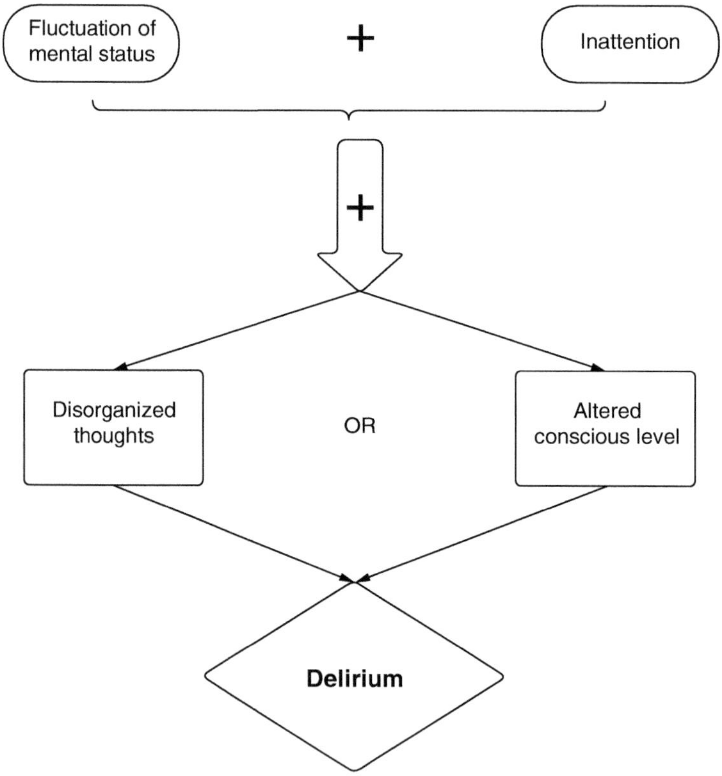

Fig. 34.1 The CAM-ICU method of delirium assessment. Presence of inattention and fluctuation of mental status with either altered conscious level or disorganized thinking indicates delirium

perform at the bedside; however, it may not be feasible in patients with cognitive deficits and those who are deeply sedated. Besides, it requires adaptation to the local language and culture.

The Intensive Care Delirium Screening Checklist (ICDSC) includes eight dichotomized items, each carrying one point. Delirium is identified by a score of 4 or more on this checklist [7].

34.4 Types of Delirium

Delirium may present with hyperactive features, characterized by restlessness, agitated behavior, and emotional lability. Hallucinations and illusions are also common. The aggressive nature of the disorder may interfere with the effective delivery of care. More difficult to diagnose, and hence less often recognized, is the hypoactive type of delirium. Patients who experience hypoactive delirium are confused, withdrawn, and apathetic. Hypoactive delirium may also be characterized by slowing down of motor activity, lethargy, and drowsiness. A validated screening tool is crucial to screen for hypoactive delirium; it may otherwise be misinterpreted as fatigue or depression. Clinical outcomes from hypoactive delirium tend to be worse compared to the hyperactive type, with higher 6-month mortality [3]. Mixed delirium is the most common type, with clinical manifestations fluctuating between the hypo- and hyperactive types.

The third type of delirium is sedation-related and rapidly reversible with a spontaneous awakening trial. Rapidly reversible, sedation-related delirium has been shown to be more benign and associated with fewer days on mechanical ventilation and in the hospital compared with delirium that persisted after cessation of sedation. This study also emphasized the importance of daily sedation hold and assessment if feasible, among patients on mechanical ventilation [8].

34.5 Pharmacological Interventions for Delirium

Several classes of medication have been evaluated in the management of delirium among critically ill patients. Most of the available evidence suggests that such therapy is largely ineffective at preventing delirium.

The HOPE-ICU trial evaluated the efficacy of haloperidol in reducing delirium among critically ill patients [9]. Haloperidol 2.5 mg intravenously thrice daily was compared to placebo among patients who were mechanically ventilated and within 72 h of admission to a mixed medical-surgical ICU. Haloperidol was discontinued after a 2-day delirium-free period, until discharge from ICU, or up to 14 days, whichever occurred earliest. In this study, the median number of days alive, not in a coma and free of delirium, was comparable between patients who received haloperidol and the control group (5 vs. 6 days $p = 0{\cdot}53$). Among the secondary outcomes, the 28-day mortality, the duration of mechanical ventilation, and the length of stay in ICU and hospital also did not differ significantly between the two groups.

The multicentric REDUCE study included critically ill patients, with a predicted ICU stay of at least 2 days which was considered to be a risk factor for delirium [10]. This RCT was conducted across 21 centers in the Netherlands. The initial design was a three-armed RCT that compared haloperidol 1 or 2 mg 8 hourly intravenously with placebo. The 1 mg dose was ceased early for futility upon the recommendation of the data and safety board. The 28-day survival, the primary outcome, was not significantly different between the haloperidol 2 mg and the placebo groups (83.3% vs. 82.7%). The incidence of delirium, the number of delirium-free and coma-free days, the duration of mechanical ventilation, and length of stay in the ICU and in hospital were also similar between the two groups.

In the MIND-USA trial, haloperidol and ziprasidone (an atypical antipsychotic drug) were compared to placebo in a three-armed trial among patients with acute respiratory failure or shock who experienced hypoactive or hyperactive delirium [11]. The maximum dose of haloperidol was 40 mg and ziprasidone 20 mg daily, intravenously. The CAM-ICU severity scale was used to evaluate the presence of delirium. In this study, delirium occurred in 48% of patients studied; the majority of patients experienced hypoactive delirium (89%). The median number of days alive and coma- and delirium-free was similar between patients in all three groups. Survival at 30 and 90 days, the duration of mechanical ventilation, ICU, and hospital stay were also similar between all three groups of patients.

Burry et al. evaluated the impact of pharmacotherapy on the duration of delirium in critically ill patients [12]. In their systematic review, they analyzed 11 studies, including 1153 patients. Multiple agents were used for delirium control, including antipsychotics, dexmedetomidine, statins, morphine, ondansetron, and the anticholinesterase inhibitor, rivastigmine. No drug, compared to placebo, reduced the number of delirium-free days or days in coma. Besides, the use of physical restraints, duration of ICU stay, cognitive outcomes, and mortality were not significantly different. Among all the agents evaluated, dexmedetomidine alone was found to shorten the duration of delirium in an RCT that included 74 patients from Australia and New Zealand. In this study, dexmedetomidine use was associated with earlier extubation and more rapid resolution of delirium. However, a large number of patients were excluded at initial screening (around 21,000 patients were screened) and hence lack external validity [13]. Table 34.1 summarizes studies that used a pharmacological approach toward delirium control in the ICU.

The AID-ICU trial was a multicenter, blinded, RCT of critically ill patients with delirium [14]. Patients were admitted to the ICU for an acute illness. Intravenous haloperidol, 2.5 mg three times daily, was administered with additional doses of 2.5 mg as needed. The maximum daily dose was 20 mg. Patients in the control

Table 34.1 Studies on pharmacological approaches toward delirium control in the ICU

Study/year	Design/ population	Intervention	Control	Outcomes
Page et al. (HOPE-ICU, 2013) [9]	RCT, critically ill patients requiring mechanical ventilation	Haloperidol 2.5 mg IV, thrice daily	Placebo	The median number of days alive, coma-free, and delirium-free was similar. No difference in the 28-day mortality, duration of ventilation, ICU and hospital LOS
van den Boogaard et al. (REDUCE, 2018) [10]	RCT, critically ill patients expected to have an ICU stay ≥2 days	Haloperidol 1 or 2 mg IV, thrice daily. The 1 mg arm was ceased prematurely for futility	Placebo	No difference in 28-day survival, incidence of delirium, delirium-free days, coma-free days, duration of ventilation, LOS in ICU and hospital
Girard et al. (MIND-USA, 2018) [11]	RCT, ICU patients with acute respiratory failure or shock with delirium	Three-armed trial; boluses of haloperidol or ziprasidone IV	Placebo	Median number days alive and coma-free and delirium-free similar in all three groups. No difference in 30- and 90-day survival, duration of ventilation, ICU and hospital LOS
Reade et al. (DahLIA, 2016) [13]	RCT, patients who were considered inappropriate to extubate due to delirium	Dexmedetomidine infusion, commenced at 0.5 μg/kg/h titrated between 0 and 1.5 μg/kg/h	Placebo	More ventilator-free hours at 7 days, earlier extubation, and more rapid resolution of delirium with dexmedetomidine
Andersen-Ranberg et al. (AID-ICU, 2022) [14]	ICU patients with delirium	Haloperidol, 2.5 mg three times daily with additional doses of 2.5 mg as needed. Maximum daily dose: 20 mg	Placebo	Mean number of days alive and out of hospital at 90 days similar. 90-day mortality lower with haloperidol

RCT randomized controlled trial, *LOS* length of stay

group received a placebo. Among the 1000 patients who were randomized, 987 were included in the final analyses; 501 received haloperidol, while 486 received placebo. The mean number of days alive and out of the hospital at 90 days was similar between the two groups (haloperidol vs. placebo: 35.8 vs. 32.9 days, adjusted mean difference 2.9 days, $p = 0.22$). The 90-day mortality was lower with haloperidol compared to placebo [36.3% vs. 43.3%, adjusted relative risk: 0.84 (0.72–0.98)]. Among the secondary outcomes, days alive and off mechanical ventilation and days alive without delirium or coma were similar between the two groups.

34.6 The Non-Pharmacological Approach

Several risk factors contribute to the occurrence of delirium in critically ill patients. Interventions directed toward mitigating these risk factors have been shown to reduce the incidence of delirium. These include reorientating patients to time and place, providing clocks to help them keep in touch with the time, spectacles and hearing aids that are used regularly [15], and early mobilization. Interventions may be minimized during sleep time, including blood draws and routine examinations that could be performed later. The patient is best addressed by their name, and information may be offered regarding the disease process in a simplified manner with positive reinforcement. Other measures that may reduce the incidence of delirium include minimization of noise levels, effective management of pain, and keeping track of drugs that may be implicated in delirium [16, 17].

A prospective observational study evaluated the efficacy of non-pharmacologic interventions bundled with nursing education and multidisciplinary intervention including intensivists, clinical pharmacists, and critical care nursing staff [18]. Sedation algorithm and mobilization protocol were combined with delirium screening performed 4 hourly using the ICDSC tool. This protocolized approach was compared with a pre-protocol phase as the control group. The adoption of the protocolized approach resulted in a significant reduction in the incidence and the duration of delirium. After controlling for risk factors including age, the APACHE II score, mechanical ventilation, and the presence of dementia, the odds of developing delirium reduced by 57% with the protocolized approach compared to the pre-protocol phase.

34.7 A "Bundled" Strategy

The PADIS guidelines recommend a multicomponent approach. The ABCDEF bundle includes assessment, prevention, and management of pain (A), both spontaneous awakening and spontaneous breathing trials (B), choice of analgesics and sedatives (C), monitoring and management of delirium (D), early mobilization and exercise (E), and engagement with family (F). Barnes-Daly et al. conducted a prospective cohort study using this bundle as part of a quality improvement initiative among patients admitted to a mixed medical-surgical ICU. Higher compliance with the bundled approach was independently associated with hospital survival on adjusted analysis. Besides, complete compliance with the bundle was associated with more days alive and free of delirium and coma [19].

Balas et al. evaluated the efficacy and safety of a similar bundled approach. In this before-after study, implementation of the bundle resulted in more ventilator-free days and a lower incidence of delirium. Besides, patients were mobilized more often during ICU stay compared to the control group [20]. Table 34.2 summarizes studies based on a bundled approach toward delirium control in the ICU.

Table 34.2 Studies on a bundled approach toward delirium control in the ICU

Study/ year	Design/ population	Intervention	Control	Outcomes
Barnes-Daly et al. (2017) [18]	Prospective cohort study of medical-surgical ICU patients	Multimodal approach using the ABDCDEF bundle	No control group	Bundle compliance associated with improved survival, more days alive and free of coma and delirium
Balas et al. 2014) [19]	Prospective, cohort, before-after study of medical-surgical ICU patients	A bundled approach of awakening and breathing coordination, monitoring and management of delirium, and early mobilization	Pre-bundle implementation group	The bundled approach resulted in 3 more days of breathing without mechanical assistance compared with the pre-intervention period. Significant reduction in incidence of delirium, higher rate of mobilization out of bed during the intervention period. No difference in self-extubation or reintubation rates

ABDCDEF bundle awakening and breathing coordination, choice of drugs, delirium monitoring and management, early mobility, and family engagement (ABCDEF) [18]

Key Points

- Although delirium is associated with adverse clinical outcomes including increased mortality, it is an oft-neglected aspect of care among critically ill patients.
- The incidence of delirium is closely related to the severity of the underlying illness and may occur in 20–80% of ICU patients.
- Delirium is difficult to detect in the absence of a concerted approach including the use of screening tools and often remains undiagnosed. The CAM-ICU and the ICDSC are sensitive screening tools that enable early detection of delirium.
- The diagnosis of the hypoactive type of delirium is more likely to be missed and carries worse clinical outcomes compared to the hyperactive type.
- No pharmacological agent has been shown to be effective in the prevention of delirium; however, pharmacotherapy may be required if the presence of delirium interferes with the delivery of care.
- A largely non-pharmacological, bundled approach is the most effective strategy in delirium management. This includes provision of adequate pain relief, avoidance of excessive sedation, and early mobilization. Patients must be given spectacles and hearing aids that they are used to, reorientated, and allowed to interact with the family as much as possible. Positive reinforcement about their progress is also an important facet of care.

References

1. Morandi A, Piva S, Ely EW, Myatra SN, Salluh JIF, Amare D, et al. Worldwide survey of the "assessing pain, both spontaneous awakening and breathing trials, choice of drugs, delirium monitoring/management, early exercise/mobility, and family empowerment" (ABCDEF) bundle. Crit Care Med. 2017;45(11):e1111–22.
2. Girard TD, Thompson JL, Pandharipande PP, Brummel NE, Jackson JC, Patel MB, et al. Clinical phenotypes of delirium during critical illness and severity of subsequent long-term cognitive impairment: a prospective cohort study. Lancet Respir Med. 2018;6(3):213–22.
3. Ely EW, Inouye SK, Bernard GR, Gordon S, Francis J, May L, et al. Delirium in mechanically ventilated patients: validity and reliability of the confusion assessment method for the intensive care unit (CAM-ICU). JAMA. 2001;286(21):2703–10.
4. Stollings JL, Kotfis K, Chanques G, Pun BT, Pandharipande PP, Ely EW. Delirium in critical illness: clinical manifestations, outcomes, and management. Intensive Care Med. 2021;47(10):1089–103.
5. Ely EW, Shintani A, Truman B, Speroff T, Gordon SM, Harrell FE, et al. Delirium as a predictor of mortality in mechanically ventilated patients in the intensive care unit. JAMA. 2004;291(14):1753–62.
6. Devlin JW, Skrobik Y, Gélinas C, Needham DM, Slooter AJC, Pandharipande PP, et al. Clinical practice guidelines for the prevention and management of pain, agitation/sedation, delirium, immobility, and sleep disruption in adult patients in the ICU. Crit Care Med. 2018;46(9):e825.
7. Bergeron N, Dubois MJ, Dumont M, Dial S, Skrobik Y. Intensive care delirium screening checklist: evaluation of a new screening tool. Intensive Care Med. 2001;27(5):859–64.
8. Patel SB, Poston JT, Pohlman A, Hall JB, Kress JP. Rapidly reversible, sedation-related delirium versus persistent delirium in the intensive care unit. Am J Respir Crit Care Med. 2014;189(6):658–65.
9. Page VJ, Ely EW, Gates S, Zhao XB, Alce T, Shintani A, et al. Effect of intravenous haloperidol on the duration of delirium and coma in critically ill patients (Hope-ICU): a randomised, double-blind, placebo-controlled trial. Lancet Respir Med. 2013;1(7):515–23.
10. van den Boogaard M, Slooter AJC, Brüggemann RJM, Schoonhoven L, Beishuizen A, Vermeijden JW, et al. Effect of haloperidol on survival among critically ill adults with a high risk of delirium. JAMA. 2018;319(7):680–91.
11. Girard TD, Exline MC, Carson SS, Hough CL, Rock P, Gong MN, et al. Haloperidol and ziprasidone for treatment of delirium in critical illness. N Engl J Med. 2018;379(26):2506–16.
12. Burry L, Hutton B, Williamson DR, Mehta S, Adhikari NK, Cheng W, et al. Pharmacological interventions for the treatment of delirium in critically ill adults. Cochrane Database Syst Rev. 2019;9(9):CD011749. https://doi.org/10.1002/14651858.CD011749.pub2.
13. Reade MC, Eastwood GM, Bellomo R, Bailey M, Bersten A, Cheung B, et al. Effect of dexmedetomidine added to standard care on ventilator-free time in patients with agitated delirium: a randomized clinical trial. JAMA. 2016;315(14):1460–8.
14. Andersen-Ranberg NC, Poulsen LM, Perner A, Wetterslev J, Estrup S, Hästbacka J, et al. Haloperidol for the treatment of delirium in ICU patients. N Engl J Med. 2022;387(26):2425–35. https://doi.org/10.1056/NEJMoa2211868.
15. McCusker J, Cole MG, Voyer P, Vu M, Ciampi A, Monette J, et al. Environmental factors predict the severity of delirium symptoms in long-term care residents with and without delirium. J Am Geriatr Soc. 2013;61(4):502–11.
16. Balas MC, Rice M, Chaperon C, Smith H, Disbot M, Fuchs B. Management of delirium in critically ill older adults. Crit Care Nurse. 2012;32(4):15–26.
17. Popeo DM. Delirium in older adults. Mt Sinai J Med. 2011;78(4):571–82.
18. Rivosecchi RM, Kane-Gill SL, Svec S, Campbell S, Smithburger PL. The implementation of a nonpharmacologic protocol to prevent intensive care delirium. J Crit Care. 2016;31(1):206–11.

19. Barnes-Daly MA, Phillips G, Ely EW. Improving hospital survival and reducing brain dysfunction at seven California community hospitals: implementing PAD guidelines via the ABCDEF bundle in 6,064 patients. Crit Care Med. 2017;45(2):171–8.
20. Balas MC, Vasilevskis EE, Olsen KM, Schmid KK, Shostrom V, Cohen MZ, et al. Effectiveness and safety of the awakening and breathing coordination, delirium monitoring/management, and early exercise/mobility bundle. Crit Care Med. 2014;42(5):1024–36.

35 Clearing the Cervical Spine in Trauma Patients

35.1 Introduction

Despite many guidelines, recommendations, and validated algorithms, clearance of cervical spine (C-spine) in neurologically obtunded patients following blunt trauma remains controversial. The incidence of C-spine injury in blunt trauma is reported to be 3.9% [1]. Failure to identify C-spine abnormalities may lead to significant disability and poor health-related quality of life (HRQL). Although C-spine clearance is an important topic, practices across the world vary significantly.

35.2 Rationale

Primary cervical immobilization with a stiff collar is considered to minimize the consequences of C-spine injuries. However, application of a hard collar may be associated with the following complications:

1. Increased intracranial pressure.
2. Difficult laryngoscopy and intubation and, hence, a risk of hypoxia.
3. Difficult central line insertion—increased rates of femoral line insertion and risk of infection.
4. Increased risk of pulmonary embolus.
5. Increased risk of infection—ventilator-associated pneumonia (VAP) and central line-associated blood stream infections (CLABSI).
6. Increased risk of pressure injuries including ulceration and necrosis.

J. Chacko et al., *Controversies in Critical Care*,
https://doi.org/10.1007/978-981-19-9940-6_35

35.3 C-Spine Clearance

Guidelines and recommendations have been proposed to evaluate the C-spine in blunt trauma.

35.3.1 National Emergency X-Radiography Utilization Study (NEXUS) Criteria

The NEXUS criteria include a set of validated parameters to enable decision-making on the appropriateness of imaging for C-spine clearance in patients who sustain blunt trauma. C-spine imaging may not be required if the patient meets all the following criteria:

- Alert and stable
- No focal neurologic deficit
- No altered level of consciousness
- Not intoxicated
- No midline spinal tenderness
- No distracting injury

The NEXUS criteria have a sensitivity of 99.6% for ruling out cervical spine injury in the original study validating the criteria (95% confidence interval, 98.6–100%). They may not be reliable in patients >65 years of age [2].

35.3.2 Canadian C-Spine Rules (CCR)

These are a set of guidelines that help the clinician decide on the appropriateness of C-spine imaging for a trauma patient in the emergency department. The patient must be alert and stable. The following rules are applied:

Is there any *high-risk* factor present that requires cervical spine imaging?

- Age ≥ 65 years
- A dangerous mechanism
- Fall from elevation >3 ft (or 5 stairs)
- Axial load to the head
- High-speed motor vehicle collision (e.g., >100 km/h or ~60 mph, rollover, ejection)
- Motorized recreational vehicles
- Bicycle collision
- Parasthesia in extremities

If a high-risk factor is present, cervical spine imaging is warranted.

Is there any *low-risk* factor present?

- Simple rear-end motor vehicle collision (excludes being hit by a high-speed vehicle, a large vehicle e.g., bus, or rollover).
- Sitting position in the emergency department.
- Ambulatory at any time since the injury.
- Delayed onset of neck pain.
- Absence of midline C-spine tenderness.

If the patient does not meet the criteria of a low-risk injury, then cervical spine imaging is warranted. If the patient meets the criteria of a low-risk injury, then a physical exam is carried out to evaluate whether the patient can rotate the neck through 45°.

- If low-risk injury and the patient can rotate the neck 45°, no C-spine imaging is required.
- If low-risk injury and the patient cannot rotate the neck 45°, C-spine imaging is required.

The original study presented 100% sensitivity for identifying "clinically important C-spine injuries" (95% confidence interval, 98%–100%) [3].

35.4 What Is the Evidence Behind Appropriate C-Spine Imaging in the Patient with Blunt Trauma?

Expeditious evaluation of the C-spine and limitation of the duration of immobilization, if appropriate, may reduce the incidence of complications and improve clinical outcomes in blunt trauma victims. Ackland et al. aimed to determine the incidence and predictors of cervical collar-related decubitus ulceration (CRU). Data were collected from a trauma registry database at a level 1 trauma center. It included 299 major trauma patients admitted over a 6-month period. Predictors of CRU including ICU admission, mechanical ventilation, necessity for MRI, and the time taken for C-spine clearance were retrospectively examined. The study concluded that the risk of CRU increased significantly for every day of Philadelphia cervical collar time. The prospect of developing decubitus ulceration increased by 66% for each day of increase in collar time. The associated increased morbidity may be reduced by measures aimed at earlier cervical spine clearance [4].

Most of the studies that have evaluated appropriate imaging in suspected C-spine injury are either prospective or retrospective cohort studies (Table 35.1).

A prospective cohort study compared the CCR and the NEXUS Low-Risk Criteria (NLC) in the evaluation of C-spine injuries. The study was conducted among 8283 patients across 9 Canadian emergency departments. This study concluded that the CCR was more sensitive than the NEXUS-NLC (99.4% vs. 90.7%, $P < 0.001$) and more specific (45.1% vs. 36.8%, $P < 0.001$) for diagnosing C-spine injury, and its use would have resulted in lower radiography rates [5].

Table 35.1 Studies evaluating different modalities of imaging in suspected C-spine injury

Author/ year	Population/design	Group 1	Group 2	Outcomes
Stiell et al. (2003) [5]	Alert trauma patients; prospective cohort study	CCR	NLC	CCR more sensitive and specific compared to NLC for cervical-spine injury
Stelfox et al. (2007) [6]	Mechanically ventilated patients with blunt injury; normal findings on HCT-recon from C1 to T1. Prospective observational study	Clinical or MRI scan	HCT-recon	C-spine immobilization for fewer days with HCT-recon. Fewer complications, shorter duration of mechanical ventilation, shorter ICU and hospital stay with HCT-recon
Schuster et al. (2005) [7]	Patients admitted to a trauma service. Analysis of prospective registry data	Patients with a negative CT of the C- spine were further evaluated with MRI for persistent pain with MRI scans		MRI imaging was negative in all cases. No neurologic deterioration was experienced by any patient; none required operative intervention
Hogan et al. (2005) [8]	Mechanically ventilated with multiple blunt injuries. Retrospective observational study	Multi-detector row CT of the cervical spine	MRI scan	In comparison with MRI scans, multi-detector row CT had predictive value of 98.9% for ligamentous injury and 100% for unstable C-spine injury
Adams et al. [9]	Patients who are under MRI spine trauma protocol. Retrospective chart review	CT scan	MRI scan	CT imaging had an overall sensitivity of 94% with a specificity of 91%. In 2/85 cases, MRI revealed ligamentous injuries that changed management

CCR Canadian C-spine rule, *NLC* NEXUS low-risk criteria (NLC), *HCT-recon* helical CT reconstruction

In a prospective study, Stelfox et al. compared two different C-spine evaluation protocols—clinical examination/MRI with helical CT reconstruction (HCT-recon) for evaluation of the C-spine in mechanically ventilated patients at a level I trauma center. Trauma patients with normal findings from C1 to T1 on HCT-recon did not require continued C-spine immobilization. The study concluded that the duration of C-spine immobilization was less when HCT-recon was used as the imaging modality in intubated polytrauma patients. It was also associated with fewer complications, fewer days of mechanical ventilation, and shorter stays in the ICU and in hospital [6].

Do MRI scans facilitate the adequacy of C-spine clearance? Schuster et al. compared detection of cervical spine injury by CT and/or magnetic resonance imaging (MRI) in a Level II community-based trauma center. The study included 2854 trauma patients, of whom 91.2% sustained blunt trauma. One hundred patients had cervical spine and/or spinal cord injuries. Eighty-five patients had a cervical spine injury diagnosed by CT. Ninety-three patients had a normal motor function on admission, and CT of the C-spine was negative for trauma; however, they had persistent pain in the region of the C-spine. These patients were further evaluated with MRI scans; however, they did not reveal evidence of clinically significant injury. The authors concluded that blunt trauma patients without motor deficits and a normal CT do not require further MRI examination for excluding C-spine injury [7].

Hogan et al. evaluated trauma patients who underwent MRI scans of the C-spine to evaluate potential cervical spine injuries. These patients had already undergone multi-detector row CT imaging that did not reveal any injury. MRI scanning was performed mainly to exclude soft tissue injury in clinically obtunded patients in whom C-spine injury could not be excluded by clinical examination. Compared with MRI scans, multi-detector row CT revealed a negative predictive value of 98.9% for ligamentous injury and 100% for unstable C-spine injury [8]. The authors concluded that normal multi-detector row CT scans of the C-spine were reliable in excluding unstable injuries, based on confirmatory findings on MRI scans.

Adams et al. evaluated the sensitivity of CT scan for spinal injuries compared to evaluation by a screening "trauma protocol" spinal MRI. The study included 97 patients who underwent MRI cervical spine trauma protocol. MRI confirmed the initial CT findings without new injuries in 83 cases. However, in two cases, the MRI identified new injuries, including a stable partial ligament tear and a T7 chance fracture with ligamental disruption that required operative fixation. The results of this study suggested that CT scan of the C-spine and axial spine is sensitive for spinal trauma, but not specific. The overall sensitivity of CT versus MRI was 94%; the specificity was 91%; and the negative predictive value was 98%. The study concluded that MRI trauma protocol should be reserved for cases when initial CT of the C-spine is suggestive of traumatic injury [9].

A retrospective analysis reviewed the use of early (<72 h from injury) limited MRI to "clear" extradural soft tissue injuries of the C-spine in ICU patients sustaining blunt trauma. The analysis included 150 patients. Forty-one patients had initial static radiographs that revealed cervical spine trauma. The study showed that a significant number of un-evaluable patients who had normal CT or plain radiography had findings that were concerning for injury on MRI of the C-spine and were treated with a semirigid cervical collar for 4–6 weeks. A limited MRI scan enabled ruling out significant C-spine injury and allowed early discontinuation of immobilization [10].

Key Points

- C-spine injury occurs in 5% of patients with blunt trauma. Reduced level of consciousness poses problems with the clearance of C-spine.
- A CT scan of the brain and C-spine should be performed in all trauma patients with traumatic brain injury and reduced level of consciousness.
- A CT scan of the brain and C-spine avoids the necessity for other imaging modalities that need transport of the critically ill patient.
- A normal CT C-spine (64 slice, 1 mm thick) suggests a negligible risk of ligamental injury (<0.1%).
- The potential benefits of C-spine clearance based on a 1 mm slice CT scan outweigh the risk of prolonged C-spine immobilization using a hard collar.
- All abnormal CT spines should be reviewed by either a neuro or orthopedic surgeon according to institutional policy.
- If the CT of the C-spine as reported by a fully qualified radiologist reveals no spinal or occipital condyle injury, the hard collar may be removed.
- A confirmed unstable C-spine injury on CT scan should be immobilized using a Miami-J collar. The collar should remain in place except when attending to hygiene needs or pressure area care [11].

References

1. Stephan K, Huber S, Häberle S, Kanz KG, Bühren V, van Griensven M, et al. Spinal cord injury—incidence, prognosis, and outcome: an analysis of the TraumaRegister DGU. Spine J. 2015;15(9):1994–2001.
2. Hoffman JR, Mower WR, Wolfson AB, Todd KH, Zucker MI. Validity of a set of clinical criteria to rule out injury to the cervical spine in patients with blunt trauma. N Engl J Med. 2000;343(2):94–9.
3. Stiell IG, Clement CM, Grimshaw J, Brison RJ, Rowe BH, Schull MJ, et al. Implementation of the Canadian C-spine rule: prospective 12 centre cluster randomised trial. BMJ. 2009;339:b4146. https://www.ncbi.nlm.nih.gov/pmc/articles/PMC2770593/. Accessed 7 Sep 2022.
4. Ackland HM, Cooper DJ, Cooper JD, Malham GM, Kossmann T. Factors predicting cervical collar-related decubitus ulceration in major trauma patients. Spine (Phila Pa 1976). 2007;32(4):423–8.
5. Stiell IG, Clement CM, McKnight RD, Brison R, Schull MJ, Rowe BH, et al. The Canadian C-spine rule versus the NEXUS low-risk criteria in patients with trauma. N Engl J Med. 2003;349(26):2510–8.
6. Stelfox HT, Velmahos GC, Gettings E, Bigatello LM, Schmidt U. Computed tomography for early and safe discontinuation of cervical spine immobilization in obtunded multiply injured patients. J Trauma. 2007;63(3):630–6.
7. Schuster R, Waxman K, Sanchez B, Becerra S, Chung R, Conner S, et al. Magnetic resonance imaging is not needed to clear cervical spines in blunt trauma patients with normal computed tomographic results and no motor deficits. Arch Surg. 2005;140(8):762–6.
8. Hogan GJ, Mirvis SE, Shanmuganathan K, Scalea TM. Exclusion of unstable cervical spine injury in obtunded patients with blunt trauma: is MR imaging needed when multi-detector row CT findings are normal? Radiology. 2005;237(1):106–13.

9. Adams JM, Cockburn MIE, Difazio LT, Garcia FA, Siegel BK, Bilaniuk JW. Spinal clearance in the difficult trauma patient: a role for screening MRI of the spine. Am Surg. 2006;72(1):101–5.
10. Albrecht RM, Kingsley D, Schermer CR, Demarest GB, Benzel EC, Hart BL. Evaluation of cervical spine in intensive care patients following blunt trauma. World J Surg. 2001;25(8):1089–96.
11. Como JJ, Diaz JJ, Dunham CM, Chiu WC, Duane TM, Capella JM, et al. Practice management guidelines for identification of cervical spine injuries following trauma: update from the eastern association for the surgery of trauma practice management guidelines committee. J Trauma. 2009;67(3):651–9.

Part V

Metabolic Support in Critical Illness

Glycemic Control in the Critically Ill

36

Uncontrolled hyperglycemia may adversely impact critically ill patients through diverse mechanisms. High glucose levels may impair the innate immune response, with abnormal glycosylation of immunoglobulins [1]. Neutrophil migration is inhibited with suppression of phagocytic activity; complement fixation and bacterial opsonization are also disrupted by uncontrolled blood glucose levels [2]. Animal models have suggested that targeting normoglycemia may attenuate hyperglycemia-induced inhibition of bacterial opsonization [3]. Furthermore, insulin may exert an anti-inflammatory effect that may ameliorate organ dysfunction in critical illness [4] (Fig. 36.1). However, aiming for tightly controlled blood glucose levels may lead to episodes of hypoglycemia that may adversely affect outcomes. Several landmark clinical trials have explored the impact of glycemic control in critically ill patients (Table 36.1).

Nearly half a century ago, Sodi-Pollares et al. described the salutary effects of a cocktail of intravenous glucose, insulin, and potassium (GIK) on the electrocardiographic signs of acute and chronic myocardial ischemia [5]. Several studies have hence explored the benefits of GIK therapy on infarct size and survival after acute myocardial infarction [6, 7].

Intravenous infusion of insulin and maintenance of blood glucose levels within a narrow target range had its roots in postoperative patients who underwent coronary artery bypass surgery. In a pioneering study, Furnary et al. studied 3554 diabetic patients who underwent coronary artery bypass surgery over a 15-year period between 1987 and 2001 [8]. Compared to subcutaneous insulin, intravenous insulin infusion resulted in significantly better control of blood glucose levels and reduced postoperative mortality.

Do meticulously controlled blood glucose levels within a narrow range influence clinical outcomes in critically ill patients?

J. Chacko et al., *Controversies in Critical Care*,
https://doi.org/10.1007/978-981-19-9940-6_36

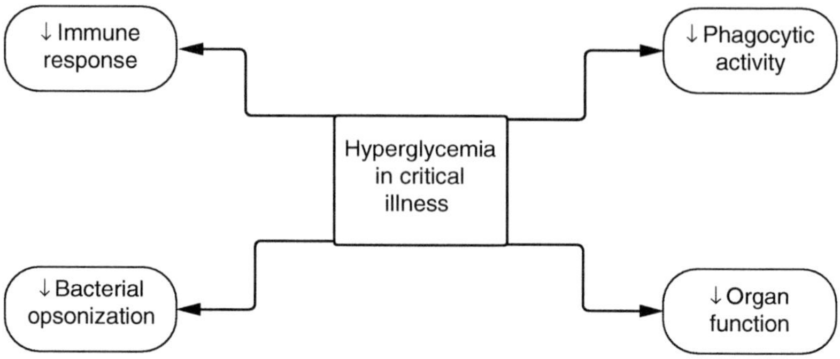

Fig. 36.1 Possible adverse effects of hyperglycemia in critically ill patients

Table 36.1 RCTs evaluating intensive insulin therapy in critically ill patients

Study/year	Population/ sample size	Blood glucose level	Control	Outcomes
Van den Berghe et al. (Leuven 1, 2001) [9]	1548 surgical ICU patients	80–110 mg/dl	Insulin commenced when blood glucose >215 mg/dl; maintained between 180 and 200 mg/dl	ICU and hospital mortality significantly less; reduced blood stream infections, less AKI requiring RRT, less blood transfusions, and reduced need for long-term ventilation and ICU care with intensive insulin therapy. Highest mortality benefit with sepsis and multiorgan failure
Van den Berghe et al. (Leuven 2, 2006) [10]	1200 medical ICU patients	80–110 mg/dl	180–200 mg/dl	In-hospital mortality similar. AKI less, time to weaning from ventilation, duration of hospital and ICU stay less with intensive insulin therapy. In-hospital mortality lower with intensive insulin therapy in patients with ICU stay >3 days
Finfer et al. (NICE-SUGAR, 2009) [11]	6104 mixed ICU patients	81–108 mg/dl	180 mg/dl or lower	90-day all-cause mortality higher, more hypoglycemic events with intensive insulin therapy. No difference in the duration of ventilation, ICU, hospital stay, requirement for RRT

RCT randomized controlled trial, *AKI* acute kidney injury, *RRT* renal replacement therapy

36.1 Review of Evidence

36.1.1 The Leuven 1 Trial—Surgical ICU Patients

One of the earliest studies on glycemic control in critically ill patients was from a surgical intensive care unit at the Catholic University of Leuven in Belgium. In this randomized controlled trial (RCT), patients were randomized to receive intensive insulin therapy to maintain a blood glucose level between 80 and 110 mg/dl in the intervention arm [9]. In the conventional arm, insulin infusion was commenced if the blood glucose level was higher than 215 mg/dl, with the maintenance of levels between 180 and 200 mg/dl. Among the 1548 patients studied, the ICU mortality was significantly lower with intensive insulin therapy compared to conventional therapy (4.6% vs. 8.0%, $p < 0.04$). The difference in mortality was predominantly evident in patients with a duration of ICU stay of more than 5 days, with the greatest mortality reduction observed in patients with a septic focus and multiorgan failure. Furthermore, intensive insulin therapy reduced the overall hospital mortality, incidence of bloodstream infections, acute kidney injury requiring renal replacement therapy, the number of red blood cell transfusions, and the incidence of critical illness polyneuropathy. Intensive insulin therapy also reduced the requirement for prolonged mechanical ventilation and intensive care.

36.1.2 The Leuven 2 Trial—Medical ICU Patients

The Leuven 1 trial revealed evidence of benefit among surgical intensive care patients, the majority being postoperative cardiac surgical patients (62.7%). Could the beneficial effects of intensive insulin therapy be replicated in a medical intensive care unit? The Leuven 2 trial included 1200 patients admitted to the medical intensive care unit, aiming for glycemic control using a similar protocol with intensive and conventional therapies [10]. In this RCT, the in-hospital mortality was not significantly different between the intensive and conventional insulin therapy groups (37.3% vs. 40.0%, $p = 0.33$). The incidence of acute kidney injury was lower with intensive insulin therapy; besides, the time to weaning from mechanical ventilation and the duration of stay in the ICU and hospital were lower with intensive insulin therapy. In-hospital mortality was lower with intensive insulin therapy in patients who stayed in the ICU for longer than 3 days and, paradoxically, higher among patients with a duration of ICU stay of less than 3 days.

36.1.3 The ANZICS NICE-SUGAR Trial

Against the background of clinical trials that revealed conflicting evidence regarding possible benefit from intensive glucose control, the NICE-SUGAR study investigators conducted a multicenter RCT across 42 ICUs in Australia, New Zealand, and North America [11]. Patients were randomized to receive intensive insulin therapy to maintain blood glucose levels between 81 and 108 mg/dl or a conventional target of 180 mg/dl or lower. The study included 3054 patients in the intensive control arm and 3050 patients in the conventional arm. Death from any cause at 90 days was significantly higher in the intensive control arm compared to the conventional arm (27.5% vs. 24.9%, OR:1.14; 95% CI, 1.02 to 1.28; $P = 0.02$). The treatment effect did not differ between medical and surgical patients. The incidence of severe hypoglycemia (blood glucose level < 40 mg/dl) was significantly higher in the intensive compared to the conventional control group (6.8% vs. 0.5%, $p < 0.001$). There was no difference in the duration of mechanical ventilation, hospital and ICU stay, or renal replacement therapy between groups. This large RCT conducted across a heterogeneous group of critically ill patients demonstrated possible harm from targeting blood glucose levels within a narrow range between 81 and 108 mg/dl.

Table 36.1 summarizes the main RCTs that have evaluated the efficacy of intensive insulin therapy in critically ill patients.

36.2 Reconciling with Conflicting Evidence

36.2.1 Time in the Target Range

Could wide variations in blood glucose levels lead to adverse outcomes? Is the duration of blood glucose levels within the target range important? In an observational study, the maintenance of a blood glucose target between 72 and 136 mg/dl for more than 70% of the time was independently associated with improved survival [12]. Reduced organ dysfunction was observed when the duration within the target range of blood glucose was more than 50%. A target blood glucose range of 70–140 mg/dl for more than 80% of the time was associated with survival among non-diabetic, critically ill patients in another observational trial [13]. It is also noteworthy that the time in the target range was as low 31% in the NICE-SUGAR trial compared to 53.1% in the Leuven 1 trial of surgical patients that showed improved survival with intensive insulin therapy [14]. The duration of blood glucose levels in the target range may thus be an important determinant of clinical outcomes.

36.2.2 Should Blood Glucose Targets Be Based on Hemoglobin A1c Levels?

The recently published CONTROLING study compared a target of 180 vs. blood glucose target range based on “usual glycemia” in a multicentric RCT

[15]. Usual glycemia was calculated based on the hemoglobin A1c (HbA1c) level using the formula:

$$\text{Usual glycemia} = (28.7 \times \text{HbA1c}) - 46.7$$

In the individualized control group, the blood glucose target was set to the usual glycemia level + 15 mg/dl or less, with a range of 111–217 mg/dl. In the conventional control group, the blood glucose level was maintained at 180 mg/dl or less. The blood glucose targets were maintained throughout the ICU stay. The all-cause mortality at 90 days was not significantly different between groups (individualized vs. conventional groups, 32.8% vs. 30.5%). No difference was observed in other clinical endpoints including the 28-day mortality, ICU length of stay, duration of vasoactive drug support, mechanical ventilation, and renal replacement therapy. On post hoc analysis, the 90-day mortality was higher among non-diabetic patients in the individualized control group, surgical patients, and patients with HbA1c levels between 5 and 6%.

36.2.3 Diabetics Vs. Non-diabetics

A more liberal target range among diabetic patients has been shown to be associated with reduced mortality in a before-and-after study [16]. Kwan et al. evaluated frequency and outcomes associated with relative hypoglycemia in 1592 critically ill diabetic patients [17]. Relative hypoglycemia was defined as a decrease in blood glucose levels below 30% of baseline levels, as estimated by HbA1c levels. The 28-day mortality was significantly higher among patients who developed relative hypoglycemia. Besides, the incidence of absolute hypoglycemia (blood glucose <70 mg/dl) was significantly higher among patients who experienced relative hypoglycemia.

Thus, the optimal target range may vary between patients with and without diabetes mellitus and need to be tailored to the clinical situation.

36.2.4 Continuous Measurement of Glucose Levels

Intermittent measurement at set time intervals may result in wide fluctuation of blood glucose levels and unidentified episodes of hypoglycemia, leading to adverse clinical outcomes [18]. Continuous subcutaneous glucose monitoring systems measure glucose levels every few minutes, might enable more efficient control, and reduce the risk of hypoglycemia [19]. Lu et al. compared glucose control using a continuous subcutaneous glucose monitoring system with conventional, intermittent point-of-care measurements [20]. Time in the target range of blood glucose between 144 and 180 mg/dl was significantly longer with continuous monitoring (51.5% vs. 29.0%, $p < 0.001$). The mean glucose level and incidence of hypoglycemia (<72 mg/dl) did not differ between groups. However, the duration of hypoglycemia was significantly lower with continuous monitoring. This study suggests that continuous subcutaneous monitoring may enable better maintenance of blood glucose within the target range with fewer episodes of hypoglycemia.

Key Points

- Tight glycemic control has failed to live up to the initial promise in real-world studies.
- Failure to maintain blood glucose levels consistently within the target range and episodes of hypoglycemia may have contributed to the adverse clinical outcomes observed.
- Time in the target range may be important to ensure efficient control.
- There is observational data that suggests hyperglycemia-associated mortality in non-diabetics; however, in diabetic patients, higher glycemic targets may be more appropriate.
- Diabetic patients may be particularly vulnerable to the adverse effects associated with relative hypoglycemia; future research should focus on optimal blood glucose range in critically ill diabetic patients.
- Continuous subcutaneous measurement of blood glucose levels may enable maintenance of blood glucose levels in the target range and lower the risk of hypoglycemia.

References

1. Turina M, Fry DE, Polk HC. Acute hyperglycemia and the innate immune system: clinical, cellular, and molecular aspects. Crit Care Med. 2005;33(7):1624–33. https://doi.org/10.1097/01.ccm.0000170106.61978.d8.
2. Jafar N, Edriss H, Nugent K. The effect of short-term hyperglycemia on the innate immune system. Am J Med Sci. 2016;351(2):201–11. https://doi.org/10.1016/j.amjms.2015.11.011.
3. Weekers F, Giulietti AP, Michalaki M, et al. Metabolic, endocrine, and immune effects of stress hyperglycemia in a rabbit model of prolonged critical illness. Endocrinology. 2003;144(12):5329–38. https://doi.org/10.1210/en.2003-0697.
4. Hansen TK, Thiel S, Wouters PJ, Christiansen JS, Van den Berghe G. Intensive insulin therapy exerts antiinflammatory effects in critically ill patients and counteracts the adverse effect of low mannose-binding lectin levels. J Clin Endocrinol Metab. 2003;88(3):1082–8. https://doi.org/10.1210/jc.2002-021478.
5. Sodi-Pallares D, Testelli MR, Fishleder BL, et al. Effects of an intravenous infusion of a potassium-glucose-insulin solution on the electrocardiographic signs of myocardial infarction. A preliminary clinical report. Am J Cardiol. 1962;9:166–81. https://doi.org/10.1016/0002-9149(62)90035-8.
6. Rogers WJ, Stanley AW, Breinig JB, et al. Reduction of hospital mortality rate of acute myocardial infarction with glucose-insulin-potassium infusion. Am Heart J. 1976;92(4):441–54. https://doi.org/10.1016/s0002-8703(76)80043-9.

7. Apstein CS, Opie LH. Glucose-insulin-potassium (GIK) for acute myocardial infarction: a negative study with a positive value. Cardiovasc Drugs Ther. 1999;13(3):185–9. https://doi.org/10.1023/a:1007757407246.
8. Furnary AP, Gao G, Grunkemeier GL, et al. Continuous insulin infusion reduces mortality in patients with diabetes undergoing coronary artery bypass grafting. J Thorac Cardiovasc Surg. 2003;125(5):1007–21. https://doi.org/10.1067/mtc.2003.181.
9. Van den Berghe G, Wouters P, Weekers F, et al. Intensive insulin therapy in critically ill patients. N Engl J Med. 2001;345(19):1359–67. https://doi.org/10.1056/NEJMoa011300.
10. Van den Berghe G, Wilmer A, Hermans G, et al. Intensive insulin therapy in the medical ICU. N Engl J Med. 2006;354(5):449–61. https://doi.org/10.1056/NEJMoa052521.
11. NICE-SUGAR Study Investigators. Intensive versus conventional glucose control in critically ill patients. N Engl J Med. 2009;360(13):1283–97. https://doi.org/10.1056/NEJMoa0810625.
12. Chase JG, Shaw G, Le Compte A, et al. Implementation and evaluation of the SPRINT protocol for tight glycaemic control in critically ill patients: a clinical practice change. Crit Care. 2008;12(2):R49. https://doi.org/10.1186/cc6868.
13. Krinsley JS, Preiser JC. Time in blood glucose range 70 to 140 mg/dl >80% is strongly associated with increased survival in non-diabetic critically ill adults. Crit Care. 2015;19:179. https://doi.org/10.1186/s13054-015-0908-7.
14. Krinsley JS, Preiser JC. Is it time to abandon glucose control in critically ill adult patients? Curr Opin Crit Care. 2019;25(4):299–306. https://doi.org/10.1097/MCC.0000000000000621.
15. Bohé J, Abidi H, Brunot V, Klich A, Klouche K, et al. CONTROLe INdividualisé de la Glycémie (CONTROLING) study group. Individualised versus conventional glucose control in critically-ill patients: the CONTROLING study-a randomized clinical trial. Intensive Care Med. 2021;47(11):1271–83. https://doi.org/10.1007/s00134-021-06526-8.
16. Krinsley JS, Preiser JC, Hirsch IB. Safety and efficacy of personalised glycemic control in critically ill patients: a 2-year before and after international trial. Endocr Pract. 2017;23(3):318–30. https://doi.org/10.4158/EP161532.
17. Kwan TN, Zwakman-Hessels L, Marhoon N, Robbins R, Mårtensson J, Ekinci E, et al. Relative hypoglycemia in diabetic patients with critical illness. Crit Care Med. 2020;48(3):e233–40.
18. Hermanides J, Vriesendorp TM, Bosman RJ, Zandstra DF, Hoekstra JB, Devries JH. Glucose variability is associated with intensive care unit mortality. Crit Care Med. 2010;38(3):838–42. https://doi.org/10.1097/CCM.0b013e3181cc4be9.
19. De Block C, Manuel-y-Keenoy B, Rogiers P, Jorens P, Van Gaal L. Glucose control and use of continuous glucose monitoring in the intensive care unit: a critical review. Curr Diabetes Rev. 2008;4(3):234–44. https://doi.org/10.2174/157339908785294460.
20. Lu M, Zuo Y, Guo J, Wen X, Kang Y. Continuous glucose monitoring system can improve the quality of glucose control and glucose variability compared with point-of-care measurement in critically ill patients. Medicine (Baltimore). 2018;97(36):e12138. https://doi.org/10.1097/MD.0000000000012138.

Vitamin C in Sepsis: End of the Debate? 37

37.1 Introduction

Oxidative stress is one of the key pathophysiological mechanisms that mediate sepsis-related tissue injury [1]. In ischemia-reperfusion injury and septic shock, there is enhanced generation of reactive oxygen species (ROS) and reactive nitrogen species (RNS), as part of the biological defense mechanism [2]. Excessive ROS activity can be harmful and is normally regulated by counterregulatory antioxidant mechanisms. However, the massive surge of ROS that often occurs in sepsis results in the overwhelming of the antioxidant defense mechanisms. Excessive ROS activity causes injury to proteins, lipids, and nucleic acids, resulting in endothelial injury and cellular and organ dysfunction [3].

37.2 ROS: Pathophysiological Mechanisms of Injury

Uncontrolled ROS activity leads to endothelial dysfunction in ischemia-reperfusion injury and sepsis. This triggers damage to the endothelial glycocalyx and cell membranes with disruption of tight intercellular junctions, resulting in increased capillary permeability [4].

Endothelial nitric oxide (eNO) is crucial in maintaining the patency of blood vessels through its vasodilator effect. The vasodilator effect of eNO is mediated through cyclic guanosine monophosphate by activation of soluble guanyl-cyclase [5]. Besides, eNO inhibits platelet aggregation and adhesion of activated platelets and leukocytes, thus maintaining vascular patency [6]. Unopposed ROS activity leads to inhibition of eNO synthetase, with reduced production of eNO and thereby loss of its vasodilator effect. The loss of the endothelial vasodilator response attenuates the effect of vasoconstrictor agents [7]. Furthermore, reduced levels of eNO lead to adhesion of leukocytes and platelets besides triggering inflammation and coagulation. Vasodilatation-induced hypotension, capillary leak, and blockage of microcirculatory blood flow ensue, leading to worsening hypoxia.

J. Chacko et al., *Controversies in Critical Care*,
https://doi.org/10.1007/978-981-19-9940-6_37

Ascorbate, the redox product of vitamin C, ameliorates oxidative stress in endothelial cells through inhibition of the generation of ROS, including superoxide, hydrogen peroxide, and peroxynitrite [8]. Ascorbate may also scavenge peroxides at high doses and increase the bioavailability of eNO. Through the generation of eNO by stimulation of eNOS, ascorbate may also tighten the endothelial barrier, thereby decreasing endothelial permeability. Ascorbate may also inhibit apoptosis [9] and promote the generation of endothelial progenitor cells [10]. Ascorbate-mediated inhibition of ROS may attenuate ischemia-reperfusion injury to the myocardium, thereby reducing the incidence of myocardial stunning and arrhythmias [11].

37.3 The Antioxidant Effect of Vitamin C in Sepsis

Vitamin C, by its antioxidant effect, may ameliorate tissue injury triggered by oxidative stress [12]. Preclinical studies have demonstrated the putative benefits of vitamin C in reversing the pathophysiological changes observed in sepsis. Vitamin C may improve the response to vasopressor agents [13]. Besides, it may augment the endothelial barrier function by mitigating the increase in vascular permeability [14], thereby enhancing microvascular blood flow [15]. Humans are unable to synthesize vitamin C [16], and levels are often low in critically ill patients [17]. Hence, biological plausibility suggests that vitamin C supplementation in critically ill septic patients may be beneficial (Fig. 37.1).

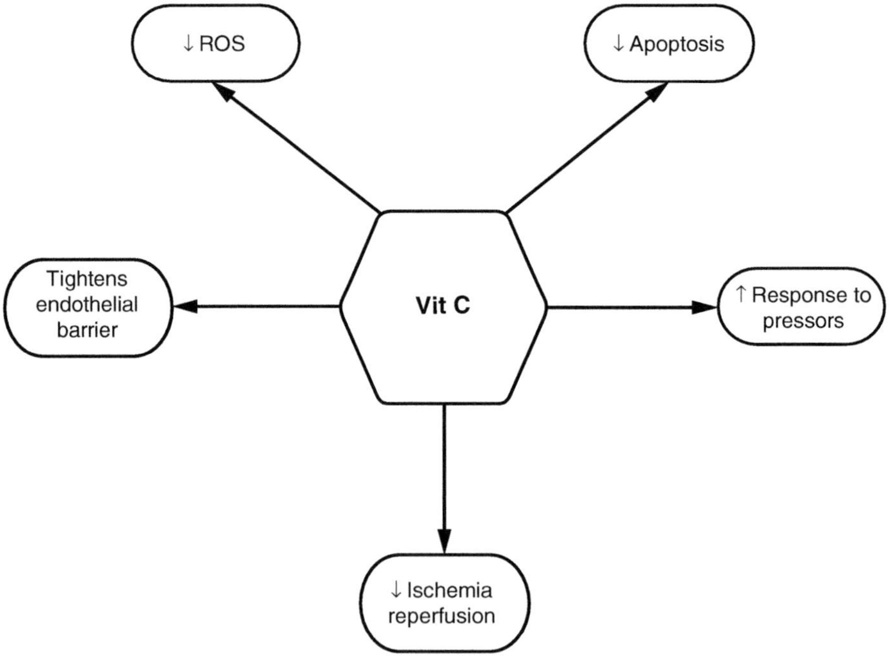

Fig. 37.1 Putative benefits of vitamin C in sepsis

37.4 Vitamin C in Sepsis: Clinical Studies

Considering the potential for clinical benefit from its antioxidant effect, several recent clinical trials have evaluated clinical outcomes using variable doses of vitamin C in patients with sepsis (Table 37.1). Vitamin C has been administered as monotherapy or as combination therapy with thiamine and hydrocortisone.

37.4.1 High-Dose Vitamin C

The LOVIT study was carried out in 35 medical-surgical ICUs in Canada, France, and New Zealand [18]. This study included patients who had suspected or proven infection and were on vasopressor support. In the intervention arm, vitamin C 50 mg/kg was administered 6 h, intravenously, for 96 h for a maximum of 16 doses. The control group received matching placebo. Thiamine and glucocorticoids were administered based on clinician judgment. The vitamin C group included 429 patients, and the control group 434 patients. The primary outcome, a composite of death or persistent organ dysfunction at 28 days, was significantly higher in the vitamin C compared to the control group (44.5% vs. 38.5%; risk ratio: 1.21; 95% CI, 1.04 to 1.40; $P = 0.01$). Among the secondary outcomes, there was no significant difference in the individual components of the composite primary outcome—mortality or persisting organ dysfunction at 28 days. The median organ dysfunction-free days were also not significantly different between groups. The SOFA scores at specific time intervals from days 1–28, 6-month survival, and health-related quality of life were also similar between the two groups. This study clearly demonstrated a lack of beneficial effect and possible harm from the use of high-dose vitamin C in patients with severe sepsis.

37.4.2 Vitamin C in Patients with Sepsis and Acute Respiratory Distress Syndrome (ARDS)

The CITRIS-ALI trial randomized 167 patients with sepsis and ARDS to receive vitamin C 50 mg/kg/6 h intravenously or placebo for 96 h [19]. The change in the mean modified SOFA scores from baseline to 96 h was similar between the two groups. The C-reactive protein and thrombomodulin levels were also similar at 168 h. On exploratory analysis without adjustment for multiple comparisons, the 28-day mortality was significantly lower in the vitamin C group (29.8% vs. 46.3%; $p = 0.03$).

37.4.3 Vitamin C as Part of Combination Therapy

Marik et al. performed an electronic health record-based, retrospective, before-after study to evaluate the efficacy of treatment with a cocktail including vitamin C,

Table 37.1 Main studies on the effect of vitamin C in sepsis

Study (year)	Type	Population	Intervention	Control	Outcomes (intervention vs. control)
Marik et al. [20] (2017)	Electronic health record -based retrospective before-after study	Primary diagnosis of severe sepsis or septic shock and a procalcitonin level 2 ng/mL	47 patients Vitamin C 1.5 g/6 h × 4 days, hydrocortisone 50 mg/6 h × 7 days, thiamine 200 mg/12 h × 4 days	47 patients Hydrocortisone 50 mg/6 h at clinician discretion	Hospital mortality lower with the Vit C cocktail: 8.5% vs. 40.4% ($P < 0.001$) Mean vasopressor duration lower: 54.9 vs. 28.4 h ($P < 0.001$)
Fowler et al. [19] (CITRIS-ALI, 2019)	Randomized controlled trial	Sepsis, ARDS	84 patients Vitamin C 50 mg/kg/6 h × 4 days	83 patients Placebo	No change in mean modified SOFA score from baseline to 96 h: 3 vs. 3.5 points; difference – 0.10; 95% CI, −1.23 to 1.03; $P = 0.86$ C-reactive protein and thrombomodulin levels similar
Fujii et al. [21] (VITAMINS, 2020)	Randomized controlled trial	Septic shock	107 patients Vitamin C 1.5 g/6 h, hydrocortisone 50 mg/6 h, thiamine 200 mg/12 h	104 patients Hydrocortisone 50 mg/6 h	No difference in the time alive and off vasopressor until day 7: 122.1 (76.3–145.4 h) vs. 124.6 h (82.1–147.0 h) $P = 0.83$); no difference in the 90-day mortality: 28.6% vs. 24.5% (hazard ratio, 1.18; 95% CI, 0.69–2.00)
Sevransky et al. [22] (VICTAS, 2021)	Randomized controlled trial	Sepsis-induced respiratory or cardiovascular dysfunction	252 patients Vitamin C 1.5 g/6 h, thiamine 100 mg/6 h, and hydrocortisone 50 mg /6 h	249 patients Placebo	No difference in the median ventilator- and vasopressor-free days: 25 (IQR, 0–29 days) vs. 26 days (IQR, 0–28 days). Median difference: −1 day (95% CI, −4 to 2 days; $P = 0.85$) 30-days mortality similar: 22% vs. 24%

Lamontagne et al. [18] (LOVIT, 2022)	Randomized controlled trial	Proven or suspected infection, on vasopressors, not longer than 24 h in ICU	429 patients Vitamin C 50 mg/kg/6 h × 96 h	434 patients Placebo	Death or persistent organ dysfunction on day 28 higher with vit C: 44.5% vs. 38.5% (risk ratio, 1.21; 95% CI, 1.04 to 1.40; $P = 0.01$) 28-days mortality: 35.4% vs. 31.6% (risk ratio, 1.17; 95% CI, 0.98 to 1.40) Persistent organ dysfunction on day 28 was similar: 9.1% vs. 6.9% risk ratio, 1.30; 95% CI, 0.83 to 2.05
Hwang et al. [23] (ATESS, 2020)	Randomized controlled trial	Septic shock	53 patients Vitamin C 50 mg/kg (max single dose: 3 g), thiamine 200 mg every 12 h × 48 h	58 patients	No difference in ΔSOFA between groups (baseline- 72 h) scores 3, (−1 to 5) vs. 3, (0–4), $p = 0.96$ No difference in mortality at 7, 28, and 90 days; no difference in ICU or hospital mortality. Shock reversal, vasopressor-free days similar

thiamine, and hydrocortisone in patients with septic shock [20]. During a 7-month period, consecutive patients with severe sepsis or septic shock and a procalcitonin level ≥ 2 ng/mL were administered vitamin C 1.5 g/h, hydrocortisone 50 mg/6 h, and thiamine 200 mg/12 h. Vasopressors were administered to target a mean arterial pressure of 65 mm Hg. The control group included consecutive patients with severe sepsis or septic shock admitted during a 7-month period preceding the intervention. During the control period, no patient received thiamine or vitamin C as part of therapy. Forty-seven patients were included in each group. The hospital mortality was significantly lower in the treatment group (8.5% vs. 40.4%, $P < 0.001$). On propensity-adjusted analysis, the odds ratio for mortality with the vitamin C cocktail was 0.13 (95% CI, 0.04–0.48; $P = 0.002$). The mean duration of vasopressor support was also significantly shorter in the intervention arm (18.3 vs. 54.9 h, $P = 0.001$). This observational study suggested possible benefits with a combination of vitamin C, thiamine, and hydrocortisone in patients with septic shock; the authors suggested further controlled trials to confirm the findings of their study.

Against the background of the Marik et al. study, the VITAMINS trial evaluated the effect of a cocktail including vitamin C, thiamine, and hydrocortisone in patients with septic shock [21]. The eligibility criteria included a primary diagnosis of septic shock with an acute increase in the SOFA score by at least two points, a lactate level >2 mmol/l and the requirement for vasopressor support for at least 2 h prior to enrollment. The combination of intravenous vitamin C 1.5 g/6 h, hydrocortisone 50 mg/6 h, and thiamine 200 mg/12 h was compared to a control group that received hydrocortisone 50 mg/6 h alone. This multicenter RCT was conducted across ten ICUs in Australia, New Zealand, and Brazil. In the primary analysis, 107 patients were included in the intervention arm; 104 were included in the control arm.

The primary outcome, the duration of time alive and vasopressor-free days until day 7, was not significantly different between the two groups [intervention group: 122.1 (76.3–145.4 h) vs. control group: 124.6 (82.1–147.0 h, $P = 0.83$)]. Among the secondary outcomes, there was no significant difference between groups in the 28-, 90-day, ICU, or hospital mortality. The duration of vasopressor-free days, mechanical ventilation-free days, and renal replacement-free days was also similar between the two groups. The SOFA score decreased by day 3 in both groups; the decrease was marginally greater in the intervention group. This study demonstrated that the combination of vitamin C, thiamine, and hydrocortisone did not lead to a more rapid resolution of septic shock compared to hydrocortisone alone.

The vitamin C cocktail was evaluated among patients with sepsis in the VICTAS trial [22]. Patients with cardiovascular or respiratory dysfunction due to suspected infection were included. In the intervention arm, patients received intravenous vitamin C 1.5 g, thiamine 100 mg, and hydrocortisone 50 mg, 6 h for up to 96 h. The treatment was commenced within 4 h of randomization. Matching placebos were administered in the control group. The trial was designed to include up to 2000 patients; however, it was prematurely stopped after the enrolment of 501 patients due to a lack of continued funding. The intervention group included 252 patients in the primary analysis, with 249 patients in the control group. The primary outcome, the ventilator- and vasopressor-free days in the first 30 days following randomization, was not significantly different between groups [intervention: 25 days (0–29 days) vs. control: 26 days (0–28 days), $p = 0.85$]. The 30-day mortality was also similar between the intervention and the control groups (22% vs. 24%). This study, although terminated early, did not reveal any difference in clinical outcomes with the use of the vitamin C cocktail in patients with sepsis with respiratory or cardiovascular dysfunction.

The findings of the South Korean, multicenter ATESS RCT were similar [23]. Patients in septic shock were randomized to receive intravenous vitamin C 50 mg/kg (maximum dose of 6 g/day) and thiamine 200 mg 12 h for 48 h or placebo. Among the 111 patients enrolled, 53 were included in the intervention group and 58 in the control group. Vasopressin infusion and hydrocortisone 200 mg/day were administered in patients who required high-dose norepinephrine. The primary outcome was Δ SOFA, the difference between the baseline and 72-h SOFA scores. No significant difference was observed in the Δ SOFA at 72 h between the intervention and the control groups [3, (− 1 to 5) vs. 3, (0–4), $P = 0.96$]. Predefined secondary outcomes, including the 7-, 28-, 90-day, hospital, and ICU mortality, were also similar between the two groups. The occurrence of shock reversal was also similar.

37.4.4 Meta-analysis of Vitamin C in Sepsis

Agarwal et al. performed a meta-analysis of RCTs that evaluated the effect of vitamin C as monotherapy or combination therapy among hospitalized patients with severe infection [24]. The authors identified 41 RCTs including 4915 patients eligible for inclusion. Low-quality evidence suggested that vitamin C may reduce in-hospital, 30-day, and early mortality. However, on sensitivity analysis including only published trials that were blinded and with a low risk of bias, the impact of vitamin C was nonsignificant. All the trials that evaluated the 90-day mortality were at low risk of bias and revealed higher mortality with vitamin C administration. There was no evidence of benefit among subgroups of patients related to cointerventions (monotherapy vs. combination therapy), the dose administered, or the type of infection. Overall, there was no evidence of improved survival in this meta-analysis.

Key Points

- Oxidative stress arising from the generation of excessive ROS may be a key trigger of sepsis-induced organ dysfunction.
- Vitamin C evokes robust antioxidant mechanisms and may mitigate the impact of oxidative stress in sepsis.
- Besides enhancing the response to vasopressor agents through inhibition of the synthesis of eNO, vitamin C may also augment endothelial barrier function and reduce vascular permeability.
- Preclinical studies had demonstrated putative benefits of vitamin C in reversing the pathophysiological changes observed in sepsis; this led to several clinical trials that explored possible clinical benefit from vitamin C administration either alone or in combination with thiamine and hydrocortisone in patients with sepsis.
- An early observational study by Marik et al. revealed reduced hospital mortality and a shorter duration of vasopressor support in patients with septic shock who were administered a cocktail of vitamin C, thiamine, and hydrocortisone.
- Subsequently, several RCTs have evaluated the benefit of vitamin C alone or in combination in patients with sepsis; however, no evidence of clinical benefit has been observed.
- The composite outcome of death or persistent organ dysfunction at 28 days was significantly higher with a high-dose vitamin C cocktail in the LOVIT study, the largest RCT so far on this topic.
- Based on the available evidence, there is no suggestion of benefit with vitamin C therapy, either alone or in combination, in patients with severe sepsis and septic shock.

References

1. Mantzarlis K, Tsolaki V, Zakynthinos E. Role of oxidative stress and mitochondrial dysfunction in sepsis and potential therapies. Oxidative Med Cell Longev. 2017;2017:5985209.
2. De Backer D, Orbegozo Cortes D, Donadello K, Vincent JL. Pathophysiology of microcirculatory dysfunction and the pathogenesis of septic shock. Virulence. 2014;5(1):73–9.
3. Biesalski HK, McGregor GP. Antioxidant therapy in critical care--is the microcirculation the primary target? Crit Care Med. 2007;35(9 Suppl):S577–83.
4. Burke-Gaffney A, Evans TW. Lest we forget the endothelial glycocalyx in sepsis. Crit Care. 2012;16(2):121.
5. Hellsten Y, Nyberg M, Jensen LG, Mortensen SP. Vasodilator interactions in skeletal muscle blood flow regulation. J Physiol. 2012;590(24):6297–305.
6. Cyr AR, Huckaby LV, Shiva SS, Zuckerbraun BS. Nitric oxide and endothelial dysfunction. Crit Care Clin. 2020;36(2):307–21.
7. Rubio-Gayosso I, Platts SH, Duling BR. Reactive oxygen species mediate modification of glycocalyx during ischemia-reperfusion injury. Am J Physiol Heart Circ Physiol. 2006;290(6):H2247–56.

8. Wilson JX, Wu F. Vitamin C in sepsis. Subcell Biochem. 2012;56:67–83.
9. Haendeler J, Zeiher AM, Dimmeler S. Vitamin C and E prevent lipopolysaccharide-induced apoptosis in human endothelial cells by modulation of Bcl-2 and Bax. Eur J Pharmacol. 1996;317(2–3):407–11.
10. Fiorito C, Rienzo M, Crimi E, Rossiello R, Balestrieri ML, Casamassimi A, et al. Antioxidants increase number of progenitor endothelial cells through multiple gene expression pathways. Free Radic Res. 2008;42(8):754–62.
11. Valls N, Gormaz JG, Aguayo R, González J, Brito R, Hasson D, et al. Amelioration of persistent left ventricular function impairment through increased plasma ascorbate levels following myocardial infarction. Redox Rep. 2016;21(2):75–83.
12. Amrein K, Oudemans-van Straaten HM, Berger MM. Vitamin therapy in critically ill patients: focus on thiamine, vitamin C, and vitamin D. Intensive Care Med. 2018;44(11):1940–4.
13. Armour J, Tyml K, Lidington D, Wilson JX. Ascorbate prevents microvascular dysfunction in the skeletal muscle of the septic rat. J Appl Physiol (1985). 2001;90(3):795–803.
14. Han M, Pendem S, Teh SL, Sukumaran DK, Wu F, Wilson JX. Ascorbate protects endothelial barrier function during septic insult: role of protein phosphatase type 2A. Free Radic Biol Med. 2010;48(1):128–35.
15. Tyml K, Li F, Wilson JX. Septic impairment of capillary blood flow requires nicotinamide adenine dinucleotide phosphate oxidase but not nitric oxide synthase and is rapidly reversed by ascorbate through an endothelial nitric oxide synthase-dependent mechanism. Crit Care Med. 2008;36(8):2355–62.
16. Drouin G, Godin JR, Pagé B. The genetics of vitamin C loss in vertebrates. Curr Genomics. 2011;12(5):371–8.
17. Carr AC, Rosengrave PC, Bayer S, Chambers S, Mehrtens J, Shaw GM. Hypovitaminosis C and vitamin C deficiency in critically ill patients despite recommended enteral and parenteral intakes. Crit Care. 2017;21(1):300.
18. Lamontagne F, Masse MH, Menard J, Sprague S, Pinto R, Heyland DK, et al. Intravenous vitamin C in adults with sepsis in the intensive care unit. N Engl J Med. 2022;386(25):2387–98.
19. Fowler AA, Truwit JD, Hite RD, Morris PE, DeWilde C, Priday A, et al. Effect of vitamin C infusion on organ failure and biomarkers of inflammation and vascular injury in patients with sepsis and severe acute respiratory failure: the CITRIS-ALI randomized clinical trial. JAMA. 2019;322(13):1261.
20. Marik PE, Khangoora V, Rivera R, Hooper MH, Catravas J. Hydrocortisone, vitamin C, and thiamine for the treatment of severe sepsis and septic shock: a retrospective before-after study. Chest. 2017;151(6):1229–38.
21. Fujii T, Luethi N, Young PJ, Frei DR, Eastwood GM, French CJ, et al. Effect of vitamin C, hydrocortisone, and thiamine vs hydrocortisone alone on time alive and free of vasopressor support among patients with septic shock: the VITAMINS randomized clinical trial. JAMA. 2020;323(5):423.
22. Sevransky JE, Rothman RE, Hager DN, Bernard GR, Brown SM, Buchman TG, et al. Effect of vitamin C, thiamine, and hydrocortisone on ventilator- and vasopressor-free days in patients with sepsis: the VICTAS randomized clinical trial. JAMA. 2021;325(8):742.
23. Hwang SY, Ryoo SM, Park JE, Jo YH, Jang DH, Suh GJ, et al. Combination therapy of vitamin C and thiamine for septic shock: a multi-Centre, double-blinded randomized, controlled study. Intensive Care Med. 2020;46(11):2015–25.
24. Agarwal A, Basmaji J, Fernando SM, Ge FZ, Xiao Y, Faisal H, et al. Parenteral vitamin C in patients with severe infection: a systematic review. NEJM Evid. 2022; https://doi.org/10.1056/EVIDoa2200105.

Part VI

The Gut and Nutrition

38 Early or Supplemental Parenteral Nutrition vs. Enteral Nutrition Alone in the Critically Ill

38.1 Introduction

Enteral nutrition (EN) alone often fails to meet nutritional targets in critically ill patients [1]. An observational study revealed that critically ill patients may receive only up to 50% of the calorie target over the first 12 days. Initiation of EN may also be prolonged by more than 60 h after ICU admission [2]. Early, aggressive enteral feeding may result in intolerance and lead to aspiration [3]. Besides, a higher incidence of gastrointestinal adverse effects including vomiting, diarrhea, bowel ischemia, and pseudo-obstruction of the colon has been reported with early EN [4]. Underfeeding may occur with EN alone and may be associated with muscle weakness and an increase in the incidence of infections and prolong the duration of mechanical ventilation [5].

38.2 The Role of Parenteral Nutrition (PN)

Conventionally, PN has been considered to be associated with a higher risk of complications compared to EN. The incidence of infectious complications may be higher with PN, as suggested by previous meta-analyses [6, 7]. The higher risk of infections may have been related to poor glycemic control with PN [8]. However, more recent randomized controlled trials (RCTs) that compared early EN vs. PN did not reveal any difference in infectious complications or mortality [4, 9].

Early, targeted nutritional support may reduce catabolism and attenuate muscle wasting besides maintaining nutritional status [10]. EN, with supplemental PN, may prevent nutritional deficit; however, such a strategy might lead to overfeeding resulting in hepatic dysfunction, nosocomial infections, and prolongation of ventilatory

J. Chacko et al., *Controversies in Critical Care*,
https://doi.org/10.1007/978-981-19-9940-6_38

support [11, 12]. Based on the available evidence, current clinical guidelines do not recommend the commencement of supplemental PN during the first week of ICU admission [13]. Several RCTs have evaluated the impact of initiating PN early or combining PN with EN to meet nutritional targets among critically ill patients.

38.3 Early or Supplemental PN and Outcomes: The Evidence

38.3.1 Early PN

Does early PN within 24 h of ICU admission in patients with short-term contraindications to EN improve clinical outcomes? Doig et al. evaluated this question among 1372 patients admitted to the ICU in a multicentric study conducted in Australia and New Zealand [14]. Patients were expected to stay in the ICU for more than 2 days. The early PN group included 686 patients with caloric targets based on the Harris-Benedict equation and a maximum limit of 35 kcal/kg/day. The protein dose was not targeted independently. The standard care group also included 686 patients; feeding was not protocolized in this group, with the attending physician choosing the route, initial dose, targets, and composition based on clinical judgment. The time to commencement of nutritional support was 2.8 days in the standard care group compared to 44 min after randomization in the early PN group. Among patients randomized to standard care, 29.2% were initiated on EN, while 27.3% were commenced on PN; 40.8% of patients did not receive feeds. The 60-day mortality, the primary outcome, was not significantly different between the two groups (early PN vs. standard care: 22.8 vs. 21.5%). The 60-day quality of life, assessed using the RAND-36 score, was significantly better in the early PN group; however, although statistically significant, the difference did not reach the magnitude set a priori as clinically meaningful. Patients who received early PN also received fewer days of mechanical ventilation and experienced less muscle wasting and fat loss compared to the standard care group. The duration of stay in ICU and hospital was not different between the two groups.

Although early PN did not improve the 60-day survival, this study suggested that loss of muscle mass may be attenuated with early PN. The authors hypothesized that improved diaphragmatic function may have resulted in a reduced requirement for mechanical ventilator support in the early PN group.

38.3.2 Supplemental PN in General ICU Patients

Considering the failure of EN alone to achieve nutritional targets in the early phase of critical illness, several RCTs have examined the efficacy of supplemental PN combined with EN in improving clinical outcomes among critically ill patients (Table 38.1).

Table 38.1 RCTs comparing the efficacy of early or supplemental PN combined with EN alone in critically ill patients

Study/year	Population	Intervention	Control	Outcomes
Doig et al. [14] (2013)	Critically ill patients with relative contraindications to EN, expected to stay in ICU for >2 days	Early PN with aim to achieve nutritional targets by day 3	Route, time of commencement, and targets, based on clinician judgment and local practice	60-day mortality, duration of ICU and hospital stay similar in both groups. 60-day QOL significantly better in the early PN group, although not considered clinically meaningful. Early PN associated with fewer days of mechanical ventilation, less muscle wasting and fat loss
Heidegger et al. [15] (2013)	Critically ill patients in whom nutritional targets could not be attained with EN alone by day 3, expected ICU stay >5 d	Supplemental PN to meet the energy target from day 4 to day 8	EN alone	Fewer infective complications from day 8 to day 28 with supplemental PN. Less antibiotic use with supplemental PN. Duration of mechanical ventilation, ICU and hospital stay, hospital mortality, not different between groups
Casaer et al. [16] (EPaNIC, 2011)	ICU patients at nutritional risk based on the NRS scale	EN supplemented with PN on day 3 to achieve 100% caloric requirement	Supplemental PN commenced on day 8 to achieve calorie target	Duration of ICU stay less, higher likelihood of being discharged alive earlier from the ICU and from the hospital with late PN. Lower incidence of nosocomial infections, reduced duration of mechanical ventilation and requirement for RRT with late PN. Cost of care less with late PN
Ridely et al. [17] (2018)	Mechanically ventilated patients with at least one organ failure; EN delivery below 80% of estimated requirement	Supplemental PN within 48–72 h of ICU admission	Usual practice	Duration of stay in hospital and the ICU, hospital mortality, and use of antibiotics not different between groups

(continued)

Table 38.1 (continued)

Study/year	Population	Intervention	Control	Outcomes
Wischmeyer et al. [19] (TOP-UP, 2017)	Patients with a BMI of <25 or >35 with acute respiratory failure, expected to require mechanical ventilation for >72 h	Supplemental PN with EN aiming for 100% nutrition goal	EN alone	Incidence of new infections similar; trend toward lower hospital mortality in the supplemental PN group. Trend toward lower ICU and hospital mortality in patients with BMI <25
Gao et al. [20] (2022)	Patients undergoing major abdominal surgery at high nutritional risk	Supplemental PN, administered from post-op among patients who underwent major abdominal surgery	Late PN from day 8 post-op	Nosocomial infections significantly lower with early supplemental PN. No difference in incidence of non-infectious complications, adverse events, or symptoms of gastrointestinal intolerance
Allingstrup et al. [21] (EAT-ICU, 2017)	Mechanically ventilated patients with expected ICU stay >3 days	EGDN aiming to meet 100% of nutritional requirements from day 1 with EN combined with PN	25 kcal/kg/day by EN	No difference in the physical quality of life at 6 months. 6-month mortality, duration of ICU and hospital stay, life support-free days at 90 days, similar

EN enteral nutrition, *PN* parenteral nutrition, *QOL* quality of life, *NRS* nutritional risk screening, *RRT* renal replacement therapy, *BMI* body mass index

Would supplemental PN be beneficial among critically ill patients in whom nutritional targets cannot be met with EN alone by day 3? Heidegger et al. studied patients who received less than 60% of their caloric requirement target from EN by day 3 of ICU admission with an expected duration of ICU stay of more than 5 days [15]. The study patients were expected to survive for more than 7 days. The energy target was calculated by indirect calorimetry or as 25 kcal/kg for women and 30 kcal/kg for men. Patients were randomized to receive supplemental PN to meet the energy target from day 4 to day 8 or to continue with EN alone. The supplemental PN group received significantly higher calories compared to patients who received EN alone between day 4 and day 8 (103% vs. 77% of target). Patients who received supplemental PN and attained caloric targets experienced significantly fewer infective complications from day 8 to day 28 compared to those who continued to receive EN alone (27% vs. 38%). The use of antibiotics was also significantly lower among patients who received supplemental PN. The duration of mechanical ventilation, duration of ICU and hospital stay, and mortality did not differ between groups.

Supplemental PN was evaluated in the EPaNIC study, a multicentric RCT conducted across seven ICUs in Belgium. Patients were randomized to the early or late PN group [16]. In the early group, EN was supplemented with PN on day 3 with the goal of achieving 100% caloric requirement. Among patients in the late group in whom EN was insufficient, supplemental PN was commenced on day 8 to achieve the calorie target. The median duration of stay in the ICU was less by 1 day in the late PN group; besides, late PN was associated with a significantly higher likelihood of being discharged alive earlier from the ICU and from the hospital. Patients in the late PN had a lower incidence of nosocomial infections and reduced duration of mechanical ventilation and renal replacement therapy. The cost of healthcare was also significantly less with the late initiation of PN. Thus, the EPaNIC study supported delayed initiation of PN, if nutritional targets could not be achieved within a week.

A pilot RCT across six centers in Australia and New Zealand evaluated a supplemental PN strategy within 48–72 h of ICU admission [17]. In the control arm, the usual practice at the study center was followed, with administration of PN only if EN delivery continued to remain insufficient. Calorie and protein delivery was significantly higher with supplemental PN during the 7-day intervention period. However, clinical and functional outcomes including the use of antibiotics, ICU and hospital stay, and mortality were similar between the two groups.

38.3.3 Supplemental PN in Under- and Overweight Subjects

Would underweight and obese critically ill patients be particularly vulnerable to the effects of undernutrition? A higher calorie intake might lead to improved outcomes among this subgroup of critically ill patients [18]. The TOP-UP pilot trial tested this hypothesis in patients with a BMI of <25 or >35 with acute respiratory failure who were expected to require mechanical ventilation for more than 72 h [19]. Patients were randomized to EN alone or supplemented with PN to achieve 100% of the nutritional target. Over the first 7 days, the supplemental PN group revealed a 26% increase in the delivery of calories and protein, compared to a 22% increase in the EN alone group. Clinical outcomes were not significantly different between the two groups in this pilot trial. The overall incidence of new infections was similar; there was a trend toward lower hospital mortality in the supplemental PN group. There was a trend toward reduced ICU and hospital mortality in the subgroup of underweight patients with BMI <25, underlining the requirement for future studies in this context. There was no increase in the incidence of nosocomial infections in supplemental PN compared with the EN-alone group.

38.3.4 Supplemental PN Following Abdominal Surgery

Enteral nutrition is often delayed following abdominal surgery and may lead to delayed wound healing, nosocomial infections, prolongation of hospital stay, and higher mortality. Would early supplemental PN lead to improved clinical outcomes in postoperative patients following abdominal surgery?

Gao et al. evaluated the impact of early supplemental PN, administered from day 3 postoperatively compared with late administration from day 8 among patients who underwent major abdominal surgery in an RCT [20]. These patients were considered to be at high nutritional risk with poor tolerance to EN. Patients in the early supplemental PN group received significantly more calories compared with the late supplemental PN group between days 3 and 7. The incidence of nosocomial infections, the primary outcome, was significantly lower with early supplemental PN. No difference was noted in the incidence of non-infectious complications, adverse events, or symptoms of gastrointestinal intolerance. In contrast to previous studies, this RCT revealed a decrease in the incidence of nosocomial infections with early supplemental PN in patients at high nutritional risk and intolerance to enteral nutrition.

38.3.5 Individualized Calorie and Protein Delivery

Most trials on nutritional support do not target the protein requirement. The EAT-ICU trial evaluated the efficacy of early goal-directed nutrition based on indirect calorimetry and 24-h urinary urea excretion to calculate the protein requirement

[21]. Based on this calculation, 100% of the nutritional requirement was administered from day 1 of the study for the entire duration of ICU stay. EN was combined with PN to meet nutritional targets. In the control group, energy requirement was calculated as 25 kcal/kg/day, and EN was commenced within 24 h of randomization. EN was stepped up gradually; if the calculated calorie goal could not be met by day 7, supplemental PN was commenced. Patients randomized to the early goal-directed nutrition arm received more calories and protein compared to the standard care arm. However, early goal-directed nutrition did not result in any improvement in the physical quality of life at 6 months. Mortality at 6 months, the duration of stay in the ICU and hospital, and life support-free days at 90 days were also similar between the two groups.

38.4 Nutritional Strategies for the Future

Most clinical studies on nutritional strategies have targeted heterogeneous groups of critically ill patients. Particularly, the premorbid nutritional state may have a crucial impact on the planning of the nutritional strategy and clinical outcomes. A more intensive nutritional strategy might benefit patients who are malnourished at the outset [22]. Patients who are underweight or obese at baseline and those expected to require prolonged supportive care in the ICU may benefit from an early, aggressive nutritional strategy [19]. A crucial component of nutritional therapy may be the provision of adequate proteins. Most RCTs have not focused on protein requirements; this could explain the relative lack of efficacy of a solely calorie-targeted nutritional approach [23]. In fact, in non-septic critically ill patients, the provision of an early, high-protein nutritional approach was associated with lower mortality compared to an early high-calorie approach [24]. In an RCT on PN that compared 0.8 g/kg compared to 1.1 g/kg of protein per day, higher protein administration was associated with greater handgrip strength at 1 week, reduced fatigue score, improved forearm muscle thickness, and higher cross-sectional area of the rectal femoris muscle assessed by ultrasonography [25].

Most nutritional research so far has been based on hardcore clinical outcomes including mortality. Future investigations should address the impact of optimizing nutritional support on improved quality of life among survivors of critical illness, including alleviation of fatigue and enhanced muscle strength. The provision of early EN and enhanced protein delivery during the early phase of critical illness needs to be evaluated in this perspective.

Key Points

- EN alone may not meet nutritional requirements, particularly during the early phase of critical illness. Pursuance of an early, aggressive EN strategy may lead to intolerance and adverse clinical outcomes.
- Prolonged underfeeding from EN alone may lead to muscle weakness and an increase in the incidence of infections. Diaphragmatic weakness may prolong the duration of mechanical ventilation.
- Earlier studies suggested that PN may be associated with more infectious complications compared to EN; however, more recent studies establish the relative safety of PN.
- Supplemental PN to mitigate the shortfall in nutritional targets has been evaluated in several RCTs. However, there is no definite indication toward an advantage with supplemental PN during the first week of critical illness.
- Early, supplemental PN may improve outcomes in subgroups of patients with a poor nutritional state at the baseline.
- Future studies should address the efficacy of fulfilling protein targets besides caloric requirements; besides, outcomes related to the quality of life after critical illness need heightened focus.

References

1. Genton L, Dupertuis YM, Romand JA, Simonet ML, Jolliet P, Huber O, et al. Higher calorie prescription improves nutrient delivery during the first 5 days of enteral nutrition. Clin Nutr. 2004;23(3):307–15.
2. Cahill NE, Dhaliwal R, Day AG, Jiang X, Heyland DK. Nutrition therapy in the critical care setting: what is "best achievable" practice? An international multicenter observational study. Crit Care Med. 2010;38(2):395–401.
3. Desachy A, Clavel M, Vuagnat A, Normand S, Gissot V, François B. Initial efficacy and tolerability of early enteral nutrition with immediate or gradual introduction in intubated patients. Intensive Care Med. 2008;34(6):1054–9.
4. Reignier J, Boisramé-Helms J, Brisard L, Lascarrou JB, Ait Hssain A, Anguel N, et al. Enteral versus parenteral early nutrition in ventilated adults with shock: a randomised, controlled, multicentre, open-label, parallel-group study (NUTRIREA-2). Lancet. 2018;391(10116):133–43.
5. Villet S, Chiolero RL, Bollmann MD, Revelly JP, Cayeux RNMC, Delarue J, et al. Negative impact of hypocaloric feeding and energy balance on clinical outcome in ICU patients. Clin Nutr. 2005;24(4):502–9.
6. Gramlich L, Kichian K, Pinilla J, Rodych NJ, Dhaliwal R, Heyland DK. Does enteral nutrition compared to parenteral nutrition result in better outcomes in critically ill adult patients? A systematic review of the literature. Nutrition. 2004;20(10):843–8.
7. Peter JV, Moran JL, Phillips-Hughes J. A metaanalysis of treatment outcomes of early enteral versus early parenteral nutrition in hospitalized patients. Crit Care Med. 2005;33(1):213–20; discussion 260–261
8. McCulloch A, Bansiya V, Woodward JM. Addition of insulin to parenteral nutrition for control of hyperglycemia. JPEN J Parenter Enteral Nutr. 2018;42(5):846–54.

9. Harvey SE, Parrott F, Harrison DA, Bear DE, Segaran E, Beale R, et al. Trial of the route of early nutritional support in critically ill adults. N Engl J Med. 2014;371(18):1673–84.
10. McClave SA, Martindale RG, Rice TW, Heyland DK. Feeding the critically ill patient. Crit Care Med. 2014;42(12):2600–10.
11. Dhaliwal R, Jurewitsch B, Harrietha D, Heyland DK. Combination enteral and parenteral nutrition in critically ill patients: harmful or beneficial? A systematic review of the evidence. Intensive Care Med. 2004;30(8):1666–71.
12. Grau T, Bonet A, Rubio M, Mateo D, Farré M, Acosta JA, et al. Liver dysfunction associated with artificial nutrition in critically ill patients. Crit Care. 2007;11(1):R10.
13. Compher C, Bingham AL, McCall M, Patel J, Rice TW, Braunschweig C, et al. Guidelines for the provision of nutrition support therapy in the adult critically ill patient: the American Society for Parenteral and Enteral Nutrition. J Parenter Enter Nutr. 2022;46(1):12–41.
14. Doig GS. Early parenteral nutrition in critically ill patients with short-term relative contraindications to early enteral nutrition: a randomized controlled trial. JAMA. 2013;309(20):2130.
15. Heidegger CP, Berger MM, Graf S, Zingg W, Darmon P, Costanza MC, et al. Optimisation of energy provision with supplemental parenteral nutrition in critically ill patients: a randomised controlled clinical trial. Lancet. 2013;381(9864):385–93.
16. Casaer MP, Mesotten D, Hermans G, Wouters PJ, Schetz M, Meyfroidt G, et al. Early versus late parenteral nutrition in critically ill adults. N Engl J Med. 2011;365(6):506–17.
17. Ridley EJ, Davies AR, Parke R, Bailey M, McArthur C, Gillanders L, et al. Supplemental parenteral nutrition versus usual care in critically ill adults: a pilot randomized controlled study. Crit Care. 2018;22(1):12.
18. Alberda C, Gramlich L, Jones N, Jeejeebhoy K, Day AG, Dhaliwal R, et al. The relationship between nutritional intake and clinical outcomes in critically ill patients: results of an international multicenter observational study. Intensive Care Med. 2009;35(10):1728–37.
19. Wischmeyer PE, Hasselmann M, Kummerlen C, Kozar R, Kutsogiannis DJ, Karvellas CJ, et al. A randomized trial of supplemental parenteral nutrition in underweight and overweight critically ill patients: the TOP-UP pilot trial. Crit Care. 2017;21(1):142.
20. Gao X, Liu Y, Zhang L, Zhou D, Tian F, Gao T, et al. Effect of early vs. late supplemental parenteral nutrition in patients undergoing abdominal surgery: a randomized clinical trial. JAMA Surg. 2022;157(5):384–93.
21. Allingstrup MJ, Kondrup J, Wiis J, Claudius C, Pedersen UG, Hein-Rasmussen R, et al. Early goal-directed nutrition versus standard of care in adult intensive care patients: the single-Centre, randomised, outcome assessor-blinded EAT-ICU trial. Intensive Care Med. 2017;43(11):1637–47.
22. Heyland DK, Dhaliwal R, Jiang X, Day AG. Identifying critically ill patients who benefit the most from nutrition therapy: the development and initial validation of a novel risk assessment tool. Crit Care. 2011;15(6):R268.
23. National Heart, Lung, and Blood Institute Acute Respiratory Distress Syndrome (ARDS) Clinical Trials Network, Rice TW, Wheeler AP, Thompson BT, Steingrub J, Hite RD, et al. Initial trophic vs full enteral feeding in patients with acute lung injury: the EDEN randomized trial. JAMA. 2012;307(8):795–803.
24. Weijs PJ, Looijaard WG, Beishuizen A, Girbes AR, Oudemans-van Straaten HM. Early high protein intake is associated with low mortality and energy overfeeding with high mortality in non-septic mechanically ventilated critically ill patients. Crit Care. 2014;18(6):701.
25. Ferrie S, Allman-Farinelli M, Daley M, Smith K. Protein requirements in the critically ill: a randomized controlled trial using parenteral nutrition. JPEN J Parenter Enteral Nutr. 2016;40(6):795–805.

Stress Ulcer Prophylaxis in the Critically Ill

39

39.1 Introduction

"Stress ulcer prophylaxis" is part of the dogma of modern intensive care protocols and is mandated in many "bundles of care." The actual prevalence of significant stress ulceration is very low, however, and there is emerging evidence that prophylactic agents are themselves associated with harm, particularly from nosocomial infection due to gastric acid suppression and subsequent colonization of the upper aerodigestive tract. Major clinical trials are currently underway to re-evaluate the place of stress ulcer prophylaxis in modern intensive care practice.

39.2 Pathophysiology and History

"Stress ulceration" with severe gastrointestinal hemorrhage was first described in 1969 in 8 of 150 consecutive critically ill patients with multiorgan failure, of whom 7 (4.7%) died [1]. In the six who had post-mortem examinations, the hemorrhage was due to lesions in the mucosa of the gastric fundus. Subsequent endoscopic studies reported between 74% and 100% of critically patients had stress-related mucosal erosions and sub-epithelial hemorrhage [2], and as a consequence, some form of "stress ulcer prophylaxis" became common practice, initially using histamine-2 receptor antagonists (H_2RAs) such as cimetidine [3] or ranitidine or cytoprotective agents such as sucralfate. More recently proton-pump inhibitors (PPI) have been increasingly used. Stress ulcer prophylaxis (SUP) was included as one of the elements of the "ventilator bundle" of the US Institute for Healthcare Improvement [4], and many studies since then have evaluated the overall "bundle" [5] without necessarily critically evaluating the individual components.

J. Chacko et al., *Controversies in Critical Care*,
https://doi.org/10.1007/978-981-19-9940-6_39

In a large prospective cohort study in 1994, 2252 consecutive patients were studied in 4 major Canadian ICUs [6]. Only 33 (1.5%) had clinically important GI bleeding, of whom 23 developed bleeding despite the use of SUP. Overall, only 30% of the cohort were prescribed SUP. The two independent risk factors were the presence of respiratory failure and coagulopathy, and only two patients without these risk factors had bleeding. Mortality was 48.5% in those with bleeding and 9.1% in those without. In the mechanically ventilated cohort, 3.7% had clinically significant bleeding. The authors conclude SUP could be safely withheld from patients unless they have coagulopathy or require mechanical ventilation.

39.3 Controversies

1. Despite increasing use of prophylactic acid-suppression drugs, the incidence of GI bleeding does not appear to have changed.

   In a period-prevalence study in 2014, conducted in 97 ICUs in 11 countries, 2.6% of 1034 patients had clinically important GI bleeding [7]. In this cohort 73% of patients received SUP, most frequently a PPI (pantoprazole). In the subset of 544 patients who were mechanically ventilated, the prevalence of clinically important bleeding was 3.1%, very similar to the 3.7% seen 20 years earlier. In the 2014 study, only two patients (0.19%) were found to have bleeding peptic ulcers on endoscopy. This is very similar to the findings from 20 years earlier. It is possible that prophylactic drugs are not targeting the real cause of GI bleeding in the critically ill.
2. At the same time, there is emerging evidence of possible harm from stress ulcer prophylaxis and particularly from the ubiquitous use of PPIs.

   Gastric acid suppression leads to bacterial colonization of the upper gastrointestinal tract and can predispose to nosocomial infections, particularly pneumonia [8]. SUP has, in particular, been associated with ventilator-associated pneumonia (VAP), with evidence in that H_2RAs may have been associated with a higher incidence of VAP [9]. Many of the trials in this analysis were older trials with lower rates of enteral feeding in critically ill patients, which led clinicians to question whether the results are applied in the modern era of early enteral feeding. A greater incidence of VAP has however been seen in the presence of H_2RAs [OR 2.8] in one more recent examination of exclusively enterally fed patients [10]. The risk of VAP with PPIs also appears to be greater than that seen with H_2RA, with an OR of 1.2 in a large observational cohort of 35,312 critically ill patients [11].

   In the community, the escalating use of PPIs has been associated with several complications, including pneumonia, osteoporotic fractures and magnesium deficiency, acute interstitial nephritis, vitamin B12 deficiency, and extensive drug-drug interactions. A meta-analysis of eight community-based observational studies with 1.9 million subjects found an increased risk of pneumonia, with a risk ratio of 1.27 [12]. There is an even stronger association with other infections such as *Clostridioides difficile*, with an odds ratio of 1.74 in one meta-analysis [13] which has led to formal warnings by drug regulatory agencies.

3. Routine SUP, particularly with PPIs, has been incorporated into many protocols and "bundles" without robust evidence and at great expense.

   To date, there is no convincing evidence to support the routine prescription of PPIs for SUP in critically ill patients, but since the adoption of many "bundles" which include SUP as a quality marker in some jurisdictions, this has become habit for clinicians in many areas and is very difficult to break. Early SUP trials in the 1970s and 1980s had significant methodological flaws and were conducted in very different clinical environments compared to the modern intensive care unit. Despite the weakness of the underlying evidence, the Surviving Sepsis Campaign suggests SUP be used in patients who have risk factors for gastrointestinal bleeding, though the 2021 *Surviving Sepsis Guidelines* have downgraded a previously strong recommendation to what is now a weak recommendation based on moderate quality evidence [14].
4. Public health concerns about over-prescribing and ongoing prescribing of PPIs.

   Many patients who were not taking acid suppression medication prior to ICU had these medications continued after discharge from ICU and even after discharge from the hospital, increasing the risk and the potential cost to the community [15].

39.4 Recent Trials

Recent major trials have looked at this ongoing controversy or are currently recruiting patients.

The PEPTIC trial [16] in Australia, New Zealand, Canada, and Ireland used a novel registry-embedded cluster crossover RCT methodology to compare 13,436 mechanically ventilated patients receiving an H_2-receptor blocker with 13,392 randomized to receive a PPI. The primary outcome was 90-day mortality, which was 17.5% (H_2-RB) vs. 18.3% (PPI) with an incidence of 1.8% vs. 1.3% of clinically significant bleeding.

Stress Ulcer Prophylaxis in the Intensive Care Unit (SUPICU) was a recent 3298 patient European RCT comparing pantoprazole with placebo [17]. The primary endpoint was a composite outcome of clinically important GI bleeding, pneumonia, *Clostridioides difficile* infection, and myocardial ischemia; there was no significant difference between groups (21.9% vs. 22.6%, RR 0.96, 95% CI 0.83–1.11). There were fewer GI bleeds in the pantoprazole group (2.5% vs. 4.2%), but many did not lead to blood transfusion, endoscopy, or any other intervention, leaving open to question the significance of this finding. The mortality was marginally higher at 90 days in the pantoprazole group compared to placebo (31.1% vs. 30.4%).

Re-Evaluating the Inhibition of Stress Erosions: Gastrointestinal Bleeding Prophylaxis in ICU (REVISE) is currently recruiting in Australia, New Zealand, and Canada [18]. This is a placebo-controlled comparison with pantoprazole in 4800 patients who are mechanically ventilated and expected to remain ventilated for ≥48 h. The primary efficacy endpoint is clinically important GI bleeding, centrally adjudicated, and the primary safety endpoint is 90-day all-cause mortality. At the time of writing, more than half (2400 patients) have been recruited. There is an interesting ethical twist to this trial, in that patients receiving pantoprazole are considered to be the control group (receiving usual care), whereas placebo is considered to be the intervention. The primary trial will be accompanied by a detailed Health Economic Analysis.

Key Points

- Based on current evidence, SUP is only indicated in high-risk patients (coagulopathic or on mechanical ventilation).
- SUP may be necessary only until enteral feeds are established, following which it should be ceased.
- Ongoing trials address the possible harms of routine SUP; the risks of SUP may well outweigh the benefits.
- In the meantime, cautious and judicious use is recommended.

References

1. Skillman JJ, Bushnell LS, Goldman H, et al. Respiratory failure, hypotension, sepsis and jaundice. A clinical syndrome associated with lethal hemorrhage from acute stress ulceration of the stomach. Am J Surg. 1969;117(4):523–30.
2. Czaja AJ, McAlhany JC, Pruitt BA. Acute gastroduodenal disease after thermal injury. An endoscopic evaluation of incidence and natural history. N Engl J Med. 1974;291(18):925–9.
3. Peura DA, Johnson LF. Cimetidine for prevention and treatment of gastroduodenal mucosal lesions in patients in an intensive care unit. Ann Intern Med. 1985;103(2):173–7.
4. Institute for Healthcare Improvement. Available at http://www.ihi.org. Accessed 27 Sep 2022
5. Zilberberg MD, Shorr AF, Kollef MH. Implementing quality improvements in the intensive care unit: ventilator bundle as an example. Crit Care Med. 2009;3791:305–9.
6. Cook DJ, Fuller HD, Guyatt GH, et al. Risk factors for gastrointestinal bleeding in critically ill patients. New Engl J Med. 1994;330(6):377–81.
7. Krag M, Perner A, Wetterslev J, et al. Prevalence and outcome of gastrointestinal bleeding and use of acid suppressants in acutely ill adult intensive care patients. Intens Care Med. 2015;41(4):833–45.
8. Plummer MP, Blaser AR, Deane AM. Stress ulceration: prevalence, pathology and association with adverse outcomes. Crit Care. 2014;18(2):213.
9. Krag M, Perner A, Wetterslev J, et al. Stress ulcer prophylaxis versus placebo or no prophylaxis in critically ill patients. A systematic review of randomised clinical trials with meta-analysis and trial sequential analysis. Intens Care Med. 2014;40(1):11–22.
10. Marik PE, Vasu T, Hirani A, et al. Stress ulcer prophylaxis in the new millennium; a systematic review and meta-analysis. Crit Care Med. 2010;38(11):2222–8.
11. MacLaren R, Reynolds PM, Allen RR. Histamine-2 receptor antagonists vs proton pump inhibitors on gastrointestinal tract hemorrhage and infectious complications in the intensive care unit. JAMA Intern Med. 2014;174(4):564–74.
12. Eom CS, Jeon CY, Lim JW, et al. Use of acid-suppressive drugs and risk of pneumonia: a systematic review and meta-analysis. CMAJ. 2011;183(3):310–9.
13. Kwok CS, Arthur AK, Anibueze CI, et al. Risk of Clostridium difficile infection with acid suppressing drugs and antibiotics: meta-analysis. Am J Gastroenterol. 2012;107(7):1011–9.

14. Evans L, Rhodes A, Alhazzani W, et al. Surviving sepsis campaign: international guidelines for management of sepsis and septic shock 2021. Intens Care Med. 2021;49(11):e1063–143. https://doi.org/10.1007/s00134-021-06506-y.
15. Farley KJ, Barned KL, Crozier TM. Inappropriate continuation of stress ulcer prophylaxis beyond the intensive care setting. Crit Care Resusc. 2013;15(2):147–51.
16. The PEPTIC Investigators. Effect of stress ulcer prophylaxis with proton pump inhibitors vs Histamine-2 receptor blockers on in-hospital mortality among ICU patients receiving invasive mechanical ventilation. JAMA. 2020;323(7):616–26. https://doi.org/10.1001/jama.2019.22190.
17. Krag M, Marker S, Perner A, et al. Pantoprazole in patients at risk for gastrointestinal bleeding in the IACU. New Engl J Med. 2018;379(23):2199–208.
18. Re-Evaluating the Inhibition of Stress Erosions: Gastrointestinal Bleeding Prophylaxis in ICU (REVISE), NCT03374800, ClinicalTrials.gov. Accessed 27 Sep 2022.

Do Tradition-Borne Fasting Practices Apply to ICU Patients with a Protected Airway?

40

40.1 Introduction

The first recorded case of possible aspiration from general anesthesia occurred in 1848, when Hannah Greener, a 15-year-old girl, underwent chloroform anesthesia for the removal of a toenail. Her surgeon, Dr. Meggison, who conducted the anesthetic, administered an extra dose of chloroform dropped through a handkerchief placed over her face. However, she began to cough and her lips turned blue. Dr. Meggison tried to revive her with water and a few drops of brandy; in spite of his best efforts, she choked and died. Subsequently, Simpson, one of the early proponents of chloroform anesthesia, extensively investigated the case. He came to the conclusion that Hannah had probably died of pulmonary aspiration that had little to do with any toxic effect of chloroform. Seven years later, John Snow recommended 6 h of fasting before chloroform anesthesia. The text books of that era followed this up and stipulated variable periods of fasting for patients undergoing procedures under anesthesia.

40.2 Fasting in the ICU

Feeding is commonly interrupted in critically ill patients for presumed intolerance, performance of investigations, and surgical procedures that may be airway or non-airway related. Fasting may occur for extended periods on a regular basis in ICU patients in spite of the airway protection offered by a cuffed endotracheal tube or a tracheostomy. Fasting prior to extubation in the ICU is a typical example. Extubation rarely takes place at a fixed time, resulting in unduly prolonged periods of fasting. It may not occur at all and may be reconsidered the following day. The fasting protocol may get repeated day after day for several days until the patient finally gets extubated, leading to a significantly reduced delivery of nutrition.

J. Chacko et al., *Controversies in Critical Care*,
https://doi.org/10.1007/978-981-19-9940-6_40

Fasting guidelines are highly variable; besides, adherence to the guidelines is also not consistent. The American Society of Anesthesiology recommends fasting for solid food of 8 h, while the European Society of Anesthesia stipulates a 6-h fasting period [1]. A UK survey revealed only 20% of institutions had clear-cut guidelines, with a relatively low adherence of 66% [2].

40.3 Possible Harmful Effects of Fasting

A large international multicenter study observed that critically ill patients were uniformly underfed, receiving an average of only 59% of the prescribed energy [3]. This was also evident in the CALORIES trial, where the calorie target was not achieved with either the enteral (62% of target) or the parenteral route (73% of target). Undernutrition may lead to an increase in the rate of nosocomial infections, besides leading to higher all-cause mortality, bloodstream infections, and prolonged ICU and hospital stay [4, 5]. Besides meeting nutritional requirements, enteral feeds maintain the integrity of the gut mucosal barrier and reduce the incidence of infections through bacterial translocation [6]. Enteral nutrition also plays an important part in modulating the stress response to critical illness [7].

40.4 Pre-procedural Fasting in Critically Ill Patients with Protected Airway

Historically, fasting has been recommended to reduce the incidence of aspiration. Traditional fasting guidelines are intended for awake, otherwise healthy patients, eating normal food who are scheduled to undergo elective surgical procedures. Do we need to religiously apply the same rigid guidelines in our ICU patients who undergo non-airway-related procedures, with their airways protected to the maximal extent possible by endotracheal intubation or tracheostomy? Unfortunately, no standard fasting guidelines exist for critically ill patients with protected airways. Malnutrition may lead to an increase in the incidence of infectious complications, which in turn may lead to prolongation of the duration of mechanical ventilation, ICU, and hospital stay [8, 9].

40.5 Is It Time to Reconsider the Duration of Fasting in ICU Patients—What Is the Evidence?

Uninterrupted enteral nutrition is an important facet of care of burns patients, who often need to undergo repeated, prolonged surgical procedures, during which significant nutritional deficits occur due to interruption of enteral feeding. In a retrospective study, Varon et al. evaluated the feasibility and safety of intraoperative feeding in burns patients. Thirty-three patients were included; 17 patients received intraoperative enteral feeds, while 16 did not. Feeding was carried out through a postpyloric tube and continued throughout the intraoperative period. No difference in mortality was observed between the two groups; besides, there was no intraoperative incidence of regurgitation or aspiration in either group. Patients who continued to be fed intraoperatively received 98% of the prescribed nutrition, compared to 70–73% among those who were not fed. The authors concluded that continued intraoperative enteral feeding in burns patients was feasible without an increase in the incidence of intraoperative regurgitation, aspiration, or increase in mortality while maintaining nutritional targets [10].

A before-after study evaluated the impact of a revised fasting guideline for patients on enteral nutrition with a protected airway (endotracheal tube or tracheostomy). The study was conducted in a mixed, general, and trauma ICU. According to the guideline, enteral nutrition was continued until the patient left the ICU for non-airway surgery and other procedures. Feeding was ceased 4 h prior to airway-related procedures. Enteral nutrition was recommenced soon after returning from theater if feasible and after 4 h following extubation. Although complete elimination of fasting was not achieved, a significant reduction in the duration of fasting was noted before and after procedures. The delivery of enteral nutrition improved with a lower calorie deficit after guideline implementation. No incidence of pulmonary aspiration was noted during the study period [11].

In a study among surgical ICU patients, 14 received continued feeding through a postpyloric tube until the commencement of the procedure. The procedures included debridement of necrotizing fasciitis, bowel surgery, and orthopedic procedures. The mean duration of interruption of feeding per procedure was only 222.4 min; an additional 4.7 h of feeding was provided through avoidance of the conventional period of NPO.

Critically ill trauma patients on invasive mechanical ventilation who underwent surgical or non-surgical procedures were the subjects of the study by Pousman et al. Enteral feeds administered through a gastric tube were continued for up to 45 min of the procedure; feeding through a small bowel feeding tube was continued until the time of commencement of the procedure. The investigators specifically evaluated the incidence of complications related to continued enteral feeding, including ventilated associated pneumonia, urinary infections, catheter-related bloodstream infections, wound infections, hypoglycemia, and intraoperative vomiting and regurgitation. There was no increase in the incidence of complications compared to a control group who underwent a conventional duration of fasting before the procedure. The authors concluded that continued feeding up until the commencement of the procedure was safe and allowed to meet nutritional targets better [12].

How about fasting prior to bedside percutaneous tracheostomy? Yeh et al. compared 10 patients who were continued on routine enteral feeding with 22 patients who were fasted according to American Society of Anesthesiology NPO guidelines

[13]. Patients who continued to be fed received higher median calories and had less calorie deficit on the day of the procedure compared to the control group. The overall incidence of complications was not different between groups, including airway-related, gastrointestinal, and infectious complications. Table 40.1 summarizes important studies that have evaluated the impact of the duration of fasting among ICU patients.

Table 40.1 Studies that have evaluated the impact of the duration of fasting among ICU patients

Study/year	Population	Intervention	Control	Findings
Varon et al. (2017) [10]	Major burns	Enteral nutrition was continued intraoperatively	No intraoperative feeding	Continued enteral feeds intraoperatively resulted in greater achievement of prescribed protein and caloric targets. No aspiration noted intraoperatively. No difference in mortality between groups
Segaran et al. (2016) [11]	ICU patients with airway protected by intubation or tracheostomy	Implementation of a fasting guideline	Before guideline implementation	A significant reduction in the duration of fasting noted before and after procedures. Lower calorie deficit after guideline implementation. No incidence of pulmonary aspiration noted during the study period
Pousman et al. (2009) [12]	Critically ill, mechanically ventilated trauma patients	Enteral nutrition until the time of the procedure, if on small bowel feeds; enteral nutrition discontinued 45 min prior to procedure, if on gastric feeds	Pre-implementation phase with an 8-h fasting protocol	Greater delivery of enteral nutrition, more rapid achievement of nutritional targets. Infective complications similar; no difference in other adverse outcomes. No difference in ICU length of stay
Yeh et al. (2015) [13]	ICU patients scheduled for bedside PDT	Enteral nutrition continued until just before the procedure; compensatory nutrition for the duration of fasting	Fasting protocol based on the ASA guidelines	No difference in the incidence of gastrointestinal, infective complications. Higher caloric delivery in the no fasting group with compensatory nutrition for the duration of interruption of feeds

Key Points

- Continuing enteral nutrition in patients with a protected airway who do not undergo airway-related procedures does not lead to an increase in the incidence of complications or adverse clinical outcomes.
- Continued feeding enables more efficient achievement of nutritional goals with a reduced incidence of nutritional deficiencies.
- Feeds are interrupted for varying periods in patients with protected airways based on an archaic belief that complications related to regurgitation and aspiration may ensue. This tradition-borne practice is based on recommendations meant for otherwise healthy patients, who eat normal food and present for elective procedures.
- The presumed higher incidence of aspiration-related complications related to continued enteral feeding in patients with protected airways is not supported by the available evidence. A shorter period of fasting allows more optimal achievement of nutritional goals; prolonged 8-h fasting or NPO from midnight may be inappropriate in critically ill patients with protected airways.
- The available evidence suggests that a reduced duration of fasting or even no routine fasting prior to general anesthesia in critically ill adult patients who have a cuffed endotracheal or tracheostomy tube in place may be safe and appropriate, especially in the context of non-airway-related and non-abdominal surgery.
- Continued feeding, in addition to improved achievement of nutritional goals, may also lead to more favorable clinical outcomes. Needless to emphasize, patients must be closely observed during and after the procedure for subclinical signs of aspiration.

References

1. López Muñoz AC, Busto Aguirreurreta N, Tomás BJ. Preoperative fasting guidelines: an update. Rev Esp Anestesiol Reanim. 2015;62(3):145–56. https://doi.org/10.1016/j.redar.2014.09.006.
2. Segaran E, Lovejoy TD, Proctor C, et al. Exploring fasting practices for critical care patients—a web-based survey of UK intensive care units. J Intensive Care Soc. 2018;19(3):188–95. https://doi.org/10.1177/1751143717748555.
3. Alberda C, Gramlich L, Jones N, et al. The relationship between nutritional intake and clinical outcomes in critically ill patients: results of an international multicenter observational study. Intensive Care Med. 2009;35(10):1728–37. https://doi.org/10.1007/s00134-009-1567-4.
4. Villet S, Chiolero RL, Bollmann MD, et al. Negative impact of hypocaloric feeding and energy balance on clinical outcome in ICU patients. Clin Nutr. 2005;24(4):502–9. https://doi.org/10.1016/j.clnu.2005.03.006.
5. Strack van Schijndel RJM, Weijs PJM, Koopmans RH, Sauerwein HP, Beishuizen A, Girbes ARJ. Optimal nutrition during the period of mechanical ventilation decreases mortality in critically ill, long-term acute female patients: a prospective observational cohort study. Crit Care. 2009;13(4):R132. https://doi.org/10.1186/cc7993.

6. Alpers DH. Enteral feeding and gut atrophy. Curr Opin Clin Nutr Metab Care. 2002;5(6):679–83. https://doi.org/10.1097/00075197-200211000-00011.
7. McClave SA, Sexton LK, Spain DA, et al. Enteral tube feeding in the intensive care unit: factors impeding adequate delivery. Crit Care Med. 1999;27(7):1252–6. https://doi.org/10.1097/00003246-199907000-00003.
8. Seron-Arbeloa C, Zamora-Elson M, Labarta-Monzon L, Mallor-Bonet T. Enteral nutrition in critical care. J Clin Med Res. 2013;5(1):1–11. https://doi.org/10.4021/jocmr1210w.
9. Marik PE, Zaloga GP. Early enteral nutrition in acutely ill patients: a systematic review. Crit Care Med. 2001;29(12):2264–70. https://doi.org/10.1097/00003246-200112000-00005.
10. Varon DE, Freitas G, Goel N, et al. Intraoperative feeding improves calorie and protein delivery in acute burn patients. J Burn Care Res. 2017;38(5):299–303. https://doi.org/10.1097/BCR.0000000000000514.
11. Segaran E, Barker I, Hartle A. Optimising enteral nutrition in critically ill patients by reducing fasting times. J Intensive Care Soc. 2016;17(1):38–43.
12. Pousman RM, Pepper C, Pandharipande P, et al. Feasibility of implementing a reduced fasting protocol for critically ill trauma patients undergoing operative and nonoperative procedures. JPEN J Parenter Enteral Nutr. 2009;33(2):176–80. https://doi.org/10.1177/0148607108327527.
13. Yeh DD, Cropano C, Quraishi SA, et al. Periprocedural nutrition in the intensive care unit: a pilot study. J Surg Res. 2015;198(2):346–50. https://doi.org/10.1016/j.jss.2015.06.039.

Part VII

Infections and Antibiotic Therapy

Multidrug-Resistant Gram-Negative Bacteria in the ICU: Do We Have Answers?

41

41.1 Introduction

Following the discovery of penicillin in 1928, and its widespread use in clinical practice from the 1940s, several new antibiotic classes were introduced. Vancomycin was introduced in 1958, followed by cephalosporins, beta-lactamase inhibitors, and quinolones. However, since the introduction of carbapenems in the 1980s, no new class of antibiotics has been added to our therapeutic armamentarium. Multidrug-resistant bacteria have, in the meantime, multiplied across the globe by several-fold. There has been an ever-increasing concern with multidrug-resistant Gram-negative bacteria in critically ill patients.

41.2 What Is Antimicrobial Resistance (AMR)? How Does It Occur?

Microorganisms may be intrinsically resistant to some antimicrobial agents, e.g., *Pseudomonas aeruginosa* is intrinsically resistant to first- and second-generation cephalosporins. Resistance genes are located mainly on plasmids that can easily transfer resistance within the same or other species, especially among Gram-negative bacteria. Acquired AMR occurs through different mechanisms (Fig. 41.1).

J. Chacko et al., *Controversies in Critical Care*,
https://doi.org/10.1007/978-981-19-9940-6_41

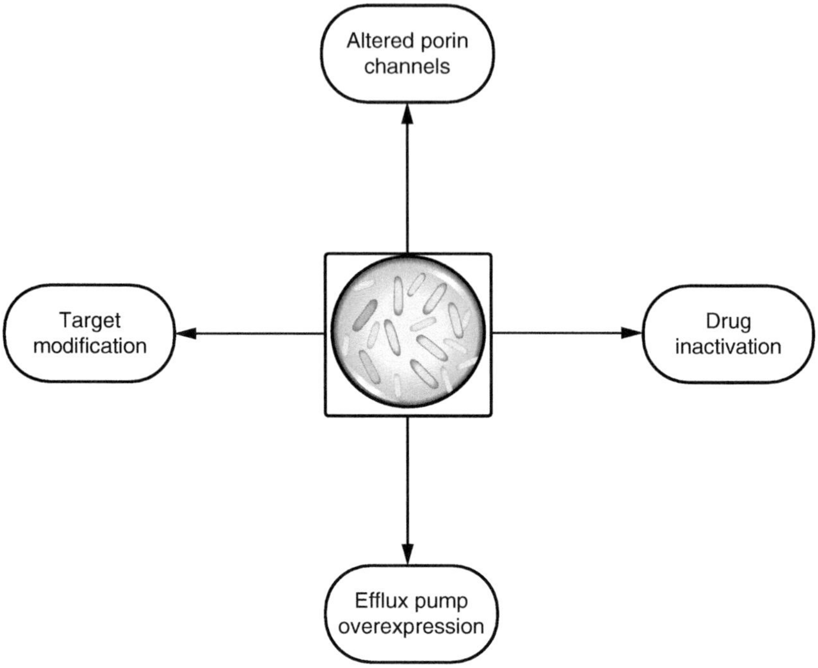

Fig. 41.1 Mechanisms of resistance in Gram-negative bacteria

41.2.1 Limitation of Drug Uptake by the Microorganism

The lipopolysaccharide cell membrane of Gram-negative bacteria acts as a barrier to the entry of antimicrobial agents. Some bacteria have large outer membranes with porin channels that allow entry of antimicrobial agents. Resistance may occur due to a decrease in the number of porin channels or from mutations that alter their affinity to antimicrobial agents [1].

41.2.2 Alteration in Drug Targets

Antimicrobial agents bind to specific targets on the bacterial cell wall, thus facilitating entry into the cell. Bacteria are capable of modifying the configuration of these targets, thus inhibiting the binding of the antimicrobial agent to the cell wall. Gram-positive bacteria develop resistance to beta-lactam antibiotics by altering the configuration of penicillin-binding proteins (PBPs) located on their cell wall. The change in the PBPs reduces binding, leading to beta-lactam resistance.

41.2.3 Inactivation of the Antimicrobial Agent

Bacteria may inactivate antimicrobial agents by degradation of the drug. The beta-lactamases inactivate antimicrobial agents through enzymatic hydrolysis. Another mechanism of drug inactivation occurs through the transfer of chemical groups including acetyl, phosphoryl, and adenyl groups, which renders the antimicrobial agent ineffective.

41.2.4 Efflux Pumps

Efflux pumps present in Gram-negative bacteria actively remove antimicrobial agents and other substances that are toxic to the bacterial cell. Biofilm resistance is mediated through efflux pumps in microorganisms including *Pseudomonas aeruginosa*, *Escherichia coli*, and *Candida albicans*.

41.3 Multidrug Resistance (MDR) and Extensive Drug Resistance (XDR)

Considering the lack of consensus in the definitions of resistance, an expert international group, as a joint initiative of the European Centre for Disease Prevention and Control (ECDC) and the Center for Disease Control and Prevention (CDC), created a standardized terminology for bacterial resistance [2]. The expert group defined multidrug resistance (MDR) as acquired resistance to at least one drug in three or more antibiotic categories. Extensive drug resistance (XDR) was defined as resistance to at least one agent in all except two or fewer categories and pan drug resistance (PDR) as resistance to all agents of all categories. Resistance testing is rarely carried out against all antibiotic categories; hence these definitions cannot be strictly applied to bedside practice. However, they are useful in the surveillance of antibiotic resistance.

The burden of AMR varies widely across countries and continents. It is difficult to assess the true incidence of resistance globally; data are scarce from many parts of the world where regular surveillance may not be undertaken. The Antimicrobial Resistance Collaborators performed a systematic analysis to evaluate the mortality and disability-adjusted life-years due to AMR. The study analyzed AMR across 204 countries and territories in 2019; an estimated 1.27 million deaths were attributable to AMR. The mortality attributable to AMR was highest in sub-Saharan Africa, followed by South Asia, and Eastern Europe. The lowest attributable mortality was observed in Australasia, followed by North Africa and the Middle East. The six leading pathogens that caused mortality from AMR included *Escherichia coli*, *Staphylococcus aureus*, *Klebsiella pneumoniae*, *Streptococcus pneumoniae*, *Acinetobacter baumannii*, and *Pseudomonas aeruginosa* [3].

41.4 Antibiotic Resistance in the ICU

Critically ill patients are especially susceptible to infection with resistant organisms. They are often treated with multiple antibiotics, leading to the evolution of resistant microbial flora. The extensive use of broad-spectrum antibiotics, often inappropriate, is closely associated with the development and transmission of drug-resistant microorganisms [4]. Patient-to-patient transmission occurs through fomites and the hands of healthcare workers. The underlying severity of illness, prolonged stay in the ICU, presence of invasive lines, and the underlying immunocompromised state that often accompanies critical illness are predisposing factors for vulnerability to resistant organisms [5].

According to the World Health Organization (WHO), antimicrobial resistance constitutes a major threat to human health [6]. A UK Government health report estimated that approximately ten million people will die yearly due to antimicrobial resistance if the current trend continues unabated [7]. Are these gross overestimates of the real-world situation, or should we be really concerned?

41.5 Gram-Negative Infections

Worldwide, Gram-negative infections represent a major challenge among critically ill patients. Common Gram-negative pathogens of concern in the ICU are MDR *Pseudomonas aeruginosa*, *Acinetobacter* spp., carbapenem-resistant *Enterobacterales* including carbapenemase producers, and extended-spectrum beta-lactamase (ESBL) producing *Enterobacterales*. ESBL-producing organisms have been observed to spread in the community and within healthcare settings [8]. In a post hoc analysis of a multicenter European surveillance study, the ICU transmission rate of non-*E. coli Enterobacterales* that produce ESBL were 3.7 times higher compared to *E. coli Enterobacterales* that produce ESBL. The main non-*E. coli Enterobacterales* producing ESBL was *K. pneumoniae* [9]. MDR *Pseudomonas aeruginosa* and *Acinetobacter* outbreaks occur frequently in ICUs; the latter may be more common [10]. Contact transmission occurs more often with *Acinetobacter*, while transmission through contaminated devices and water occurs more commonly with *Pseudomonas aeruginosa* infections. In fact, handwashing areas were reservoirs of infection for carbapenemase-producing and carbapenem-resistant *Enterobacterales* in a surveillance study [11]. Water-free hand hygiene resulted in a reduction in the transmission of Gram-negative organisms in a study from five ICUs in the Netherlands [12].

41.6 MDR Gram-Negative Infections in the ICU and Outcomes

Infections caused by resistant bacterial strains may lead to adverse outcomes twice as high compared to similar infections caused by susceptible strains [13]. Do MDR Gram-negative infections among critically ill patients lead to adverse clinical outcomes?

ESBL-producing *Enterobacterales* infections have been shown to be associated with higher rates of treatment failure and mortality in patients with bacteremia compared to infection with non-ESBL producers [14]. In a prospective cohort study, infection with MDR Gram-negative organisms in the ICU resulted in a 38% in-hospital mortality, which was significantly higher compared to infections with sensitive organisms. A longer ICU and hospital stay was also observed in patients who developed infections with MDR organisms [15]. The prospective, multicenter, CRACKLE-2 cohort study evaluated hospitalized patients with carbapenem-resistant *Klebsiella pneumoniae* infections from 71 hospitals in 8 countries. The unadjusted 30-day mortality was high and ranged between 12% and 28% in different regions [16]. Bloodstream infection with carbapenem-resistant *Klebsiella pneumoniae* was associated with significantly higher mortality compared to infection with susceptible strains in a retrospective study [17]. The emergence of resistance to third-generation cephalosporins in *Enterobacter* spp. is also associated with increased mortality, prolongation of hospital stay, and increased cost of care [18].

Different types of beta-lactamases are produced by Gram-negative bacteria rendering them resistant to the commonly available antibiotics (Table 41.1).

Considering the lack of new agents to combat these organisms, several older antibiotics, including colistin and fosfomycin, have been repurposed with renewed utility in the treatment of resistant infections with Gram-negative bacteria in critically ill patients. Combinations of drugs with reduced sensitivity have also been resorted to in the face of a lack of availability of more effective therapy. However, infection with carbapenem-resistant *Enterobacteriaceae*, *Pseudomonas aeruginosa*, and *Acinetobacter baumannii* continues to be of serious concern among the critically ill. Several newer antibiotics have undergone clinical evaluation and introduced into clinical practice recently, with increased potency against MDR Gram-negative bacteria (Table 41.2).

Table 41.1 The Ambler classification of beta-lactamases

Beta-lactamase type	Characteristics
Class A	Penicillinases, narrow and extended- spectrum beta-lactamases, carbapenemases including *Klebsiella pneumoniae* carbapenemase (KPC)
Class B	Metallo-beta-lactamases
Class C	Cephalosporinases
Class D	Oxa-type enzymes

Table 41.2 Newer antibiotic agents potentially effective against MDR Gram-negative organisms

Antibiotic	Type/spectrum	Clinical use
Ceftolozane/tazobactam	Ceftolozane is a third-generation cephalosporin with enhanced efficacy against PBPs. Lower MIC against *Ps. aeruginosa* compared to usual agents. Tazobactam inhibits Amp C and ESBLs	Intra-abdominal and complicated UTI. May be effective against carbapenem-resistant *Ps. aeruginosa*
Ceftazidime/avibactam	Ceftazidime is a third-generation cephalosporin. Avibactam is a non-beta-lactam type beta-lactamase inhibitor. Protects against class A and C beta-lactamases. Not effective against class B beta-lactamases, including metallo-lactamases	Complicated UTI, intra-abdominal infections, nosocomial pneumonias
Meropenem/vaborbactam	Vaborbactam is a beta-lactamase inhibitor with no intrinsic anti-bacterial activity. Inhibits beta-lactamases that neutralize meropenem. Effective against type A beta-lactamases, including KPC	Complicated UTI, intra-abdominal infections, nosocomial and community-acquired pneumonia
Plazomicin	Aminoglycoside with activity against carbapenem-resistant *Enterobacteriaceae*	Resistant Gram-negative infection in combination with meropenem, colistin, and fosfomycin
Eravacycline	New derivative of doxycycline with broader spectrum of activity. Effective against beta-lactamase producers and efflux pump-related bacterial resistance. Effective against a wide spectrum of Gram-negative organisms, except *Ps. aeruginosa* and *B. cenocepacia*. Effective against carbapenem-resistant *A. baumannii*	Complicated intra-abdominal infections. Enables switch from intravenous to oral therapy if appropriate

ESBL extended-spectrum beta-lactamase; *UTI* urinary tract infection; *KPC Klebsiella pneumoniae* carbapenemase

41.7 Ceftolozane/Tazobactam

Ceftolozane is a third-generation cephalosporin with a distinctive side-chain that confers it with enhanced efficacy against penicillin-binding proteins. Ceftolozane has a much lower minimum inhibitory concentration (MIC) against *Pseudomonas aeruginosa* compared to ceftazidime, imipenem, and ciprofloxacin. The addition of tazobactam enables inhibition of Amp C and ESBLs. Following the ASPECT-cIAI [19] and ASPECT-cUTI [20] trials, ceftolozane/tazobactam has been approved for clinical use in complicated intra-abdominal infections (cIAI) and complicated urinary tract infections (cUTI). Ceftolozane/tazobactam may be efficacious against infections caused by carbapenem-resistant *Pseudomonas aeruginosa*. It may also have a future role against ESBL-producing *Enterobacteriaceae*. A recently completed randomized controlled trial (RCT) compared 3 g ceftolozane/tazobactam with 1 g meropenem in patients with ventilator-associated pneumonia (VAP), for 8–14 days. Clinical cure and microbiological eradication rates were comparable between the two agents in this non-inferiority trial. This combination may be a viable treatment option for VAP caused by Gram-negative organisms [21].

41.8 Ceftazidime/Avibactam

Avibactam is a non-beta-lactam type of beta-lactamase inhibitor that offers protection against class A and C beta-lactamases when used in combination with ceftazidime, a third-generation cephalosporin. Ceftazidime-avibactam is effective against most carbapenemase and OXA-48 producers, including *Klebsiella pneumoniae* carbapenemase (KPC). However, it is not effective against class B beta-lactamases, including metallo-lactamases. In an RCT in patients with complicated urinary tract infection (cUTI), the ceftazidime/avibactam combination was non-inferior to doripenem for the primary endpoints of clinical and microbiological cure [22]. Ceftazidime/avibactam combined with metronidazole was non-inferior to meropenem in complicated intra-abdominal infections (cIAI) in another RCT [23].

41.9 Meropenem/Vaborbactam

Vaborbactam is a novel beta-lactamase inhibitor which has no intrinsic antibacterial activity; however, it inhibits beta-lactamases that neutralize meropenem. The meropenem/vaborbactam combination has a potent effect against type A beta-lactamases, including KPC. In the TANGO-I trial, meropenem/vaborbactam was shown to be superior to piperacillin/tazobactam in cUTI, including acute pyelonephritis. The meropenem/vaborbactam combination was also compared with the best available alternative therapy in carbapenem-resistant *Enterobacterales* infections [24]. The infections included cUTIs, hospital and community-acquired pneumonia, and bacteremia. The study was stopped early due to demonstrated superiority of meropenem/vaborbactam therapy. However, meropenem/vaborbactam may not be effective against OXA-type carbapenemase-producing *A. baumannii* and *P. aeruginosa* that acquire resistance by porin changes and efflux mechanisms. The European Medicines Agency has currently approved meropenem/vaborbactam in the treatment of c-UTI, c-IAI, hospital-acquired pneumonia (HAP), VAP, and other infections due to aerobic Gram-negative organisms.

41.10 Plazomicin

Plazomicin is a new aminoglycoside that shares a common mechanism of action by the inhibition of bacterial protein synthesis. Similar to other aminoglycosides, lung penetration is poor and elimination is through the kidneys. It has good in vitro activity against carbapenem-resistant *Enterobacteriaceae*; however, the efficacy is much less against carbapenem-resistant *A. baumannii* and *P. aeruginosa*. In the phase 3 EPIC trial, plazomicin was demonstrated to be superior to meropenem in c-UTI [25]. Plazomicin and colistin were compared in combination with other drugs in the treatment of blood-stream infections, HAP, and VAP. All-cause mortality with combination therapy, including plazomicin, was lower compared to colistin [21]. Plazomicin may be a therapeutic option in resistant Gram-negative infections in combination with meropenem, colistin, or fosfomycin.

41.11 Eravacycline

Eravacycline is a novel derivative of tigecycline with a broader spectrum of activity. It is not susceptible to beta-lactamases and efflux channel mechanisms that confer resistance to Gram-negative bacteria. In vitro studies have demonstrated a wide spectrum of activity against Gram-negative bacteria, except *Pseudomonas aeruginosa* and *Burkholderia cenocepacia*. Particularly noteworthy is the superior efficacy against carbapenem-resistant *A. baumannii*. In an RCT, eravacycline was compared with ertapenem in cIAI. Clinical cure was comparable with both drugs, establishing non-inferiority compared to ertapenem [26]. In cUTI, eravacycline did not achieve non-inferiority compared to levofloxacin and ertapenem [27]. Eravacycline has a high bioavailability on oral administration, enabling switch from intravenous to oral therapy if appropriate.

Key Points

- There has been increasing concern with MDR Gram-negative infections in critically ill patients. A recent report estimated that approximately ten million people may die every year due to infections with resistant organisms if the current trend continues.
- The ECDC and the CDC introduced standard definitions for multidrug-resistant, extensively drug-resistant, and pan-drug-resistant organisms in 2012; although these definitions enable uniform surveillance metrics, their bedside utility remains questionable.
- Critically ill patients are particularly prone to MDR infections. They are often treated with several antibiotics during the course of acute illness, leading to the evolution of resistant microbial flora. Widespread, inappropriate use of broad-spectrum antibiotics is closely associated with the development and transmission of drug-resistant microorganisms.
- MDR Gram-negative infections have been associated with adverse clinical outcomes, including increased mortality, longer duration of ICU stay, and addition to the cost of healthcare.
- In the face of increasingly resistant Gram-negative bacteria, the antibiotic cupboard appears relatively bare. The newly available agents are derivatives of the existing class of antibiotics; no new class of antibiotic has been introduced into clinical practice in more than three decades.
- It is of utmost importance to use these drugs only when there is no viable alternative; bacteria evolve and develop resistance to any new antibiotic they are exposed.

References

1. Kumar A, Schweizer HP. Bacterial resistance to antibiotics: active efflux and reduced uptake. Adv Drug Deliv Rev. 2005;57(10):1486–513.
2. Magiorakos AP, Srinivasan A, Carey RB, Carmeli Y, Falagas ME, Giske CG, et al. Multidrug-resistant, extensively drug-resistant and pandrug-resistant bacteria: an international expert proposal for interim standard definitions for acquired resistance. Clin Microbiol Infect. 2012;18(3):268–81.
3. Antimicrobial Resistance Collaborators. Global burden of bacterial antimicrobial resistance in 2019: a systematic analysis. Lancet Lond Engl. 2022;399(10325):629–55.
4. Luyt CE, Bréchot N, Trouillet JL, Chastre J. Antibiotic stewardship in the intensive care unit. Crit Care Lond Engl. 2014;18(5):480.
5. Bassetti M, Righi E, Vena A, Graziano E, Russo A, Peghin M. Risk stratification and treatment of ICU-acquired pneumonia caused by multidrug- resistant/extensively drug-resistant/ pandrug-resistant bacteria. Curr Opin Crit Care. 2018;24(5):385–93.
6. Antimicrobial resistance [Internet]. [cited 2022 Aug 9]. Available from: https://www.who.int/news-room/fact-sheets/detail/antimicrobial-resistance
7. de Kraker MEA, Stewardson AJ, Harbarth S. Will 10 million people die a year due to antimicrobial resistance by 2050? PLoS Med. 2016;13(11):e1002184.
8. Zahar JR, Blot S, Nordmann P, Martischang R, Timsit JF, Harbarth S, et al. Screening for intestinal carriage of extended-spectrum Beta-lactamase-producing Enterobacteralesin critically ill patients: expected benefits and evidence-based controversies. Clin Infect Dis. 2019;68(12):2125–30.
9. Gurieva T, Dautzenberg MJD, Gniadkowski M, Derde LPG, Bonten MJM, Bootsma MCJ. The transmissibility of antibiotic-resistant Enterobacterales in intensive care units. Clin Infect Dis. 2018;66(4):489–93.
10. Wieland K, Chhatwal P, Vonberg RP. Nosocomial outbreaks caused by Acinetobacter baumannii and Pseudomonas aeruginosa: results of a systematic review. Am J Infect Control. 2018;46(6):643–8.
11. De Geyter D, Blommaert L, Verbraeken N, Sevenois M, Huyghens L, Martini H, et al. The sink as a potential source of transmission of carbapenemase-producing Enterobacterales in the intensive care unit. Antimicrob Resist Infect Control. 2017;6:24.
12. Hopman J, Tostmann A, Wertheim H, Bos M, Kolwijck E, Akkermans R, et al. Reduced rate of intensive care unit acquired Gram-negative bacilli after removal of sinks and introduction of "water-free" patient care. Antimicrob Resist Infect Control. 2017;6:59.
13. Cosgrove SE, Carmeli Y. The impact of antimicrobial resistance on health and economic outcomes. Clin Infect Dis. 2003;36(11):1433–7.
14. Melzer M, Petersen I. Mortality following bacteraemic infection caused by extended spectrum beta-lactamase (ESBL) producing E. coli compared to non-ESBL producing *E. coli*. J Infect. 2007;55(3):254–9.
15. Siwakoti S, Subedi A, Sharma A, Baral R, Bhattarai NR, Khanal B. Incidence and outcomes of multidrug-resistant Gram-negative bacteria infections in intensive care unit from Nepal- a prospective cohort study. Antimicrob Resist Infect Control. 2018;26(7):114.
16. Wang M, Earley M, Chen L, Hanson BM, Yu Y, Liu Z, et al. Clinical outcomes and bacterial characteristics of carbapenem-resistant Klebsiella pneumoniae complex among patients from different global regions (CRACKLE-2): a prospective, multicentre, cohort study. Lancet Infect Dis. 2022;22(3):401–12.
17. Ben-David D, Kordevani R, Keller N, Tal I, Marzel A, Gal-Mor O, et al. Outcome of carbapenem resistant Klebsiella pneumoniae bloodstream infections. Clin Infect Dis. 2012;18(1):54–60.

18. Cosgrove SE. The relationship between antimicrobial resistance and patient outcomes: mortality, length of hospital stay, and health care costs. Clin Infect Dis. 2006;15(42 Suppl 2):S82–9.
19. Solomkin J, Hershberger E, Miller B, Popejoy M, Friedland I, Steenbergen J, et al. Ceftolozane/tazobactam plus metronidazole for complicated intra-abdominal infections in an era of multidrug resistance: results from a randomized, double-blind, phase 3 trial (ASPECT-cIAI). Clin Infect Dis. 2015;60(10):1462–71.
20. Wagenlehner FM, Umeh O, Steenbergen J, Yuan G, Darouiche RO. Ceftolozane-tazobactam compared with levofloxacin in the treatment of complicated urinary-tract infections, including pyelonephritis: a randomised, double-blind, phase 3 trial (ASPECT-cUTI). Lancet Lond Engl. 2015;385(9981):1949–56.
21. Koulenti D, Song A, Ellingboe A, Abdul-Aziz MH, Harris P, Gavey E, et al. Infections by multidrug-resistant Gram-negative bacteria: What's new in our arsenal and what's in the pipeline? Int J Antimicrob Agents. 2019;53(3):211–24.
22. Wagenlehner FM, Sobel JD, Newell P, Armstrong J, Huang X, Stone GG, et al. Ceftazidime-avibactam versus Doripenem for the treatment of complicated urinary tract infections, including acute pyelonephritis: RECAPTURE, a phase 3 randomized trial program. Clin Infect Dis. 2016;63(6):754–62.
23. Qin X, Tran BG, Kim MJ, Wang L, Nguyen DA, Chen Q, et al. A randomised, double-blind, phase 3 study comparing the efficacy and safety of ceftazidime/avibactam plus metronidazole versus meropenem for complicated intra-abdominal infections in hospitalised adults in Asia. Int J Antimicrob Agents. 2017;49(5):579–88.
24. Wunderink RG, Giamarellos-Bourboulis EJ, Rahav G, Mathers AJ, Bassetti M, Vazquez J, et al. Effect and safety of meropenem-Vaborbactam versus best-available therapy in patients with carbapenem-resistant Enterobacterales Infections: the TANGO II randomized clinical trial. Infect Dis Ther. 2018;7(4):439–55.
25. Wagenlehner FME, Cloutier DJ, Komirenko AS, Cebrik DS, Krause KM, Keepers TR, et al. Once-daily Plazomicin for complicated urinary tract infections. N Engl J Med. 2019;380(8):729–40.
26. Solomkin J, Evans D, Slepavicius A, Lee P, Marsh A, Tsai L, et al. Assessing the efficacy and safety of Eravacycline vs ertapenem in complicated intra-abdominal infections in the investigating Gram-negative infections treated with Eravacycline (IGNITE 1) trial: a randomized clinical trial. JAMA Surg. 2017;152(3):224–32.
27. Bassetti M, Peghin M, Vena A, Giacobbe DR. Treatment of infections due to MDR Gram-negative bacteria. Front Med. 2019;16(6):74.

Empirical Antibiotic Therapy: De-escalation Demystified

42

ICUs act as the hotbeds of bacterial resistance, with a highly susceptible population, prone to infection due to impaired defense mechanisms, and often requiring invasive interventions involving breach of anatomical barriers. The highest incidence of hospital-acquired infections occurs in ICUs [1]. The high incidence of nosocomial infection, combined with widespread, often injudicious antibiotic use, results in the emergence of resistant microorganisms among critically ill patients. More than 60% of patients are treated with antibiotics during their ICU stay [2]. Hemodynamic compromise often occurs in septic patients, leading to inadequate drug levels at the focus of infection; besides, suboptimal infection control practices among healthcare workers foster the emergence of resistant strains. Prudent choice of agents and administration for an optimal duration are the cornerstones of rational antimicrobial therapy in critically ill patients.

Early, effective antimicrobial therapy is one of the foundations of the treatment of critically ill patients with sepsis. However, adherence to this practice may have led to the extensive use of broad-spectrum antibiotics as empirical therapy, with adverse consequences, including an increase in the incidence of resistant organisms. The strategy of de-escalation is an important facet of antibiotic stewardship programs and recommended by clinical guidelines [3]. It aims to cut down the use of broad-spectrum antibiotics and enable focused therapy with narrower spectrum agents once identification and antibiotic sensitivities are available. Although such a strategy is laudable in an ideal world, several constraints may preclude tangible benefits.

J. Chacko et al., *Controversies in Critical Care*,
https://doi.org/10.1007/978-981-19-9940-6_42

42.1 De-escalation and the Use of Multiple Antimicrobial Agents

The principle of de-escalation implies the use of multiple antimicrobial agents as empirical therapy. The initial therapy with a "pivotal" agent in combination with a "companion" drug (e.g., carbapenem and aminoglycoside) may be de-escalated to monotherapy, or initial single-agent therapy may be substituted at a later stage by another agent, presumed to have a reduced spectrum of coverage. The use of multiple agents, as de-escalation demands, may be far from ideal, as it may compound the adverse impact on the gut microbiome [4]. Colonization with resistant strains may occur within the first 1–3 days of treatment with broad-spectrum agents [5], rendering de-escalation ineffective; besides, antibiotic-induced disruption of the gut microbiome may last for up to weeks after cessation of therapy [5].

Contrary to conventional wisdom, broad-spectrum antibiotics may have a less detrimental effect on the gut microbiota compared to agents that are considered to have a narrower spectrum. Imipenem has a limited impact on the gut microbiota [6]; however, piperacillin-tazobactam and ceftriaxone, the antibiotics often chosen as part of a de-escalation strategy, may be more damaging to the microbiota [7]. The more deleterious effect with narrower spectrum antibiotics may be related to the extent of biliary excretion, anti-anaerobic activity, and the level of accumulation in the gastrointestinal tract [11].

42.2 De-escalation and Emergence of Bacterial Resistance

The proponents of de-escalation recommend it as a practice that would help reduce the emergence of resistant organisms. However, there is conflicting evidence from available studies.

A prospective observational study assessed the intestinal carriage of imipenem-resistant Gram-negative bacteria in the ICU. Patients were screened for rectal colonization of imipenem-resistant gram-negative bacteria. In this study, prior treatment with imipenem was the most common risk factor for rectal colonization with imipenem-resistant Gram-negative bacteria. The rate of colonization increased with time, increasing from 5.9% after 1–3 days of imipenem to 7.8% thereafter. Thus, even short-term exposure to imipenem constituted a major risk factor for the development of resistance [8]. De-escalation has been shown to be associated with more prolonged antibiotic therapy; this may be borne out of a misconception that a longer duration of treatment with narrow-spectrum antibiotics may be acceptable.

De Bus et al. evaluated the emergence of antibiotic resistance with a de-escalation strategy. Antibiotic prescriptions were classified as de-escalation, continuation of the same antibiotics, or escalation. Anti-pseudomonal penicillins were prescribed on 478 occasions; of these, 12 (25%) were classified as de-escalation. On day 14, the emergence of resistance to the initial beta-lactam agent was comparable between de-escalation and continuation of the same antibiotics (30.6% vs. 23.5%, $p = 0.22$). This study did not reveal any impact of de-escalation on the emergence of resistant strains [9]. However, the results from a retrospective study by Yew et al. contrast with these findings. In a cohort of 300 patients, they compared patients who underwent carbapenem de-escalation with those who did not. The duration of therapy was shorter in the de-escalation group, with similar rates of clinical success based on predefined criteria in both groups. The incidence of carbapenem-resistant *Acinetobacter baumannii* was significantly lower in the de-escalation group [10].

42.3 De-escalation and the Duration of Antibiotic Therapy

De-escalation revolves around the substitution of broad-spectrum antibiotics with drugs with a narrower spectrum or less ecological influence or cessation of one or more agents of an empirical combination. The latter may be to cease double cover or stop coverage for pathogens considered likely at the commencement of empirical therapy but were not isolated on cultures. The appropriate early cessation of all antibiotic therapy, if an infective origin is ruled out, is not considered de-escalation according to this definition [11]. Thus, unnecessarily prolonged antibiotic therapy may continue after the cessation of one of the agents of an initial empirical combination, while still complying with a de-escalation protocol. A strategy of de-escalation has indeed been shown to prolong the total duration of antibiotic therapy [12]. A strong link exists between a longer duration of therapy and the emergence of resistant strains, besides the adverse impact on the microbiome. There is often a trend toward the continuation of antibiotic treatment toward fulfilling a complete "course." This practice may be based on unfounded fears of the development of antimicrobial resistance with short-term treatment. Besides, antibiotics are generally considered relatively safe and may be continued for a few extra days to ensure complete eradication of infection. The primary aim of antibiotic therapy is to diminish the number of bacteria at the focus of infection, thereby preventing local or systemic spread. A short course of therapy is sufficient for most severe infections, especially after adequate source control. In community-acquired pneumonia, and complicated intra-abdominal infection following source control, 5–7 days of antibiotics is reasonable [13]. If a short course of 5–7 days is considered appropriate, the policy of switching to a new drug for just a couple of days following identification of the organism, purely to comply with a de-escalation protocol may well be superfluous.

42.4 Scoring Antibiotics to Guide De-escalation

Ranking of antibiotics based on their spectrum of activity is essential to define and guide de-escalation. A French expert group could not reach a consensus on the ecological consequences of broad-spectrum antibiotics, including piperacillin-tazobactam, ticarcillin-clavulanic acid, fourth-generation cephalosporins, and third-generation antipseudomonal cephalosporins [14]. Besides, they failed to agree on the optimal time to de-escalation or the duration of antibiotic therapy that may be categorized as de-escalation. Meanwhile, a numerical scoring system based on the antimicrobial spectrum proposed by a US group contrasted with the French classification [15]. These studies underscore challenges in decision-making regarding what may constitute a de-escalation strategy.

42.5 Evidence for De-escalation

De-escalation has so far failed to demonstrate a reduced emergence of resistant strains, and there is a lack of evidence for clinical outcome benefit (Table 42.1). On the contrary, it may lead to inappropriately prolonged therapy. Several factors may offset potential benefits with the use of a de-escalation strategy (Fig. 42.1).

Table 42.1 Key studies on de-escalation of empirical antibiotic therapy

Study/year	Design	De-escalation	Control	Outcomes
De Bus et al. [9] (2016)	Prospective observational study	De-escalation from empirical beta-lactams	Continued empirical therapy or escalation	Duration of treatment significantly longer with de-escalation compared with continued therapy. No difference between de-escalation and continued therapy in mortality, emergence of resistant strains, or selective overgrowth of MDR strains
De Bus et al. [16] (DIANA, 2020)	Prospective observational study	Initial empirical therapy de-escalated within 3 days	Continued empirical therapy, or change other than de-escalation	Unadjusted 28-day mortality not different between de-escalation and continued therapy. Clinical cure rates higher with de-escalation
Leone et al. [17] (2014)	Multicenter RCT	De-escalation of empirical therapy	Continued empirical therapy	Median duration of ICU stay longer with de-escalation. Superinfections more with de-escalation. Duration of antibiotic therapy longer with de-escalation compared to continued empirical therapy. 90-day mortality similar
Lakbar et al. [7] (2020)	Systematic review of 20 observational studies and one RCT	De-escalation of empirical therapy	No de-escalation	Lower overall mortality with de-escalation variable results regarding duration of antibiotic therapy

MDR multidrug-resistant, *RCT* randomized controlled trial

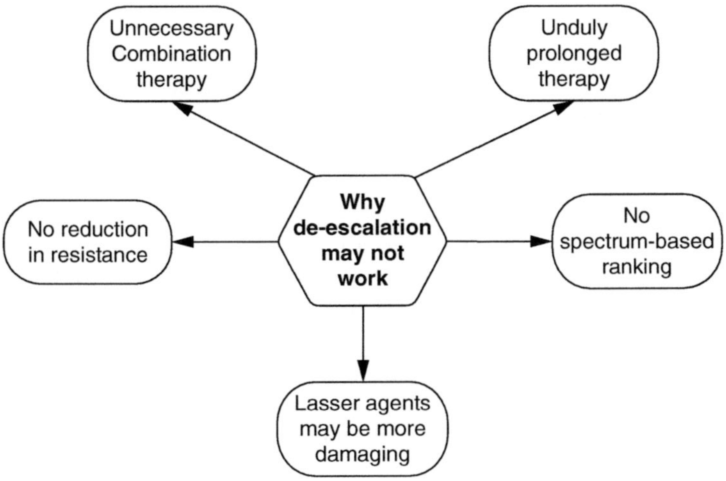

Fig. 42.1 Factors contributing to the failure of a de-escalation strategy

The DIANA study evaluated de-escalation practices from 152 ICUs across 28 countries. This prospective observational study included 1495 patients. De-escalation was defined as either the cessation of one or more antibiotics from an initial empirical combination or the substitution of an antibiotic with the intent to narrow down the spectrum of coverage, within 3 days of initiation of therapy. De-escalation was carried out in only 16% of patients; most patients were continued on the same agents (63%), while a change of antibiotic without the intent to de-escalate occurred in 22% of patients. The unadjusted 28-day mortality was 15.8% with de-escalation compared to 19.4% of patients who were continued on the same therapy; the difference was not statistically significant (RR: 0.83, 95% CI, 0.60–1.14; $p = 0.27$). Clinical cure, defined as survival with the resolution of all signs and symptoms related to infection, occurred more often among patients who underwent de-escalation compared to those who did not [16]. Although the authors performed adjusted analysis for confounders, it is plausible that de-escalation may have been carried out mostly among patients who were clinically improving. In contrast, the sicker cohort that did not show improvement or worsened could likely have been continued on the same or even escalated therapy, with predictably poor outcomes.

Leone et al. compared a strategy of de-escalation with continued empirical antibiotic treatment in patients with severe sepsis in a randomized controlled trial (RCT) [17]. The primary outcome, the median duration of ICU stay, was longer in the de-escalation group [9 (5–22) vs. 8 (4–15) days, $p = 0.71$]. A strategy of de-escalation failed to meet the preset noninferiority criteria. Among the secondary outcomes, superinfections were more common with de-escalation (16% vs. 11%, $p = 0.03$). Besides, the duration of antibiotic therapy was also higher with de-escalation compared with continued empirical therapy. The 90-day mortality was similar between the two groups. The sole RCT on de-escalation vs. continued empirical therapy, this study had several limitations. It was unblinded and underpowered, with differences in the baseline characteristic between the two groups, including age, the SAPS II score, and lung as the source of infection. Besides, the authors did not report on the appropriateness of the initial empirical antibiotic therapy.

Lakbar et al. identified 20 observational studies and one RCT that evaluated de-escalation in critically ill patients. The only RCT was by Leone et al., described above. Fourteen of 20 observational studies did not reveal a mortality difference between the de-escalation compared to a non-de-escalation strategy. None of the studies reported an increase in mortality with de-escalation. Overall, lower mortality was observed with de-escalation (relative risk: 0.71; 95% CI, 0.63–0.80); however, there was substantial heterogeneity between studies ($I^2 = 49\%$). The duration of treatment was assessed in six studies; the duration of treatment was similar between de-escalation and no de-escalation in three studies. Two studies reported an increase in the duration of treatment with a de-escalation policy, while one reported a decrease in the duration [7].

Key Points

- Although de-escalation of antibiotics is a commendable approach toward reducing the emergence of resistant strains, there are several impediments to meaningful execution in the real world.
- A de-escalation policy may lead to undue prolongation of therapy and continued treatment with one or more agents of the initial empirical combination beyond the optimal duration.
- There is a lack of consensus on the ranking of the spectrum of antibiotics and their impact on the microbiota.
- Although we assume that narrow spectrum agents may have less impact on the gut microbiota, this may not necessarily be true; for example, imipenem may be less damaging than piperacillin-tazobactam and ceftriaxone.
- Antibiotic de-escalation may not offer an advantage when the duration of therapy is expected to be 5–7 days, in infections such as pneumonia, abdominal infections with adequate source control, and uncomplicated urinary infection. Antibiotic sensitivities are usually available by day 3; a switch to a new antibiotic at this stage may only represent a second hit on the microbiota. If a more prolonged course of treatment is deemed necessary, early de-escalation is important.
- There is no strong evidence to support the reduced emergence of resistant organisms with the implementation of a de-escalation protocol. Studies on clinical outcomes are few with conflicting results.
- Early cessation of antibiotic therapy must form part of the de-escalation strategy in future guidelines.

References

1. Vincent JL, Bihari DJ, Suter PM, Bruining HA, White J, Nicolas-Chanoin MH, et al. The prevalence of nosocomial infection in intensive care units in Europe. Results of the European prevalence of infection in intensive care (EPIC) study. EPIC international advisory committee. JAMA. 1995;274(8):639–44.
2. Borg MA. Bed occupancy and overcrowding as determinant factors in the incidence of MRSA infections within general ward settings. J Hosp Infect. 2003;54(4):316–8.
3. Rhodes A, Evans LE, Alhazzani W, Levy MM, Antonelli M, Ferrer R, et al. Surviving sepsis campaign: international guidelines for Management of Sepsis and Septic Shock: 2016. Intensive Care Med. 2017;43(3):304–77.
4. De Waele JJ, Schouten J, Beovic B, Tabah A, Leone M. Antimicrobial de-escalation as part of antimicrobial stewardship in intensive care: no simple answers to simple questions—a viewpoint of experts. Intensive Care Med. 2020;46(2):236–44.
5. Bhalodi AA, van Engelen TSR, Virk HS, Wiersinga WJ. Impact of antimicrobial therapy on the gut microbiome. J Antimicrob Chemother. 2019;74(Suppl 1):i6–15.
6. Woerther PL, Lepeule R, Burdet C, Decousser JW, Ruppé É, Barbier F. Carbapenems and alternative β-lactams for the treatment of infections due to extended-spectrum β-lactamase-producing Enterobacteriaceae: what impact on intestinal colonisation resistance? Int J Antimicrob Agents. 2018;52(6):762–70.
7. Lakbar I, De Waele JJ, Tabah A, Einav S, Martin-Loeches I, Leone M. Antimicrobial De-escalation in the ICU: from recommendations to level of evidence. Adv Ther. 2020;37(7):3083–96.
8. Armand-Lefèvre L, Angebault C, Barbier F, Hamelet E, Defrance G, Ruppé E, et al. Emergence of imipenem-resistant gram-negative bacilli in intestinal Flora of intensive care patients. Antimicrob Agents Chemother. 2013;57(3):1488–95.
9. De Bus L, Denys W, Catteeuw J, Gadeyne B, Vermeulen K, Boelens J, et al. Impact of de-escalation of beta-lactam antibiotics on the emergence of antibiotic resistance in ICU patients: a retrospective observational study. Intensive Care Med. 2016;42(6):1029–39.
10. Lew KY, Ng TM, Tan M, Tan SH, Lew EL, Ling LM, et al. Safety and clinical outcomes of carbapenem de-escalation as part of an antimicrobial stewardship programme in an ESBL-endemic setting. J Antimicrob Chemother. 2015;70(4):1219–25.
11. Tabah A, Bassetti M, Kollef MH, Zahar JR, Paiva JA, Timsit JF, et al. Antimicrobial de-escalation in critically ill patients: a position statement from a task force of the European Society of Intensive Care Medicine (ESICM) and European Society of Clinical Microbiology and Infectious Diseases (ESCMID) critically ill patients study group (ESGCIP). Intensive Care Med. 2020;46(2):245–65.
12. Tabah A, Cotta MO, Garnacho-Montero J, Schouten J, Roberts JA, Lipman J, et al. A systematic review of the definitions, determinants, and clinical outcomes of antimicrobial De-escalation in the intensive care unit. Clin Infect Dis. 2016;62(8):1009–17.
13. De Waele JJ, Martin-Loeches I. Optimal duration of antibiotic treatment in Gram-negative infections. Curr Opin Infect Dis. 2018;31(6):606–11.
14. Weiss E, Zahar JR, Lesprit P, Ruppe E, Leone M, Chastre J, et al. Elaboration of a consensual definition of de-escalation allowing a ranking of β-lactams. Clin Microbiol Infect. 2015;21(7):649.e1–10.
15. Madaras-Kelly K, Jones M, Remington R, Hill N, Huttner B, Samore M. Development of an antibiotic spectrum score based on veterans affairs culture and susceptibility data for the purpose of measuring antibiotic de-escalation: a modified Delphi approach. Infect Control Hosp Epidemiol. 2014;35(9):1103–13.

16. De Bus L, Depuydt P, Steen J, Dhaese S, De Smet K, Tabah A, et al. Antimicrobial de-escalation in the critically ill patient and assessment of clinical cure: the DIANA study. Intensive Care Med. 2020;46(7):1404–17.
17. Leone M, Bechis C, Baumstarck K, Lefrant JY, Albanèse J, Jaber S, et al. De-escalation versus continuation of empirical antimicrobial treatment in severe sepsis: a multicenter non-blinded randomized noninferiority trial. Intensive Care Med. 2014;40(10):1399–408.

Is It the End of the Road for Inhaled Antibiotic Therapy in Ventilator-Associated Pneumonia?

43

43.1 Introduction

Ventilator-associated pneumonia (VAP) caused by multidrug-resistant bacteria continues to be a major cause of morbidity and mortality in our ICUs. We have a limited choice of antibiotics to combat the resistant bacterial flora prevalent in many units. Besides, most systemically administered antibiotics fail to attain therapeutic concentrations in the lung. This has led many clinicians to resort to aerosolized antibiotics, often as an adjuvant to systemic therapy in the treatment of VAP. The use of inhaled antibiotics is based on a sound rationale, with the possibility of delivering a high concentration of the drug to the target site. Furthermore, the emergence of resistant organisms may also be reduced with the preservation of the gut flora. An added advantage may be to cut down the duration of systemic antibiotics and perhaps, even use inhaled antibiotics as monotherapy.

Inhaled antibiotic therapy is by no means a new therapeutic modality; a 1975 study of ICU patients used polymyxin B in the atomized form or by endotracheal instillation in intubated patients as prophylaxis against pneumonia [1]. Predictably, such unlimited, universal, largely prophylactic therapy resulted in a high level of polymyxin resistance and high mortality. A global survey conducted in 2017 revealed that 63.4% of 261 ICUs used inhaled antibiotics, mainly for VAP and ventilator-associated tracheobronchitis (VAT) [2].

43.2 Why the Inhaled Route?

High levels of antibiotics concentration are attained in the lung when administered through the inhaled route. Animal studies have demonstrated substantially higher pulmonary concentrations in the lung by the inhaled compared with the intravenous route [3]. Studies among patients with VAP have also revealed concentrations considerably higher than the minimum inhibitory concentration (MIC) of the causative

J. Chacko et al., *Controversies in Critical Care*,
https://doi.org/10.1007/978-981-19-9940-6_43

pathogen. Besides, as systemic absorption is limited, the plasma levels remain much lower compared with intravenous administration [4]. Low systemic concentrations might reduce overall antibiotic exposure and minimize the emergence of resistant strains [5]. Toxic effects resulting from intravenous administration may also be lower with inhaled administration. The incidence of acute kidney injury may be lower with inhaled compared to intravenous administration of colistin [6].

There are several potential drawbacks and limitations of inhaled antibiotic therapy. Respiratory complications, including bronchospasm and worsening of hypoxia, may occur. Pneumonia may lead to bacteremia; the relative lack of a systemic effect would render inhaled therapy ineffective in this situation. Besides, the efficacy of aerosol delivery to the less ventilated regions of the lung including areas of consolidation or collapse may be suboptimal. The filter at the expiratory port of the ventilator may occlude, leading to interference with ventilation and serious complications, including hypoxia and cardiac arrest. Although adverse effects are often highlighted in clinical guidelines [7, 8], the actual incidence may be less than 1%, with most events being mild and easily reversible [9]. Intravenous formulations, in general, are unsuitable for inhalational delivery. Inhalational preparations must be nonpyrogenic, and preservative-free, with a pH between 4 and 8 and osmolality of 150–200 mOsm/l [10].

43.3 Mode of Delivery

43.3.1 Particle Size, Nebulizer Type

Larger particles tend to impact against the lumen of the respiratory tract as the direction of gas flow changes along the proximal airways. Such impaction leads to the deposition of particles in the large proximal airways leading to a lack of effectiveness. The optimal particle size for enhanced distal deposition ranges between 0.5 and 5 μm [11]. Jet, ultrasonic, and vibrating mesh nebulizers are commonly used in clinical practice. Jet nebulizers are the least preferred as they require an external source of compressed gas that interferes with ventilator settings. Besides, a substantial residual volume of the solution remains in the nebulizing chamber at the end of treatment, leading to inefficiency. Ultrasonic nebulizers are effective; however, they generate heat that may cause the degradation of heat-sensitive drugs. Vibrating mesh nebulizers are generally preferred for the delivery of inhaled antibiotics. A high-frequency (150–300,000 cycles per second) vibrating mesh pumps the solution through conical outlets. Mesh nebulizers are easy to use, do not interfere with ventilator settings, and leave behind the least residual volume. Vibrating mesh nebulizers may be breath-activated with nebulization synchronized to the inspiratory phase. This mechanism prevents the ventilator bias flow from carrying the aerosol

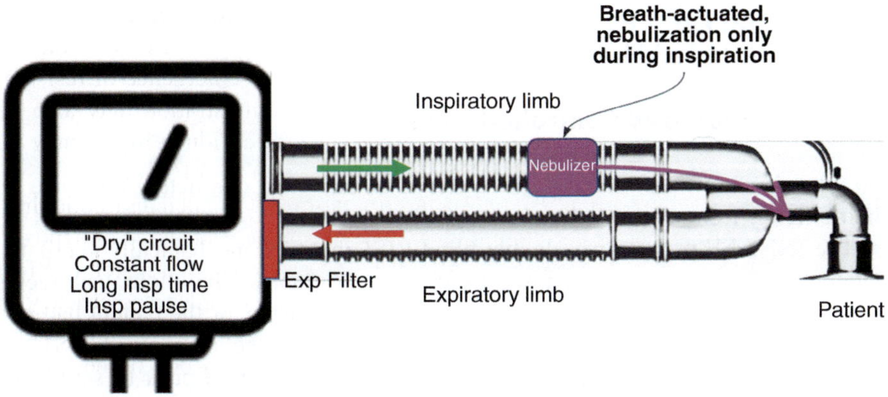

Fig. 43.1 Ventilator setup for nebulization. A dedicated "dry" circuit in a constant flow mode, long inspiratory time, and an inspiratory pause is preferred. The nebulizer is placed in the inspiratory limb. Breath-activated delivery, synchronized with the inspiratory phase, will prevent aerosol passage into the expiratory limb and wasteful deposition of particles in the circuit

into the expiratory limb during the expiratory phase, with wasteful drug deposition in the circuit [12] (Fig. 43.1). Ultrasonic and jet nebulizers are placed in the inspiratory limb, about 15–40 cm upstream to the Y-piece of the circuit; vibrating mesh nebulizers are placed immediately proximal to the Y-piece or distal to the Y-piece in a breath-activated device.

43.3.2 Circuit and Ventilator Setup

Humidification of gas flow increases particle size of the aerosol due to water absorption, leading to reduced efficacy. Heat and moisture exchanger filters completely occlude aerosol delivery and hence, must be removed prior to nebulization. It may be ideal to assign a separate "dry" circuit for the duration of nebulization, provided the duration of nebulization is less than 30 min [7]. A low, constant flow ventilation mode is preferred to optimize aerosolization. Volume control-assist control mode with a tidal volume of 7–9 ml/kg, respiratory rate of 12/min, and inspiratory:expiratory ratio of 1:1, with the addition of an end-inspiratory pause, enables efficient aerosolization [13]. Pressure-controlled ventilation with a decelerating flow pattern is not ideal for effective nebulization. Patient-ventilator asynchrony may lead to inefficient therapy; hence, an appropriate level of sedation may be required prior to nebulization to control asynchronous breaths. The duration of nebulization should be restricted to <60 min to prevent adverse events arising from interruption of heating and humidification of the inspired gas for a protracted period [14].

43.4 What Does Evidence Suggest Regarding the Efficacy of Inhaled Therapy?

43.4.1 Randomized Controlled Trials

Do inhaled antibiotics really work? There is scant, often conflicting evidence on their efficacy from controlled trials.

The INHALE prospective, double-blind RCT included mechanically ventilated patients with pneumonia diagnosed by chest radiography. The etiological agents were multidrug-resistant (MDR) Gram-negative organisms, or the patient had two risk factors for such infection. The clinical pulmonary infection score (CPIS) was ≥6, and impaired oxygenation was present in the 48-h period prior to screening. Patients were randomly assigned to receive 400 mg amikacin or saline by the inhaled route twice daily for 10 days, in addition to standard intravenous antibiotic therapy. A breath-activated, vibrating mesh nebulizer that aerosolizes the drug during the initial 75% of the inspiratory cycle was used in this study. A total of 725 patients were randomized, 362 to receive amikacin and 363 to placebo. Among these patients, 712 received at least one dose of the study drug. The primary endpoint, survival at 28–32 days, was analyzed in 508 patients; there was no significant difference between the inhaled administration of amikacin compared with placebo (amikacin vs. saline: 75% vs. 77%; odds ratio 0·841, 95% CI 0·554–1·277; $p = 0{\cdot}43$). Treatment-related adverse events were also similar between the two groups [15].

Kollef et al. conducted a randomized controlled trial (RCT) in patients with VAP due to Gram-negative bacteria. Inhalational antibiotic therapy was carried out with amikacin, 300 mg, and fosfomycin, 120 mg, delivered twice daily for 10 days or until extubation, using a vibrating mesh nebulizer [16]. Nebulization was carried out for 12 min, with a special formulation suitable for aerosol delivery. The control group received a placebo. Both groups of patients also received intravenous meropenem or imipenem as Gram-negative cover for 7 days. A total of 143 patients were included in the study, with 71 in the inhalational and 72 in the placebo group. Change in the CPIS from baseline, the primary outcome, was not significantly different between the two groups. The hierarchical secondary endpoints of being alive and clinically cured and alive and ventilator-free at day 14 were similar between groups. Compared to the placebo group, the inhaled therapy group had fewer positive cultures on days 3 and 7, although this did not translate to a clinical benefit. This RCT did not reveal any clinical benefit or improvement in the CPIS using adjuvant inhaled therapy with amikacin and fosfomycin compared with standard intravenous antibiotic therapy alone.

Would inhaled antibiotics be effective in cardiothoracic surgical patients who develop hospital-acquired pneumonia or VAP in the postoperative period?

Hassan et al. evaluated patients with nosocomial pneumonia caused by MDR Gram-negative bacilli following cardiothoracic surgery in an RCT [17]. Patients were diagnosed as having hospital-acquired pneumonia or VAP using predefined criteria. Intravenous piperacillin-tazobactam was administered to all patients. In the inhalational therapy group, amikacin 400 mg twice daily was administered as nebulization; in the control group, amikacin 20 mg/kg was administered intravenously. The primary outcome was clinical cure on day 7, defined as normalization of temperature, WBC count <10,000/ml, absence of purulent secretions, improved radiological infiltrates, and a PaO_2/FiO_2 ratio of >250 in patients with VAP. Clinical cure on day 7 was significantly higher with inhaled therapy. Inhaled therapy was associated with a shorter ICU stay, fewer days on mechanical ventilation, and a more rapid clinical cure. Nephrotoxicity was also lower in the inhaled therapy group. This study revealed improvement in clinical outcomes with the use of aerosolized compared with intravenous amikacin in combination with intravenous piperacillin/tazobactam in nosocomial pneumonia post-cardiothoracic surgery. Table 43.1 summarizes main RCTs that evaluated the efficacy of inhaled antibiotic therapy in VAP.

In contrast to the equivocal results in VAP, the use of inhaled antibiotics has met with relative success in ventilator-associated tracheobronchitis (VAT). In a double-blind RCT, mechanically ventilated patients with VAT, defined as the production of ≥2 ml of purulent secretions during a 4-h period, with a positive gram stain, were assigned to inhaled antibiotic or placebo. Compared with the placebo group, the inhaled group had reduced signs of ongoing respiratory infection by the Centers for Disease Control National Nosocomial Infection Survey VAP criteria and the CPIS. Besides, bacterial resistance was also lower with inhaled therapy [18]. In another RCT, mechanically ventilated patients with evidence of respiratory infection based on purulent secretions and a CPIS ≥6 were included. The use of inhaled antibiotics resulted in significantly greater elimination of the pathogen based on culture and gram stain, compared with placebo. The emergence of bacterial resistance was higher in the placebo arm. The use of inhaled antibiotics also led to a reduction in the Clinical Pulmonary Infection Score [5].

Table 43.1 Main RCTs that have evaluated the efficacy of inhaled antibiotics

Study/year	Inhalational antibiotic group	Control group	Outcomes
Niederman et al. [15] (INHALE, 2020)	Amikacin, 400 mg twice daily for 10 days, combined with standard intravenous antibiotics	Standard intravenous antibiotics alone	Survival at 28–32 days not different; adverse events similar
Kollef et al. [16] (2017)	Amikacin, 300 mg, and fosfomycin, 120 mg, twice daily for 10 days or until extubation + intravenous meropenem or imipenem	Placebo + intravenous meropenem or imipenem	Change in the CPIS similar; clinical cure, and alive and ventilator-free similar at day 14; fewer positive cultures at days 3 and 7 in the inhalational group
Hassan et al. [17] (2018)	Amikacin 400 mg twice daily. Intravenous piperacillin-tazobactam	Intravenous piperacillin-tazobactam alone	Clinical cure on day 7 significantly higher, nephrotoxicity lower, with inhalational therapy

CPIS Clinical pulmonary infection score

43.4.2 Meta-analyses

Zampieri et al. performed a meta-analysis comparing the combination of intravenous and aerosolized antibiotics with intravenous administration alone in the treatment of VAP [19]. The antibiotics used included gentamicin, amikacin, tobramycin, ceftazidime, and colistin. The likelihood of clinical cure was significantly higher with combined therapy; however, there was no significant difference in microbiological cure rates, ICU or hospital mortality, ventilation days, and ICU length of stay. In another meta-analysis, intravenous colistin was compared with adjunctive inhaled colistin therapy. This study reported a significantly higher clinical response, microbiological eradication, and infection-related mortality. There was no difference in the overall mortality or nephrotoxicity [20]. Liu et al. compared the efficacy of intravenous-inhaled combination of colistin with IV colistin alone in their meta-analysis. They observed a greater clinical response, a higher rate of eradication of the pathogen, and reduced all-cause mortality with the inhaled-intravenous combination [21].

43.4.3 The Future

Considering the relative lack of evidence to support inhaled therapy, should we persist with this treatment modality? The Infectious Diseases Society of America and the American Thoracic Society recommend the use of inhaled antibiotics only as a last resort to treat refractory VAP, unresponsive to conventional systemic antibiotic therapy [8]. Perhaps we need to reassess the endpoints of inhalational therapy. It is plausible that the use of the inhaled route could potentially reduce the duration of systemic therapy, thereby reducing the emergence of resistant strains. The dosing needs standardization; the currently employed dosing may well be inadequate, and a higher dose, particularly of colistin, may be required for an optimal response [22]. Patients with more severe illness may potentially benefit; future studies should specifically target subgroups of patients based on the severity of illness. The ideal mode of aerosol delivery needs further research; vibrating mesh nebulizers, synchronized with the inspiratory phase, may be superior compared to jet and ultrasonic nebulizers. It may also be appropriate to target drug levels by distal lung lavage to ensure adequate drug delivery at the site of infection [23].

Key Points

- The use of inhaled antibiotics is based on a sound physiological rationale, with the potential to deliver a high concentration of the drug at the site of infection. Besides, delivery by nebulization may alleviate systemic adverse effects, including nephrotoxicity.
- Inhalational therapy is likely to fail in the presence of bacteremia, considering the lack of a systemic effect. Besides, adverse effects may occur, including respiratory complications and prolongation of the duration of mechanical ventilation.

- Although the optimal modality of delivery is not established, vibrating mesh nebulizers may offer optimal particle size. Besides, in contrast to jet nebulizers, the residual, unused volume is significantly reduced. Synchronization with the inspiratory phase prevents the passage of aerosol into the expiratory limb and wasteful deposition in the ventilator circuit.
- RCTs and meta-analyses on the topic provide conflicting results regarding the efficacy of inhaled therapy; considering the lack of robust evidence, most guidelines recommend inhaled antibiotics only as a last resort in intractable cases and infection with MDR organisms.
- Future research should focus on the optimal dosing; more meaningful endpoints, including efficacy in subgroups of patients with more severe illness, and the likelihood of reducing the emergence of resistant strains should also be considered.

References

1. Feeley TW, Du Moulin GC, Hedley-Whyte J, Bushnell LS, Gilbert JP, Feingold DS. Aerosol polymyxin and pneumonia in seriously ill patients. N Engl J Med. 1975;293(10):471–5.
2. Alves J, Alp E, Koulenti D, Zhang Z, Ehrmann S, Blot S, et al. Nebulization of antimicrobial agents in mechanically ventilated adults in 2017: an international cross-sectional survey. Eur J Clin Microbiol Infect Dis. 2018;37(4):785–94.
3. Goldstein I, Wallet F, Nicolas-Robin A, Ferrari F, Marquette CH, Rouby JJ. Lung deposition and efficiency of nebulized amikacin during Escherichia coli pneumonia in ventilated piglets. Am J Respir Crit Care Med. 2002;166(10):1375–81.
4. Boisson M, Jacobs M, Grégoire N, Gobin P, Marchand S, Couet W, et al. Comparison of intrapulmonary and systemic pharmacokinetics of colistin methanesulfonate (CMS) and colistin after aerosol delivery and intravenous administration of CMS in critically ill patients. Antimicrob Agents Chemother. 2014;58(12):7331–9.
5. Palmer LB, Smaldone GC. Reduction of bacterial resistance with inhaled antibiotics in the intensive care unit. Am J Respir Crit Care Med. 2014;189(10):1225–33.
6. Abdellatif S, Trifi A, Daly F, Mahjoub K, Nasri R, Ben LS. Efficacy and toxicity of aerosolised colistin in ventilator-associated pneumonia: a prospective, randomised trial. Ann Intensive Care. 2016;6(1):26.
7. Ehrmann S, Chastre J, Diot P, Lu Q. Nebulized antibiotics in mechanically ventilated patients: a challenge for translational research from technology to clinical care. Ann Intensive Care. 2017;7(1):78.
8. Kalil AC, Metersky ML, Klompas M, Muscedere J, Sweeney DA, Palmer LB, et al. Management of Adults with Hospital-acquired and Ventilator-associated Pneumonia: 2016 clinical practice guidelines by the Infectious Diseases Society of America and the American Thoracic Society. Clin Infect Dis. 2016;63(5):e61–111.
9. Ehrmann S, Roche-Campo F, Bodet-Contentin L, Razazi K, Dugernier J, Trenado-Alvarez J, et al. Aerosol therapy in intensive and intermediate care units: prospective observation of 2808 critically ill patients. Intensive Care Med. 2016;42(2):192–201.
10. Bassetti M, Luyt CE, Nicolau DP, Pugin J. Characteristics of an ideal nebulized antibiotic for the treatment of pneumonia in the intubated patient. Ann Intensive Care. 2016;6(1):35.
11. Brain JD, Valberg PA. Deposition of aerosol in the respiratory tract. Am Rev Respir Dis. 1979;120(6):1325–73.

12. Gowda AA, Cuccia AD, Smaldone GC. Reliability of vibrating mesh technology. Respir Care. 2017;62(1):65–9.
13. Dhand R. Maximizing aerosol delivery during mechanical ventilation: go with the flow and go slow. Intensive Care Med. 2003;29(7):1041–2.
14. Rello J, Rouby JJ, Sole-Lleonart C, Chastre J, Blot S, Luyt CE, et al. Key considerations on nebulization of antimicrobial agents to mechanically ventilated patients. Clin Microbiol Infect. 2017;23(9):640–6.
15. Niederman MS, Alder J, Bassetti M, Boateng F, Cao B, Corkery K, et al. Inhaled amikacin adjunctive to intravenous standard-of-care antibiotics in mechanically ventilated patients with Gram-negative pneumonia (INHALE): a double-blind, randomised, placebo-controlled, phase 3, superiority trial. Lancet Infect Dis. 2020;20(3):330–40.
16. Kollef MH, Ricard JD, Roux D, Francois B, Ischaki E, Rozgonyi Z, et al. A randomized trial of the amikacin Fosfomycin inhalation system for the adjunctive therapy of Gram-negative ventilator-associated pneumonia: IASIS trial. Chest. 2017;151(6):1239–46.
17. Hassan NA, Awdallah FF, Abbassi MM, Sabry NA. Nebulized versus IV amikacin as adjunctive antibiotic for hospital and ventilator-acquired pneumonia postcardiac surgeries: a randomized controlled trial. Crit Care Med. 2018;46(1):45–52.
18. Palmer LB, Smaldone GC, Chen JJ, Baram D, Duan T, Monteforte M, et al. Aerosolized antibiotics and ventilator-associated tracheobronchitis in the intensive care unit. Crit Care Med. 2008;36(7):2008–13.
19. Zampieri FG, Nassar AP, Gusmao-Flores D, Taniguchi LU, Torres A, Ranzani OT. Nebulized antibiotics for ventilator-associated pneumonia: a systematic review and meta-analysis. Crit Care. 2015;7(19):150.
20. Valachis A, Samonis G, Kofteridis DP. The role of aerosolized colistin in the treatment of ventilator-associated pneumonia: a systematic review and metaanalysis. Crit Care Med. 2015;43(3):527–33.
21. Liu D, Zhang J, Liu HX, Zhu YG, Qu JM. Intravenous combined with aerosolised polymyxin versus intravenous polymyxin alone in the treatment of pneumonia caused by multidrug-resistant pathogens: a systematic review and meta-analysis. Int J Antimicrob Agents. 2015;46(6):603–9.
22. Honore PM, Redant S, Stoll T, Preseau T, Moorthamers S, Kaefer K, et al. Study conclude that adjunctive inhaled antibiotics were not associated with reduced mortality: we are not sure! J Crit Care. 2022;67:227–8.
23. Niederman MS. Adjunctive nebulized antibiotics: what is their place in ICU infections? Front Med. 2019;8(6):99.

Duration of Antibiotic Therapy in the Critically Ill

44

44.1 Introduction

Antibiotic therapy is often continued for an extended period, beyond the optimal duration in critically ill patients. Although there is emphasis on early administration and choice of appropriate antibiotics in septic patients, the evidence regarding duration of treatment is sparse. Ideally, the duration of antibiotic therapy should maximize clinical efficacy while reducing the risks of untoward effects including *Clostridioides difficile* infection, toxicity, the emergence of resistant strains, and increased cost of healthcare. The duration of antibiotic prescription in septic patients may be highly variable among clinicians, ranging from 3 to 5 days to more than 10 days depending on the clinical circumstances [1].

What is the available evidence regarding the optimal duration of antibiotic therapy in critically ill patients with suspected or proven infection?

44.2 Duration of Antibiotic Therapy: Intra-Abdominal Infections

Conventionally, antibiotics are prescribed for 7–14 days in patients with complicated intra-abdominal infections, after resolution of the systemic inflammatory response. However, once source control is achieved, the duration of antibiotic therapy may be curtailed, depending on the clinical response; a short duration of therapy of 3–5 days may suffice following source control [2]. Several recent studies have evaluated the optimal duration of antibiotic therapy following complicated intra-abdominal infections.

A French multicenter study included patients who underwent intra-abdominal surgery with evidence of pus collection in the peritoneal cavity [3]. Source control was achieved with appropriate surgical intervention. On postoperative day 8, patients were randomized to the cessation of antibiotic therapy or continued

J. Chacko et al., *Controversies in Critical Care*,
https://doi.org/10.1007/978-981-19-9940-6_44

administration for 15 days. The 8-day antibiotic regimen included 120 patients and the 15-day regimen, 116 patients. The number of antibiotic-free days from day 8 to 28 was significantly more in patients who were randomized to the shorter antibiotic regimen (15 (6–20) vs. 12 (6–13) days, $P < 0.0001$). Mortality at 45 days was 9.1% with the 8-day compared with 13.6% in the 15-day regimen; the difference was not statistically significant. The duration of stay in the ICU and hospital, the emergence of multidrug-resistant bacteria, and re-exploration rates were also similar between the two groups. This study suggested that a shorter, 8-day antibiotic regimen, compared to a 15-day regimen, is safe and effective following surgery for intra-abdominal infections once source control was achieved.

The STOP-IT trial also evaluated the efficacy of a short-course antibiotic therapy in intra-abdominal infection following source control [4]. Patients were randomized to receive 4 days of antibiotic therapy after source control (short-course) or continued therapy until 2 days after resolution of the systemic inflammatory response (control). The primary outcome was a composite of surgical-site infection, recurrent infection, or death within 30 days of the source control intervention. Fifty-six of 257 patients (21.8%) suffered the primary outcome in the short-course antibiotic therapy group compared to 58 of 260 patients (22.3%) in the control group; the difference was not statistically significant. The incidence of the individual components of the composite primary outcome was also similar between groups. The median duration of antibiotic treatment was significantly lower with short-course treatment compared to the control arm [4.0 (4.0–5.0) vs. 8.0 (5.0–10.0 days)].

A single-center, retrospective study evaluated the duration of antibiotic therapy and outcomes in patients with complicated intra-abdominal infections [5]. In the short-duration therapy group, antibiotics were administered for 7 days or less; in the longer-duration therapy group, antibiotics were administered for more than 7 days. The primary outcome was treatment failure, defined as a composite of recurrent infection, secondary extra-abdominal infection, and all-cause hospital mortality. Two-hundred and forty patients were included in the study, with 103 in the short and 137 in the longer duration treatment groups. Treatment failure occurred in significantly fewer patients in the short-duration therapy group (39% vs. 63%, $P < 0.001$). On logistic regression analysis, longer duration therapy was associated with treatment failure; however, it was not associated with mortality.

44.3 Duration of Antibiotic Therapy: Ventilator-Associated Pneumonia

Ventilator-associated pneumonia (VAP) is among the commonest nosocomial infections in critically ill patients. The diagnosis of VAP is often unclear; besides, clinicians may be under pressure to prescribe antibiotics early, considering the perceived adverse outcomes associated with delayed treatment. Many patients initially diagnosed with possible VAP may not, in fact, have pneumonia and undergo inappropriately prolonged antibiotic treatment [6]. A shorter duration of antibiotic administration has favorable effects on bacterial ecology and the emergence of resistant strains [7].

What does the available evidence suggest regarding the duration of antibiotic therapy for VAP?

In their landmark trial, Chastre et al. compared 8 vs. 15 days of antibiotic therapy for VAP in 51 French ICUs [8]. In this study, 197 patients were randomized to receive an 8-day antibiotic course; 204 patients received a 15-day course. The 28-day mortality was similar between the 8- and 15-day treatment groups (18.8% vs. 17.2%; 90% CI, −3.7% to 6.9%). The incidence of recurrent infection was similar between groups. Mechanical ventilation-free days, organ failure-free days, and duration of ICU stay were also not significantly different. However, patients allocated to the shorter regimen had significantly more antibiotic-free days (13.1 vs. 8.7 days, $P < 0.001$). Among patients who had infection with non-fermenting Gram-negative bacteria including *Pseudomonas aeruginosa*, the recurrence rate was higher with the shorter duration of antibiotic therapy. Among patients with recurrent infection, multidrug-resistant organisms were less frequent with a shorter duration of treatment.

Hendrik et al. specifically evaluated the efficacy of a shorter duration of antibiotic therapy in VAP caused by non-fermenting Gram-negative bacteria against the background of the previous study by Chastre et al. [9]. In a retrospective analysis, the authors analyzed data on patients who underwent treatment for VAP in a surgical and trauma ICU. Overall, 452 episodes of VAP were observed during the study period. Infection with non-fermenting Gram-negative bacilli occurred in 154 patients; 127 patients underwent antibiotic treatment for 9 or more days, while 27 patients were treated for 3–8 days. In contrast to the Chastre et al. study, the authors observed no significant difference in the rate of recurrent infection between patients who underwent short compared to a longer duration of antibiotic treatment in VAP caused by non-fermenting Gram-negative bacilli (22% vs. 34%; $P = 0.27$). The mortality rate was also not significantly different between the two groups. However, this study is limited by its retrospective design; besides, it is possible that sicker patients received a longer duration of treatment, as the decision to cease therapy was based entirely on clinician judgment.

An 8-day compared to a 15-day antibiotic therapy was evaluated for early-onset VAP in 13 ICUs in France [10]. Patients who developed VAP within the first 8 days of ventilation were randomized to the 8- or 15-day antibiotic regimen. All included patients received beta-lactams for 8 or 15 days; an aminoglycoside was administered until day 5 of treatment. The study included 225 patients: 109 in the 15-day regimen and 116 in the 8-day regimen. The primary outcome was clinical cure on day 21. Clinical cure occurred in 92/109 (84.4%) patients in the 15-day regimen and 99/116 (85.3%) patients in the 8-day regimen, demonstrating equivalence between the two regimens. The 21-day mortality was also comparable between both patient cohorts.

In a retrospective study, an ultra-short antibiotic course of 1–3 days was compared with >3 days of treatment in patients with suspected VAP [11]. Patients were on an FiO_2 of ≤ 0.4 or less and a PEEP level of ≤ 5 cm H_2O on the day of commencement of antibiotics and for the following two days. Sensitivity analyses were performed using propensity scores to match patients in both cohorts. Among 1290 patients with suspected VAP who remained on minimal, stable ventilator settings,

259 received antibiotics for 1–3 days; 1031 patients received antibiotics for >3 days. Hospital mortality, duration of mechanical ventilation, and hospital length-of-stay were not significantly different between the two groups of patients. The median duration from commencement of antibiotic treatment to extubation and hospital discharge was longer among patients who received >3 days of antibiotics. This study underlines the importance of early cessation of antibiotics in patients who are initially suspected to have VAP but may have experienced an alternate, non-infective event.

44.4 Duration of Antibiotic Therapy: Gram-Negative Bacteremia

The optimal duration of antibiotic therapy for patients with Gram-negative bacteremia is unclear. Yahav et al. evaluated the duration of antibiotic therapy and outcomes in patients with Gram-negative bacteremia who were afebrile and hemodynamically stable [12]. Patients were randomized to a 7-day or 14-day treatment regimen. The primary focus of infection was urinary in the majority (68%) of patients. Patients with an uncontrolled source were excluded from the trial. The primary outcome, assessed at 90 days, was a composite of all-cause mortality, relapse of infection, remote complications, and readmission or prolonged hospitalization of more than 14 days. The primary outcome occurred in 45.8% of patients in the 7-day treatment group and 48.3% of patients in the 14-day treatment group; the difference was not statistically significant. Besides, there was no significant difference in the incidence of new infections, development of bacterial resistance, or duration of stay in hospital between the two groups.

Chotiprasitsakul et al. compared outcomes of patients between a short-course (6–10 days) compared to prolonged-course (11–16 days) of antibiotic therapy in patients with Enterobacteriaceae bacteremia [13]. In this retrospective cohort study, 1:1 propensity score matching, followed by regression analysis, was carried out to evaluate all-cause mortality at 30 days after cessation of antibiotic treatment. No difference in mortality was observed between the two treatment groups; a trend toward reduced emergence of multidrug-resistant Gram-negative bacteria was observed with the shorter course of treatment. Table 44.1 summarizes important clinical trials that compare short vs. prolonged duration of antibiotic therapy among critically ill patients.

Table 44.1 Clinical trials that compare short vs. prolonged duration of antibiotic therapy in critically ill patients

Study/year	Design/population	Short duration	Prolonged duration	Outcomes
Montravers et al. [3] (DURAPOP, 2018)	RCT; intra-abdominal sepsis with pus collection, after source control	7 days post-operatively	15 days	More antibiotic-free days from day 8 to 28 with the shorter antibiotic regimen. 45-day mortality, duration of stay in the ICU and hospital, emergence of MDR bacteria, and re-exploration rates similar
Sawyer et al. [4] (STOP-IT, 2015)	RCT; intra-abdominal infection after source control	4 days after source control	Until 2 days after resolution of SIRS	The composite primary outcome of surgical site infection, recurrent infection, mortality within 30 days of source control, not different. Individual components of the composite outcome not different. Duration of treatment significantly less in the short-course group
Smith et al. [5] (2017)	Retrospective study; complicated abdominal infection	7 days or less	More than 7 days	Treatment failure (composite of recurrent infection, secondary extra-abdominal infection, all-cause hospital mortality) less common with short duration therapy. Longer duration of antibiotics associated with treatment failure on regression analysis
Chastre et al. [8] (2003)	RCT; patients with VAP	8 days	15 days	28-day mortality, recurrent infections, mechanical ventilation-free days, organ failure-free days, ICU LOS, not different. More antibiotic-free days with short-course treatment. MDR organisms less frequent with shorter duration treatment. Increase in the incidence of recurrent infection among patients infected with non-fermenting Gram-negative bacilli

(continued)

Table 44.1 (continued)

Study/year	Design/population	Short duration	Prolonged duration	Outcomes
Hendrik et al. [9] (2007)	Retrospective observational study; patients who underwent treatment for VAP for infection with non-fermenting Gram-negative bacilli. Surgical and trauma ICU	3–8 days	≥ 9 days	No increase in the rate of recurrent infection among patients infected with non-fermenting Gram-negative bacilli. No difference in mortality between groups
Capellier [10] (2012)	RCT; patients with VAP within 8 days of mechanical ventilation	8 days	15 days	No difference in clinical cure rates and the 21-day mortality
Klompas et al. [11] (2016)	Retrospective study; patients with suspected VAP	1–3 days	>3 days	Hospital mortality, duration of ventilation, hospital LOS, not different. Median duration from antibiotic commencement to extubation and hospital discharge longer with >3 days of antibiotic treatment
Yahav et al. [12] (2019)	RCT; patients with Gram-negative bacteremia and hemodynamically stable	7 days	14 days	Composite 90-day outcome including all-cause mortality, relapse of infection, remote complications, readmission, or hospitalization >14 days, not different. No difference in the incidence of new infections, bacterial resistance, and duration of hospital stay
Chotiprasitsakul et al. [13] (2018)	Retrospective cohort study; patients with Enterobacteriaceae bacteremia	6–10 days	11–16 days	No difference in the 30-day all-cause mortality after propensity matching; trend toward reduction in the emergence of MDR Gram-negative bacteria with a shorter course

RCT randomized controlled trial, *MDR* multi-drug resistant, *SIRS* systemic inflammatory response syndrome, *LOS* length of stay, *VAP* ventilator-associated pneumonia

44.5 Procalcitonin to Guide the Duration of Antibiotic Therapy

Procalcitonin (PCT) is often used by clinicians to decide on the duration of antibiotic therapy in septic patients. However, the utility of PCT in this situation is controversial. An RCT from the Netherlands included critically ill patients with proven or suspected sepsis. In the PCT-guided group, antibiotics were continued until the PCT level had reduced to 20% of baseline or 0·5 μg/l; in the control arm, the duration of treatment was guided by local protocols. The median duration of therapy was significantly lower in the PCT-guided group. Furthermore, the 1-year mortality was also lower in the PCT-guided treatment arm [14]. However, a multicentric RCT from 11 Australian ICUs revealed contrasting findings. This RCT included patients with bacterial infection or sepsis with an expected ICU stay of more than 24 h. A cutoff PCT value of <0.10 ng/ml was used to cease antibiotic therapy; in the standard care arm, the duration of treatment was based on clinician judgment. The overall median duration of antibiotic therapy was similar in the PCT-guided and standard care groups. The 90-day all-cause mortality was not significantly different between the two groups. On logistic regression analysis, the initial PCT level was not a predictor of mortality; however, a slow reduction in PCT levels was an independent predictor of hospital and 90-day mortality [15]. Meta-analyses comparing PCT-guided compared to standard care do not support the utility of PCT levels to guide the duration of antibiotic therapy. PCT guidance may not minimize mortality or reduce the duration of mechanical ventilation [16, 17].

Key Points

- Limiting exposure to antibiotics to an optimal duration is one of the cornerstones of treatment of infections in critically ill patients. Although there is emphasis on early, appropriate antibiotic administration, there is a relative lack of focus on the duration of therapy. An unnecessarily long duration of therapy may result in *Clostridioides difficile* infection, toxicity, the emergence of resistant strains, and an increase in the cost of healthcare.
- VAP is often difficult to diagnose; a significant number of patients who are initially suspected to have VAP may have experienced a non-infective, alternate event. Continued vigilance at the bedside may enable cessation of therapy at an early stage. There is reasonably strong evidence to support antibiotic therapy for a week or less in patients with VAP.
- Source control is all-important in complicated intra-abdominal infections. Once source control is achieved, an extended duration of therapy is unnecessary; in fact, treatment failure may be less common with a shorter duration of therapy.

- In Gram-negative bacteremia, a shorter duration of therapy of 7–10 days has been shown to be as effective as more prolonged therapy.
- PCT may be a useful biomarker of bacterial infection; although some studies support its use to reduce the duration of antibiotic therapy, the evidence has generally been inconclusive.

References

1. Results of ESCAVO's survey on antibiotic use in sepsis. Escavo. 2019 [cited 2022 Jul 10]. https://escavo.com/2019/07/18/antibiotic-use-in-sepsis-survey/
2. Schein M, Assalia A, Bachus H. Minimal antibiotic therapy after emergency abdominal surgery: a prospective study. Br J Surg. 1994;81(7):989–91.
3. Montravers P, Tubach F, Lescot T, Veber B, Esposito-Farèse M, et al. For the DURAPOP trial group. Short-course antibiotic therapy for critically ill patients treated for postoperative intra-abdominal infection: the DURAPOP randomised clinical trial. Intensive Care Med. 2018;44(3):300–10.
4. Sawyer RG, Claridge JA, Nathens AB, Rotstein OD, Duane TM, Evans HL, et al. Trial of short-course antimicrobial therapy for intraabdominal infection. N Engl J Med. 2015;372(21):1996–2005.
5. Smith SE, Rumbaugh KA, May AK. Evaluation of a short course of antimicrobial therapy for complicated intra-abdominal infections in critically ill surgical patients. Surg Infect. 2017;18(6):742–50.
6. Nussenblatt V, Avdic E, Berenholtz S, Daugherty E, Hadhazy E, Lipsett PA, et al. Ventilator-associated pneumonia: overdiagnosis and treatment are common in medical and surgical intensive care units. Infect Control Hosp Epidemiol. 2014;35(3):278–84.
7. Bottery MJ, Pitchford JW, Friman VP. Ecology and evolution of antimicrobial resistance in bacterial communities. ISME J. 2021;15(4):939–48.
8. Chastre J, Wolff M, Fagon JY, Chevret S, Thomas F, Wermert D, et al. Comparison of 8 vs 15 days of antibiotic therapy for ventilator-associated pneumonia in adults: a randomized trial. JAMA. 2003;290(19):2588–98.
9. Hedrick TL, McElearney ST, Smith RL, Evans HL, Pruett TL, Sawyer RG. Duration of antibiotic therapy for ventilator-associated pneumonia caused by non-fermentative Gram-negative bacilli. Surg Infect. 2007;8(6):589–97.
10. Capellier G, Mockly H, Charpentier C, Annane D, Blasco G, Desmettre T, et al. Early-onset ventilator-associated pneumonia in adults randomized clinical trial: comparison of 8 versus 15 days of antibiotic treatment. PLoS One. 2012;7(8):e41290.
11. Klompas M, Li L, Menchaca JT, Gruber S, for the CDC Prevention Epicenters Program. Ultra short course antibiotics for patients with suspected ventilator-associated pneumonia but minimal and stable ventilator settings. Clin Infect Dis. 2016:ciw870.
12. Yahav D, Franceschini E, Koppel F, Turjeman A, Babich T, Bitterman R, et al. Seven versus 14 days of antibiotic therapy for uncomplicated Gram-negative bacteremia: a noninferiority randomized controlled trial. Clin Infect Dis. 2019;69(7):1091–8.
13. Chotiprasitsakul D, Han JH, Cosgrove SE, Harris AD, Lautenbach E, Conley AT, et al. Comparing the outcomes of adults with Enterobacteriaceae bacteremia receiving short-course versus prolonged-course antibiotic therapy in a multicenter, propensity score-matched cohort. Clin Infect Dis. 2018;66(2):172–7.

14. de Jong E, van Oers JA, Beishuizen A, Vos P, Vermeijden WJ, Haas LE, et al. Efficacy and safety of procalcitonin guidance in reducing the duration of antibiotic treatment in critically ill patients: a randomised, controlled, open-label trial. Lancet Infect Dis. 2016;16(7):819–27.
15. Shehabi Y, Sterba M, Garrett PM, Rachakonda KS, Stephens D, Harrigan P, et al. Procalcitonin algorithm in critically ill adults with undifferentiated infection or suspected sepsis. A randomized controlled trial. Am J Respir Crit Care Med. 2014;190(10):1102–10.
16. Andriolo BN, Andriolo RB, Salomão R, Atallah ÁN. Effectiveness and safety of procalcitonin evaluation for reducing mortality in adults with sepsis, severe sepsis or septic shock. Cochrane Database Syst Rev. 2017;18(1):CD010959.
17. Arulkumaran N, Khpal M, Tam K, Baheerathan A, Corredor C, Singer M. Effect of antibiotic discontinuation strategies on mortality and infectious complications in critically ill septic patients: a meta-analysis and trial sequential analysis. Crit Care Med. 2020;48(5):757–64.

Selective Digestive Decontamination: Helpful or Harmful?

45

45.1 Introduction

Selective decontamination of the digestive tract (SDD) is an infection control measure which has remained an ongoing source of controversy since it was first described in the ICU in trauma patients in 1984 [1]. The aim of SDD is to reduce the mortality of critically ill patients by preventing hospital-acquired infection by altering the balance of potentially pathogenic and normal gastrointestinal flora and specifically to eradicate aerobic gram-negative bacilli and pathogenic yeasts from the digestive tract while maintaining normal populations of gram-positive and anaerobic bacteria. Multiple clinical trials and reviews have confirmed a positive benefit on the incidence of both ventilator-associated pneumonia and mortality [2], and SDD is standard practice in some parts of the world, particularly the Netherlands. Despite the absence of evidence, there are ongoing concerns elsewhere about the development of antibiotic resistance, however, which has prevented the widespread introduction of SDD into practice.

45.2 Pathophysiology, History, and Controversy

SDD was originally described in immunocompromised hematology patients [3] and in trauma patients [1, 4] and was extended to critically ill ICU patients in the 1980s [5, 6]. SDD is the application of topical non-absorbable antibiotics and antifungal agents to the upper gastrointestinal tract of patients receiving mechanical ventilation via an endotracheal tube [7]. While exact compositions have varied, SDD regimens usually consist of an oral paste and enteral suspension of an aminoglycoside (e.g., tobramycin), peptide antibiotic (e.g.,

J. Chacko et al., *Controversies in Critical Care*,
https://doi.org/10.1007/978-981-19-9940-6_45

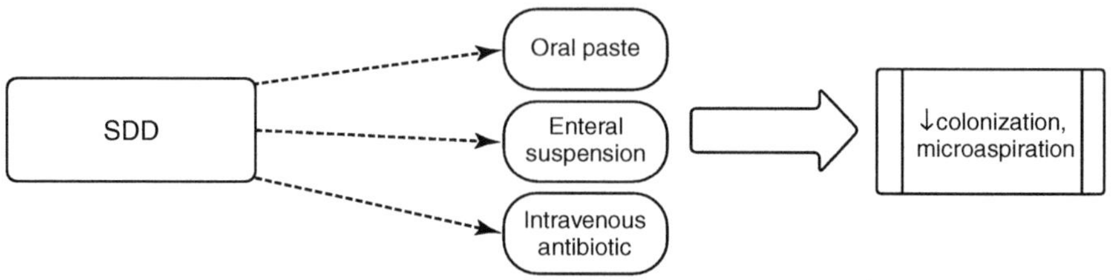

Fig. 45.1 The components of selective digestive decontamination (SDD). SDD aims to prevent colonization of the gastrointestinal tract and reduce the incidence of micro-aspiration

polymyxin B/colistin), and an antifungal (e.g., amphotericin or nystatin), combined with a short course of intravenous third generation cephalosporin (e.g., cefotaxime) or fluoroquinolone (e.g., ciprofloxacin) [7]. The principal aim of SDD is to prevent the development of ventilator-associated pneumonia caused by pathogenic gram-negative bacteria and secondary overgrowth with yeasts from the upper gastrointestinal tract, and the mechanism by which SDD prevents infection is primarily by the prevention of gastric colonization by these organisms with subsequent micro-aspiration into the lungs (Fig. 45.1).

Despite the evidence of benefit, international guideline panels have been reluctant to recommend SDD [8], despite at least 36 randomized controlled trials (RCTs) that have consistently demonstrated a reduction in hospital-acquired infections. The greatest concern limiting the uptake of SDD is that the use of SDD will lead to an increase in antibiotic resistance. The association between overuse of antibiotics and the emergence of infections due to multi-resistant organisms (especially methicillin-resistant *Staphylococcus aureus* and vancomycin-resistant *Enterococcus*) is well established, and these organisms are highly prevalent in many hospitals. Broad-spectrum antibiotics are also associated with an increased prevalence of *Clostridioides difficile* and multi-resistant *Enterobacteriaceae* and *Pseudomonas aeruginosa* due to alterations in intestinal flora. While many SDD trials report antibiotic resistance in study patients or short-term studies of ICU ecology [9], none of these trials has simultaneously studied the microbiological ecology of the whole ICU during and particularly after the introduction of SDD. Much of the existing data on the impact of SDD on antibiotic resistance patterns comes from the Netherlands which has an atypical and low prevalence of endemic bacterial resistance. Consequently, the applicability of data from the Netherlands to countries where antibiotic resistance is more prevalent is unclear. There are many isolated examples, however, where a program of SDD was actually introduced in order to deal with an outbreak of resistance. One longer-term Dutch study followed up patients for a mean of 7 years in five Dutch ICUs and documented tobramycin resistance decreasing while colistin resistance remained unchanged (and very low) over time [10].

A systematic review looking specifically at the emergence of resistance in SDD trials [11] found no increase in colonization or infection with methicillin-resistant *Staphylococcus aureus* (OR 1.46, 95% CI 0.90–1.68) or vancomycin-resistant *Enterococcus* (OR 0.63, 95% CI 0.39–1.02), no difference in development of aminoglycoside (OR 0.73, 95% CI 0.51–1.05) or quinolone resistance (OR 0.52, 95% CI 0.16–1.68) and a significant decrease in polymyxin (OR 0.58, 95% CI 0.46–0.72) and third-generation cephalosporin resistance (OR 0.33, 95% CI 0.20–0.52). Thus, despite concerns that SDD might increase the prevalence of antibiotic-resistant organisms, there is no such evidence from published clinical trials. The use of SDD is actually associated with a *reduction* in overall antibiotic use, with less "wild type" antibiotic prescribing [12], and overall, the amount of drug used in SDD is miniscule compared to overall hospital antibiotic use.

One other barrier to the uptake of SDD has been a perception that it is difficult or messy to deliver [13], with a lack of any commercially prepared and tested formulations of the study drugs. As a consequence, in most trials SDD has been prepared locally, either in hospital pharmacies or at the bedside, increasing the overall difficulty of delivering the intervention. Nurses who actually administer SDD do not have concerns, however, and emphasize that oral hygiene is a core element of intensive care nursing.

45.3 Recent Trials

Table 45.1 summarizes important recent trials that have evaluated the efficacy of SDD among ICU patients.

1. Plantinga and colleagues performed an individual patient data meta-analysis of six trials performed since 2000 [14]. These six trials, all performed in countries with low levels of antibiotic resistance, included data on 17,884 ICU admissions (including both SDD and selective oral decontamination only). The adjusted OR for hospital mortality was 0.82 (95%CI 0.72–0.93) for SDD compared to control. The effects on hospital mortality were not modified by type of ICU admission.
2. Ecological Effects of Decolonisation Strategies in Intensive Care (RGNOSIS) [15] was the first trial specifically in ICUs with higher levels of endemic resistance, conducted in 13 European ICUs where at least 5% of bloodstream infections were caused by extended spectrum β-lactamase-producing *Enterobacteriaceae*. In a three-arm cluster crossover trial, patients were randomized to 2% chlorhexidine mouthwash/1% chlorhexidine gel, selective oral decontamination, or SDD. The primary outcome was the new onset of ICU-acquired bloodstream infection caused by multidrug-resistant gram-negative bacteria. There was no significant reduction, but the overall incidence was lower than predicted (between 1.2% and 2.1% of included patients).
3. The Australian Selective Decontamination of the Digestive Tract in the Intensive Care Unit (SuDDICU) trial [16] was a cluster crossover trial in 19 ICUs which

Table 45.1 Important recent studies evaluating the impact of selective digestive decontamination in the ICU

Study/year	Type/design	Intervention	Control	Outcomes
Plantinga et al. (2018) [14]	Individual patient meta-analysis of six RCTs in countries with low levels of antibiotic resistance	SOD or SDD	Standard care or placebo	Improved ICU and hospital survival with both SDD and SOD. SDD more effective than SOD
Wittekamp et al. (2018) [15]	Three-arm cluster crossover trial. ICUs included had moderate to high levels of antibiotic resistance	Each ICU assigned randomly to 3 separate 6-month intervention periods with CHX 2%, SOD, or SDD	Standard care including daily CHX 2% body wash and hand hygiene improvement program	CHX mouthwash, SOD, or SDD not associated with reductions in ICU-acquired bloodstream infections due to multidrug-resistant gram-negative bacteria
Myburgh et al. (SuDDICU, 2022) [16]	Cluster crossover trial in 19 ICUs. Mechanically ventilated patients, two 12-month intervention periods	SDD combined with usual care	Usual care alone	In-hospital mortality, duration of mechanical ventilation, duration of ICU and hospital stay similar between groups. Fewer new cultures of resistant organisms and significantly fewer new bloodstream infections. No overall increase in resistance rates
Hammond et al. (2022) [17]	Meta-analysis of 32 RCTs	SDD	Standard care or placebo	SDD associated with lower hospital mortality. Beneficial effect confined to studies that used intravenous antibiotics. Reduced incidence of VAP and ICU-acquired bacteremia with SDD

SOD selective oral decontamination, *SDD* selective digestive decontamination, *CHX* chlorhexidine, *RCT* randomized controlled trial, *VAP* ventilator-associated pneumonia

delivered either SDD in addition to usual care or usual care alone to mechanically ventilated patients for two 12-month intervention periods, associated with a contemporaneous ecology study of all patients in the ICU at the time, whether ventilated or not. Of 5982 patients, the hospital mortality was 27% in the SDD arm and 29.1% in the standard care arm (OR 0.91, 95%CI 0.82–1.02). SDD was associated with significantly fewer new cultures of resistant organisms and significantly fewer new bloodstream infections, and the whole-of-ICU ecology study did not demonstrate any increase in resistance rates in the ICUs. SuDDICU was the first trial to use an SDD product prepared commercially according to Good Manufacturing Practice (GMP) standards with full chemical and microbiological stability testing.

4. To match the publication of SuDDICU, Hammond and colleagues conducted an updated systematic review and meta-analysis of all SDD trials to date in October 2022 [17]. In 30 trials with 24,034 patients, the risk ratio (RR) for mortality was 0.91 with SDD compared to standard care (95% CI 0.82–0.99) with a 99.3% posterior probability that SDD reduced hospital mortality. This was specifically seen in trials which included the IV component of SDD (RR 0.84). The use of SDD was associated with a significant decrease in the incidence of ventilator-associated pneumonia (RR 0.44) and ICU-acquired bacteremia (RR 0.68).

Key Points

- It is clear from evidence to date that SDD works as an infection control strategy,
- Ventilated patients treated with SDD have a significantly lower incidence of ventilator-associated pneumonia and ICU-acquired bloodstream infections, with an absolute mortality benefit of about 2% and a risk ratio of 0.9.
- There is no evidence that SDD increases antimicrobial resistance rates, but the evidence in trials is not sufficiently robust to draw firm conclusions.
- Before SDD is widely adopted internationally, there is a need for further research specifically in environments with high endemic resistance, and there needs to be commercial engagement with ready availability of drug in an easy-to-administer formulation.

References

1. Stoutenbeek CP, van Saene HKF, Miranda DR, Zandstra DF. The effect of selective decontamination of the digestive tract on colonisation and infection rate in multiple trauma patients. Intensive Care Med. 1984;10:185–92.
2. Minozzi S, Pifferi S, Brazzi L, et al. Topical antibiotic prophylaxis to reduce respiratory tract infections and mortality in adults receiving mechanical ventilation. Cochrane Database Syst Rev. 2021;1(1):CD000022.
3. Schimpff SC. Infection prevention during profound granulocytopenia. New approaches to alimentary canal microbial suppression. Ann Intern Med. 1980;93:358–61.
4. Stoutenbeek CP, van Saene HK, Little RA, Whitehead A. The effect of selective decontamination of the digestive tract on mortality in multiple trauma patients: a multicenter randomized controlled trial. Intensive Care Med. 2007;33:261–70.

5. van Saene HK, Stoutenbeek CP, Hart CA. Selective decontamination of the digestive tract (SDD) in intensive care patients: a critical evaluation of the clinical, bacteriological and epidemiological benefits. J Hosp Infect. 1991;18:261–77.
6. Vandenbroucke-Grauls CM, Vandenbroucke JP. Effect of selective decontamination of the digestive tract on respiratory tract infections and mortality in the intensive care unit. Lancet. 1991;338:859–62.
7. de Jonge E, Schultz MJ, Spanjaard L, et al. Effects of selective decontamination of digestive tract on mortality and acquisition of resistant bacteria in intensive care: a randomised controlled trial. Lancet. 2003;362:1011–6.
8. Evans L, Rhodes A, Alhazzani W, et al. Surviving sepsis campaign: international guidelines for management of sepsis and septic shock 2021. Intensive Care Med. 2021;47:1181–247.
9. Oostdijk EAN, de Smet AMGA, Blok HEM, et al. Ecological effects of selective decontamination on resistant gram-negative bacterial colonization. Am J Respir Crit Care Med. 2010;181:452–7.
10. Daneman N, Sarwar S, Fowler RA, Cuthbertson BH. Effect of selective decontamination on antimicrobial resistance in intensive care units: a systematic review and meta-analysis. Lancet Infect Dis. 2013;13:328–41.
11. Wittekamp BHJ, Oostdijk EAN, de Smet AAMGA, Bonten MJM. Colistin and tobramycin resistance during long-term use of selective decontamination strategies in the intensive care unit: a *post hoc* analysis. Crit Care. 2015;19:113.
12. de Smet AMGA, Kluytmans JAJW, Cooper BS, et al. Decontamination of the digestive tract and oropharynx in ICU patients. N Engl J Med. 2009;360:20–31.
13. Cuthbertson BH, Campbell MK, MacLennan G, et al. Clinical stakeholders' opinions on the use of selective decontamination of the digestive tract in critically ill patients in intensive care units: an international delphi study. Crit Care. 2013;17:R266.
14. Plantinga NL, de Smet A, Oostdijk EAN, et al. Selective digestive and oropharyngeal decontamination in medical and surgical ICU patients: individual patient data meta-analysis. Clin Microbiol Infect. 2018;24:505–13.
15. Wittekamp BH, Plantinga NL, Cooper BS, et al. Decontamination strategies and bloodstream infections with antibiotic-resistant microorganisms in ventilated patients: a randomized clinical trial. JAMA. 2018;320:2087–98.
16. The SuDDICU Investigators for the Australian and New Zealand Intensive Care Society Clinical Trials Group. Effect of selective decontamination of the digestive tract on hospital mortality in critically ill patients receiving mechanical ventilation: a randomized clinical trial. JAMA. 2022;328(19):1911–21. https://doi.org/10.1001/jama.2022.17927.
17. Hammond NE, Myburgh J, Seppelt I, et al. Association between selective decontamination of the digestive tract and in-hospital mortality in intensive care unit patients receiving mechanical ventilation a systematic review and meta-analysis. JAMA. 2022;328(19):1922–34. https://doi.org/10.1001/jama.2022.19709.

Part VIII

Organizational Challenges in the ICU

Which Organizational Structure to Pursue? The Open vs. Closed ICU Debate

46

46.1 Introduction

Who should be the formal decision-maker in the ICU? The question continues to arouse passionate interest among clinicians who care for critically ill patients in many parts of the world. When Bjorn Ibsen established his pioneering intensive care facility at the Kommunehospitalet, Copenhagen, in 1953, he had sought the primary caregivers to hand over the responsibility of their patients. Although the closed model is followed in many countries, considering the level of specialization and widespread use of interventional treatment modalities, there is perhaps increasing onus on the primary clinician to be the arbitrator of care. Should definitions of ICU models continue to be cast in stone in today's world?

46.2 Definitions

The following definitions are commonly followed.

Open ICU (low intensity): Patients are admitted under the care of another specialty physician or surgeon, with intensivists available for consultation and management as deemed necessary.

Closed ICU (high intensity): Critically ill patients are admitted and managed by a fully trained intensivist. The main features, advantages, and possible drawbacks of different organizational systems are summarized in Table 46.1.

J. Chacko et al., *Controversies in Critical Care*,
https://doi.org/10.1007/978-981-19-9940-6_46

Table 46.1 Main features, advantages, and disadvantages of an open vs. closed ICU system

	Open ICU	Closed ICU
Advantages	• No requirement for a dedicated intensivist; cost-effective in resource-poor settings • A dedicated clinician takes care of the patient from admission to discharge; may offer better continuity of care • Familiarity with patient; easier to build rapport and trust with patients and families • Fewer handovers—less chance of information loss and misunderstanding	• Focused critical care skills required • Better coordination • Efficient use of critical care resources • Well-defined leadership • Cohesive treatment strategy • Better end-of-life care and clear communication with families
Disadvantages	• May create confusion as to who is in charge—multiple cooks • System-specific approach—can miss the bigger picture • Disjointed treatment strategy and mixed messages can decrease family satisfaction	• Need for trained intensivist round-the-clock—staffing challenges • Multiple handovers and transfer of care—recipe for misunderstanding and loss of continuity of care • Higher likelihood of conflict between specialists and the ICU teams; differences and disagreement over limitation of care

46.3 What Is the Global Trend?

Many hospitals around the world, especially in the USA, still include open ICUs. According to a survey conducted in 2007, among 1265 ICUs across 75 countries, only 17% were open ICUs, whereas 83% were closed ICUs [1]. North America had the lowest (63%) proportion of closed ICUs, while western Europe had the highest (89%). In Canada, out of 111 ICUs across 9 provinces, 85% reported a closed format model in 2015 [2]. In 2016, across Asia, 216 out of 335 ICUs worked on a closed format [3]. In Australia, New Zealand, and the UK, the majority of ICUs are modeled on a closed format. Comparative studies between a dedicated, intensivist-driven approach and specialist-centered care are important to evaluate the impact of focused care on outcomes. A survey of 69 ICUs was carried out to characterize the organizational structure, processes of care, use of protocols, and standardized outcomes in a large sample of ICUs from the USA. Adherence to a structured approach with daily care plan review and a lower bed-to-nurse ratio were associated with lower annual ICU mortality. Besides, the study showed that improved communication within the ICU team might result in improved clinical outcomes among ICU patients [4].

46.4 What Does Evidence Suggest?

The evidence base behind the optimal ICU organizational structure is limited by a paucity of controlled clinical trials. Besides, the patient population involved in most observational studies is heterogeneous in nature, with variable severity of illness at baseline that may have confounded the results. Several observational studies and systematic reviews have addressed the question regarding the optimal ICU setup.

46.5 Observational Studies

Does staffing by dedicated intensivists affect specific quality indicators in the ICU?

A retrospective, 1-year cohort study evaluated specific quality measures before and after the implementation of 24-h ICU coverage by dedicated intensivists according to the Leapfrog staffing standards. The study was conducted in a 15-bed mixed medical-surgical community ICU. The study evaluated the outcomes of 1113 patients during the pre-implementation phase and 1068 patients after the implementation of structured staffing. Dedicated intensivist-led care resulted in a significantly lower ICU length of stay (LOS). Besides, the incidence of ventilator-associated pneumonia (VAP) and central venous catheter-related bloodstream infections were significantly lower. Furthermore, there was a substantial reduction in the cost of care and a calculated 105% return on investment in ICU physician staffing [5].

Does the conversion of an open ICU model with admitting physicians directing care compared with a closed structure with critical care specialists directing care, impact clinical outcomes? This question was addressed in a 10-bedded medical ICU of a 600-bedded university hospital in the USA. In this before-after study design, 124 patients were evaluated in the open format and 121 after switching to the closed format. The actual to predicted mortality rates based on APACHE II scores were analyzed. The severity of illness based on the APACHE II score was significantly higher during the closed ICU phase. However, the actual compared to predicted mortality was lower after transition to a closed ICU structure. The nursing staff were also supportive and felt more confident with a closed ICU format [6].

A retrospective cohort study examined the relationship between intensivist staffing and select process-based quality indicators in the intensive care unit. The study was conducted across 29 academic hospitals in the USA and included 861 patients who required prolonged mechanical ventilation in the ICU. This study revealed that high-intensity staffing with physicians trained in critical care medicine resulted in increased utilization of evidence-based quality indicators. Specifically, staffing by trained physicians was associated with a higher rate of prophylaxis against deep vein thrombosis, sedation interruption, spontaneous breathing trials, and improved glycemic control. Particularly striking was the 64% increase in sedation interruption and 40% increase with the use of intensive insulin therapy aimed at glycemic control. Consistently high quality of care was observed with an intensivist-driven model of care [7].

One of the key components of a structured ICU is the availability of trained nursing staff and the nurse-to-patient ratio. Sakr et al. conducted an international, multicenter, observational study aimed to estimate the impact of various facets of ICU organization on outcomes in a large cohort of ICU patients from different geographic regions. The study was conducted across 1265 ICUs in 75 countries. Despite the heterogeneous nature of ICUs and hospitals across various countries, a high nurse-to-patient ratio was independently associated with a lower in-hospital mortality. A nurse-to-patient ratio of more than 1:1.5 on the study day was independently associated with a lower risk of in-hospital death [1].

Does continued care by the same physician impact outcomes among ICU patients?

A retrospective cohort study from the UK included 80,122 patients across 130 ICUs in 128 hospitals. All the ICUs followed a closed model; the study aimed to evaluate the relationship between intensivist cover pattern, including the number of days of continuous cover by the same intensivist, the physician staffing during night shifts, and the daily handover patterns. The authors could not find a relationship between hospital mortality and the number of days of continuous cover by the same intensivist, or the grade of physician staffing during night shifts. Surprisingly, the presence of an intensivist during handover seemed to be associated with increased mortality. However, among the 130 units studied, only 9 did not have intensivist participation during handovers, questioning the relevance of this finding [8].

46.6 Meta-Analyses That Compare Staffing Structure in the ICU

Pronovost et al., in a meta-analysis, aimed to evaluate the impact of an organized ICU structure, staffed by dedicated intensivists on clinical outcomes. The authors compared two different organizational structures. ICUs with no intensivist, or a need-based consultation, were compared with closed ICUs following intensivist-directed care. Twenty-six observational studies were included in the meta-analysis. The hospital mortality was lower with a closed ICU structure (relative risk, 0.71, 95% CI, 0.62–0.82). The ICU mortality also followed a similar trend (relative risk: 0.61, 95% CI, 0.50–0.75). Furthermore, a closed ICU structure reduced the hospital and ICU LOS in the majority of included studies [9].

Another meta-analysis included 52 observational studies comparing high-intensity staffing with an intensivist-led team or mandatory intensivist consultation with low-intensity staffing (open model). Similar to the meta-analysis by Pronovost et al., the authors observed a lower hospital and ICU mortality with a high-intensity staffing structure. Besides, high-intensity staffing was associated with significantly lower ICU mortality and reduced LOS in hospital and the ICU. The most profound impact of high-intensity coverage was observed in surgical and medical-surgical ICUs compared with ICUs that cared for medical patients alone. Interestingly, 24-h intensivist coverage, compared with daytime-only coverage, did not seem to influence hospital or ICU mortality [10].

46.7 Closed ICU and Conflicts

When decision-making and overall responsibility of care shifts to the intensivist's domain, differences of opinion may occur; this may lead to the primary caregiver feeling disempowered. A sense of loss of ownership of the patient may be particularly perceived by surgeons who perform complex procedures in niche areas of care. In a cross-sectional survey in the USA, the experience of surgeons regarding their conflict with intensivists and nurses regarding goals of care was assessed. The study included 2100 surgeons of various specialties, including vascular, neurologic, and cardiothoracic surgery. This survey revealed regular conflict between surgeons and critical care clinicians regarding goals of care for patients, particularly among those with poor postoperative outcomes. The conflict rate was higher with relatively less experienced surgeons working in a closed ICU. The study also suggested that surgeons who acted as primary care providers had fewer conflicts with the ICU team compared to those who worked within the constraints of a closed unit [11].

46.8 ICU Structure and Family Satisfaction

Do the organization and staffing structure of the ICU impact the satisfaction level of family members?

Family satisfaction was compared between a neuro ICU and the medical intensive care unit (MICU) of an academic medical center during a contemporaneous period. The neuro ICU was staffed by residents, fellows, and intensivists from the neurology and neurosurgery training programs and functioned as an open unit. The MICU was staffed by intensivists and fellows from an internal medicine background and functioned as a closed unit. Family satisfaction was evaluated using a survey tool that sought participants to rate satisfaction based on specific aspects of their ICU experience. The participants rated a significantly better experience regarding respect and compassion they received in the MICU compared to the neuro ICU. In the neuro ICU, dissatisfaction arose from inadequate levels of communication and lack of inclusion in decision-making and overall care. This study demonstrated that family experience and satisfaction might be superior in a structured ICU setup working on a closed model with round-the-clock involvement of intensivists as primary caregivers [12].

The available evidence supports an intensivist-driven model of care in critically ill patients (Table 46.2). However, there are no multicenter prospective studies that firmly establish the superiority of a closed system. Observational studies may be confounded by heterogeneous patient populations and the absence of a control group. Besides, the outcome benefits of an intensivist-driven model of care are not firmly established. Critics of a closed system point to drawbacks, including the requirement for multi-layered handoffs at admission and discharge from the ICU, that could lead to errors and adverse events [13].

Table 46.2 Main studies that have evaluated the model of ICU care: open vs. closed systems

Study/year	Design	Outcomes
Favoring closed ICU model		
Parikh et al. (2012) [5]	Before-after cohort study	• Change from open to closed model • Shorter ICU LOS, improved quality measures, lower incidence of VAP and CLABSI, with overall decrease in ICU cost
Kahn et al. (2007) [7]	Retrospective cohort study	• Improved quality of care associated with increased use of evidence-based indicators such as sedation interruption and management of blood glucose levels
Pronovost et al. (2002) [9]	Meta-analysis	• Included 26 studies • Closed ICU associated with lower mortality and shorter LOS
Wilcox et al. (2013) [8]	Meta-analysis	• Included 52 studies • High-intensity ICU staffing associated with decreased ICU and hospital mortality, and decreased LOS
Carson et al. (1996) [6]	Before-after cohort study	• Nurses in closed ICUs more likely to feel confident about intensivist judgment compared to those in open ICUs
Olson et al. (2013) [11]	Cross-sectional survey	• Surgeons working in open ICUs less likely to have conflict with intensivists compared to those in closed ICUs
Hwang et al. (2014) [12]	Survey of families	• More families reported satisfaction with closed medical ICUs compared with a neuro-science ICU. The favorable responses related to courtesy, respect, and compassion shown by staff
Favoring open ICU model		
Checkley et al. (2014) [4]	Survey	• Failed to detect an improvement in mortality across 69 centers in the USA with a closed format • Study limited to US context and generalizing these findings is not ideal

LOS length of stay, *VAP* ventilator-associated pneumonia, *CLABSI* central line-associated bloodstream infection

Key Points

- Although there is reasonable evidence to support the closed over the open ICU format, terminologies are not meant to be followed rigidly; a collaborative approach toward patient care would enable optimization of patient outcomes.
- A team of trained intensivists offering co-ordinated care would likely improve clinical outcomes, family satisfaction, and enhance confidence among nursing staff.
- Intensivists responsible for overall care are more likely to provide a holistic approach compared to patient management by individual physicians who may be more focused on their area of expertise.
- Focused bedside care is the basic tenet of the care of critically ill patients. Critically ill patients need constant attention in clinical situations that change dramatically over time and require tailored therapy by the bedside.

- Primary care providers often have other duties to perform, including running busy outpatient departments and performance of specialized interventions; they may not be able to dedicate time to offer bedside care to unstable patients in the ICU.
- A structured ICU pattern with intensivists at the helm has been shown to improve communication and family satisfaction. Besides, the round-the-clock presence of intensivists leads to greater confidence among the nursing team in clinician judgment and enhances teamwork.
- The choice of the ICU model would largely depend on local circumstances, the availability of trained staff, and the receptiveness of the local physician community to a closed model of care.

References

1. Sakr Y, Moreira CL, Rhodes A, Ferguson ND, Kleinpell R, Pickkers P, et al. The impact of hospital and ICU organizational factors on outcome in critically ill patients: results from the extended prevalence of infection in intensive care study. Crit Care Med. 2015;43(3):519–26.
2. Holodinsky JK, Hebert MA, Zygun DA, Rigal R, Berthelot S, Cook DJ, et al. A survey of rounding practices in Canadian adult intensive care units. PLoS One. 2015;10(12):e0145408.
3. Arabi YM, Phua J, Koh Y, Du B, Faruq MO, Nishimura M, et al. Structure, organization, and delivery of critical care in Asian ICUs. Crit Care Med. 2016;44(10):e940–8.
4. Checkley W, Martin GS, Brown SM, Chang SY, Dabbagh O, Fremont RD, et al. Structure, process, and annual ICU mortality across 69 centers: United States critical illness and injury trials group critical illness outcomes study. Crit Care Med. 2014;42(2):344–56.
5. Parikh A, Huang SA, Murthy P, Dombrovskiy V, Nolledo M, Lefton R, et al. Quality improvement and cost savings after implementation of the leapfrog intensive care unit physician staffing standard at a community teaching hospital. Crit Care Med. 2012;40(10):2754–9.
6. Carson SS, Stocking C, Podsadecki T, Christenson J, Pohlman A, MacRae S, et al. Effects of organizational change in the medical intensive care unit of a teaching hospital: a comparison of "open" and "closed" formats. JAMA. 1996;276(4):322–8.
7. Kahn JM, Brake H, Steinberg KP. Intensivist physician staffing and the process of care in academic medical centres. Qual Saf Health Care. 2007;16(5):329–33.
8. Wilcox ME, Harrison DA, Short A, Jonas M, Rowan KM. Comparing mortality among adult, general intensive care units in England with varying intensivist cover patterns: a retrospective cohort study. Crit Care. 2014;18(4):491.
9. Pronovost PJ, Angus DC, Dorman T, Robinson KA, Dremsizov TT, Young TL. Physician staffing patterns and clinical outcomes in critically ill patients: a systematic review. JAMA. 2002;288(17):2151–62.
10. Wilcox ME, Chong CAKY, Niven DJ, Rubenfeld GD, Rowan KM, Wunsch H, et al. Do intensivist staffing patterns influence hospital mortality following ICU admission? A systematic review and meta-analyses. Crit Care Med. 2013;41(10):2253–74.
11. Paul Olson TJ, Brasel KJ, Redmann AJ, Alexander GC, Schwarze ML. Surgeon-reported conflict with intensivists about postoperative goals of care. JAMA Surg. 2013;148(1):29–35.
12. Hwang DY, Yagoda D, Perrey HM, Tehan TM, Guanci M, Ananian L, et al. Assessment of satisfaction with care among family members of survivors in a neuroscience intensive care unit. J Neurosci Nurs. 2014;46(2):106–16.
13. Starmer AJ, Spector ND, Srivastava R, West DC, Rosenbluth G, Allen AD, et al. Changes in medical errors after implementation of a handoff program. N Engl J Med. 2014;371(19):1803–12.

Adverse Events in the ICU: Building and Sustaining an Organizational Culture of Patient Safety

47

More than two decades ago, the Institute of Medicine highlighted the need to create safer health care systems. Medical errors were found to be the eighth most common cause of hospital mortality in the USA according to this report [1]. Errors leading to adverse outcomes are prone to occur in patient care environments that provide multifaceted care, employing life-support systems including ICUs, emergency departments, and operation theaters [2]. The patient population involved have complex underlying disease processes with limited physiological reserves and often require multiple interventions, making them particularly vulnerable to errors [1]. Adverse events or critical incidents have been variously defined. They represent unintended events consequent to failure of healthcare management, including human, organizational, or equipment error that lead to actual patient harm or have the potential to cause harm [3].

47.1 Incidence of Adverse Events

There is wide variation in the incidence of adverse events in ICUs, with some studies reporting such events in up to 20–31% of admissions [4, 5]. The high variability of adverse events reported may be due to differences in study settings, the presence of inherent safety systems, and a culture of transparency that may encourage reporting. However, adverse events are known to occur more commonly in high-acuity settings compared to other areas of the hospital where the level of care is less labor-intensive [6].

Are errors that lead to adverse events and potential patient harm, especially in vulnerable areas of healthcare, preventable? Does reporting adverse events improve patient safety?

J. Chacko et al., *Controversies in Critical Care*,
https://doi.org/10.1007/978-981-19-9940-6_47

47.2 Types of Adverse Events

Several studies have evaluated the nature and types of adverse events and their impact on patient outcomes in critically ill patients. A prospective observational study analyzed adverse events in the multidisciplinary and coronary care ICUs of a tertiary academic hospital [7]. Patients were followed up until transfer from the ICU, discharge, or death. Data regarding the patients and the staff involved were anonymized. An adverse event was defined as any injury that occurred due to medical management. The study reported 120 adverse events in 1490 patient-days (80.5/1000 patient-days). Of these, 104 were classified as severe or significant and 16 as life-threatening or fatal. The most common adverse events were respiratory (19%), nosocomial infections (15%), cardiovascular (12%), or skin and soft tissue-related (9%). Fifty-six adverse events (47%) were drug-related; among these 19 (33.9%) were considered preventable. Serious medical errors, defined as errors that caused harm or had the potential to do so, were observed on 223 occasions (149.7/1000 patient-days). Of these, 24 (11%) were deemed to be potentially life-threatening. Among the serious medical errors, 78% were drug-related. This study revealed that serious medical errors that result in patient harm or have the potential to do so are common among critically ill patients. Most of the errors emanated from failure to perform a plan of action as intended.

A retrospective cohort study evaluated adverse events in 49,447 admissions to 30 ICUs over a 3-year period [8]. Among these patients, 25.4% of ICU admissions experienced at least one documented adverse event (45.3/1000 hospital-days). The most common adverse events included respiratory-related complications (9.5/100 admissions) and nosocomial infections (8.8/100 admissions). Other reported events related to surgery, hemorrhagic incidents, delirium, complications related to fluid management, drug-related events, and decubitus ulcers. Less common adverse events included anesthesia-related, endocrine, and metabolic complications.

Harris et al. assessed the impact of a new card-based system on patient safety event reports in three ICUs in the USA. In this before-after study, the introduction of the new reporting system led to a significantly higher number of reports compared to the pre-existing web-based system of reporting. The authors analyzed the types of errors reported under the card-based system. The most common errors (33.6%) related to the conduct, administration, or interpretation of diagnostic tests, therapeutic interventions not related to the administration of medication, and procedure-related adverse events. These were collectively termed events related to "test, treatment, and procedure." The second most common type of error was related to the administration of medication (28.9%). Other adverse events reported included laboratory events, complications related to intravenous lines, equipment errors, delays and errors involving blood product administration, events related to patient behavior and psychiatric management, surgical complications, and falls [9].

Molina et al. analyzed adverse events over a 1-year period in a 12-bedded ICU from a university hospital in Colombia [10]. A total of 48 patients experienced 178 adverse events during the study period. The most common adverse events noted included pressure ulcers, equipment-related complications, skin and soft tissue injuries, hypotensive episodes due to drug error, nosocomial pneumonias, hemorrhage related to surgical procedures, respiratory system-related events, and surgical site infections. Most of the adverse events were considered preventable.

Does the type of adverse events differ between medical compared to surgical ICUs? Sinopoli et al. compared characteristics and outcomes from adverse events between medical and surgical ICUs in a prospective observational study conducted over a 2-year study period [11]. The incidence of adverse events was relatively higher among surgical patients. The authors observed no significant difference between the characteristics of adverse events reported between medical and surgical patients. A significant difference between the two groups of patients was noted only in 3 of 11 domains. Events related to device or equipment, lines, tubes, or drains were more common in surgical patients; however, events related to computerized clinician order entry were more common among medical patients. Physical injury occurred in 15%, while prolonged ICU stay was observed in 10% of patients. Less than 2% of cases resulted in a fatal outcome.

Chacko et al. evaluated the type and frequency of critical incidents in a multidisciplinary ICU in India [2]. During the 33-month study period, 280 adverse events were reported among 1918 patients admitted to the ICU, with a frequency of 3.4 incidents per 100 patient-days. Airway-related incidents were the most common (32.8%), followed by line-related (21.8) and drug-related (15%) incidents [2].

47.3 Outcomes Related to Adverse Events

Adverse events commonly occur in the ICU setting; the frequency of events may be substantially higher considering the likelihood of underreporting. It is important to evaluate the outcomes of patients who experience adverse events. Studies that evaluate incidence and outcomes of adverse events in the ICU are depicted in Table 47.1.

Cantor et al. retrospectively studied adult patients who were admitted to the ICU at The Ottawa Hospital in Canada over a 5-year period [12]. Adverse events occurred in 6070/17,173 (35.4%) patients admitted during the study period. The in-hospital mortality rate was significantly higher in patients who experienced adverse events compared to those who did not (26.2% vs. 18.4%, $P < 0.001$). After control of variables including age, gender, and comorbidity score by multivariable logistic regression, adverse events resulted in a 13% higher hospital mortality (adjusted OR = 1.13, 95% CI: 1.04–1.22). Furthermore, the duration of stay in ICU and hospital was also significantly longer in patients who experienced adverse events.

Baker et al. studied adverse events in 20 acute care hospitals in Canada, including community and teaching hospitals [13]. Adverse events were noted in 7.5/100 hospital admissions [95% confidence interval (CI) 5.7–9.3]. On review of 858 case records, 1133 adverse events were noted. Death, disability at discharge, or prolonged stay in hospital was observed in 401 (46.7%) of cases. Overall, 255 case records revealed one or more adverse events that were considered to have resulted from medical management and were likely to be preventable. Most adverse events did not lead to physical impairment or disability. Permanent disability was noted in

Table 47.1 Studies evaluating the incidence and outcomes of adverse events in the ICU

Author/year	Study type	Study population	Event rate	Outcomes
Cantor et al. (2022) [12]	Observational	17,173 ICU patients	6070 (35.4%)	Higher mortality with adverse events (26.2% vs. 18.4%, $P < 0.001$). Longer stay in hospital and ICU
Baker et al. (2004) [13]	Chart review	3745 acute care patients	1527 (40.8%) 7.5/100 hospital admissions	Permanent disability in 15/289 (5.2%) adverse events; mortality: 46 (15.9%)
Danielis et al. (2020) [14]	Retrospective observational	9355 ICU patients	1.7/100 ICU admissions; 2.86 incidents/1000 ICU days	Not available
Chacko et al. (2007) [2]	Prospective observational	1918 ICU patients	3.4 incidents per 100 patient-days	Adverse outcomes in 11.4%. Major physiological change in 3.6% of incidents, minor physiological change in 6.4%
Sinopoli et al. (2007) [11]	Prospective observational	765 ICU patients	1582 incidents	Physical injury, prolonged length of stay in 10% Death in 2%

15/289 (5.2%) adverse events, while 46 (15.9%) resulted in death. Based on the judgment of physician reviewers, the 255 patients who experienced adverse events required 1521 extra days in hospital due to these events.

An Italian study analyzed adverse events from four ICUs of an academic hospital over a 4-year period [14]. The adverse events rate was 1.7/100 ICU admissions with 2.86 incidents/1000 ICU days. The most common adverse events were related to medication or intravenous fluids (21.9%) and resources and organizational management (21.9%). This was followed by malfunction of equipment (8.1%), events related to clinical processes or procedures (11.3), and documentation error (8.8%). Medication errors commonly arose from incorrect dosing, route of administration, infusion rates, and administration of wrong medication.

Adverse outcomes following critical incidents were also uncommon in the study by Chacko et al.; 88.6% of incidents did not lead to harm. Some degree of harm occurred in 11.4% of incidents; a minor physiological change occurred in 6.4%, and a major physiological change in 3.6% of incidents. Four deaths were attributed to critical incidents, all associated with airway-related incidents [2].

47.4 Are Adverse Events Preventable?

Although there is increased awareness of the importance of reporting in recent years, the incidence of adverse events appears to be largely unchanged. This is perhaps due to increased reporting arising from an improved safety culture; however, there is plenty of room to improve in reducing harm from adverse events in critically ill patients. The key to improved patient safety would be to address lacunae in organizational systems that lead to errors. Long shifts without adequate breaks in between may contribute to lapses resulting from overwork. Interns who worked 24-h shifts or longer were more likely to commit serious errors compared to shorter shifts [15]. Diagnostic and medication errors were particularly likely during long work shifts. The study suggested that shortening the duration of shifts may enable the reduction of serious errors in the ICU.

A conceptual model aimed to improve physician compliance with five evidence-based recommendations during central venous catheter insertion [16]. These included handwashing, use of barrier precautions, skin preparation with chlorhexidine, avoidance of the femoral vein, and expeditious removal of unnecessary catheters. This multi-pronged strategy resulted in significantly fewer catheter-related bloodstream infections during an 18-month period. A lower incidence of such infections could result in reduced morbidity and cost of care. Forster et al. identified 56 adverse events in a study including 207 patients. One in five adverse events was considered preventable. The preventable adverse events related to nosocomial infections (35%), therapeutic errors (22%), and procedure-related complications (26%). Surgical complications were least likely to be preventable. An optimal strategy should focus on identifying preventable errors and the incorporation of system-based measures aimed to reduce such errors. A safer ICU environment calls for exploring the trigger for adverse events, regular system reviews, and revision of processes that culminated in, or contributed to, adverse events. The impact of system modifications must also be monitored to ensure efficacy and improved patient safety.

Key Points

- Adverse events commonly occur in the ICU setting. The underlying severity of illness, with the requirement for multi-faceted support systems, makes critically ill patients particularly vulnerable to treatment-related errors.
- Commonly reported adverse events in critically ill patients include those related to airway management, drug errors, intravenous fluid administration, procedure-related errors, and nosocomial infections.
- Although deleterious clinical outcomes are uncommon, adverse events have been associated with an increase in hospital mortality and length of stay.

- A significant proportion of adverse events may be preventable. Corrective measures should be aimed at establishing system-based strategies that enhance patient safety. The onus must be on the prevention of a recurrence of adverse events and not on apportioning blame.
- Identification of adverse events is the first important step toward creating a safe patient environment. Emphasis must be laid on a transparent system that encourages reporting without the fear of punishment or reprimand. An anonymized system that does not require details of the patient or staff involved may facilitate reporting of adverse events.
- Human errors may be triggered by distractions, haste, fatigue, and working under stressful situations, while staff inexperience aggravates the possibility of error. Adequate training is of crucial importance in the management of critically ill patients, who are particularly prone to adverse consequences, given their limited physiological reserves.
- It is also important to identify and follow up on "near-misses," as they offer valuable experience to learn from and act toward improving patient safety.

References

1. Institute of Medicine (US) Committee on Quality of Health Care in America. In: Kohn LT, Corrigan JM, Donaldson MS, editors. To Err is human: building a safer health system [Internet]. Washington, DC: National Academies Press (US); 2000. http://www.ncbi.nlm.nih.gov/books/NBK225182/. Accessed 29 May 2022.
2. Chacko J, Raju HR, Singh MK, Mishra RC. Critical incidents in a multidisciplinary intensive care unit. Anaesth Intensive Care. 2007;35(3):382–6.
3. Pagnamenta A, Rabito G, Arosio A, Perren A, Malacrida R, Barazzoni F, et al. Adverse event reporting in adult intensive care units and the impact of a multifaceted intervention on drug-related adverse events. Ann Intensive Care. 2012;2(1):47.
4. Bracco D, Favre JB, Bissonnette B, Wasserfallen JB, Revelly JP, Ravussin P, et al. Human errors in a multidisciplinary intensive care unit: a 1-year prospective study. Intensive Care Med. 2001;27(1):137–45.
5. Osmon S, Harris CB, Dunagan WC, Prentice D, Fraser VJ, Kollef MH. Reporting of medical errors: an intensive care unit experience. Crit Care Med. 2004;32(3):727–33.
6. Sauro KM, Machan M, Whalen-Browne L, Owen V, Wu G, Stelfox HT. Evolving factors in hospital safety: a systematic review and meta-analysis of hospital adverse events. J Patient Saf. 2021;17(8):e1285–95.
7. Rothschild JM, Landrigan CP, Cronin JW, Kaushal R, Lockley SW, Burdick E, et al. The critical care safety study: the incidence and nature of adverse events and serious medical errors in intensive care. Crit Care Med. 2005;33(8):1694–700.
8. Sauro KM, Soo A, Quan H, Stelfox HT. Adverse events among hospitalized critically ill patients: a retrospective cohort study. Med Care. 2020;58(1):38–44.
9. Harris CB, Krauss MJ, Coopersmith CM, Avidan M, Nast PA, Kollef MH, et al. Patient safety event reporting in critical care: a study of three intensive care units. Crit Care Med. 2007;35(4):1068–76.

10. Molina FJ, Rivera PT, Cardona A, Restrepo DC, Monroy O, Rodas D, et al. Adverse events in critical care: search and active detection through the trigger tool. World J Crit Care Med. 2018;7(1):9–15.
11. Sinopoli DJ, Needham DM, Thompson DA, Holzmueller CG, Dorman T, Lubomski LH, et al. Intensive care unit safety incidents for medical versus surgical patients: a prospective multicenter study. J Crit Care. 2007;22(3):177–83.
12. Cantor N, Durr KM, McNeill K, Thompson LH, Fernando SM, Tanuseputro P, et al. Increased mortality and costs associated with adverse events in intensive care unit patients. J Intensive Care Med. 2022;37(8):1075–81.
13. Baker GR. The Canadian adverse events study: the incidence of adverse events among hospital patients in Canada. Can Med Assoc J. 2004;170(11):1678–86.
14. Danielis M, Bellomo F, Farneti F, Palese A. Critical incidents rates and types in Italian intensive care units: a five-year analysis. Intensive Crit Care Nurs. 2021;62:102950.
15. Landrigan CP, Rothschild JM, Cronin JW, Kaushal R, Burdick E, Katz JT, et al. Effect of reducing interns' work hours on serious medical errors in intensive care units. N Engl J Med. 2004;351(18):1838–48.
16. Pronovost PJ, Goeschel CA, Colantuoni E, Watson S, Lubomski LH, Berenholtz SM, et al. Sustaining reductions in catheter related bloodstream infections in Michigan intensive care units: observational study. BMJ. 2010;340:c309.

48 How Effective Are Rapid Response Systems?

48.1 Introduction

Hospitalized patients frequently experience unanticipated deterioration of their clinical status, often leading to adverse clinical outcomes including mortality [1, 2]. A serious adverse event represents an unintended injury that occurs due to delayed or inappropriate management leading to death or disability [3]. A significant number of adverse events in hospitalized patients may be preventable through early recognition of decline in the clinical status and intervention through rescue measures. Failure to rescue represents the inability to prevent clinical deterioration and death, occurring as a result of complications arising from the underlying illness or therapeutic interventions [4]. Adverse events, including cardiac arrests, are commonly preceded by antecedents that are either unnoticed or not addressed in a timely manner [5]. Early recognition of abnormal vital signs may offer a window of opportunity to rescue deteriorating patients from potential complications. Rapid response systems are built around the concept of early recognition of warning signs followed by expeditious intervention. Rapid response teams (RRTs), in contrast to code blue teams, evaluate patients at an early stage of deterioration before cardiac or respiratory arrest occurs. Unexpected clinical worsening usually results from sepsis, respiratory or cardiac failure, hypotension, arrhythmias, or altered conscious level [6].

The Joint Commission in the USA mandates hospitals to introduce rapid response systems to improve patient safety [7]. The American Heart Association (AHA) also recommends establishment of rapid response systems to provide timely care to patients who are at risk of deterioration in general care settings [8].

J. Chacko et al., *Controversies in Critical Care*,
https://doi.org/10.1007/978-981-19-9940-6_48

48.2 Key Components of Rapid Response Systems

The efficacy of rapid response systems depends on three key elements of care, including (1) early identification of patients at risk of deterioration (2), prompt reporting to the responder team, and (3) expeditious intervention by the RRT to enable rescue. Identification and reporting represent the afferent limb, while the RRT intervention represents the efferent limb of the loop of care centered around rapid response systems (Fig. 48.1).

48.2.1 Identification of Patients at Risk of Deterioration

Medical and nursing staff play a crucial role in the timely recognition of early warning signs. The National Patient Safety Agency report in the UK highlighted the failure to recognize clinical deterioration as a key factor that leads to hospital mortality. Nursing workload and a suboptimal nurse to patient ratio may have an adverse impact on the ability to identify patients who develop abnormal vital signs that require prompt action [9].

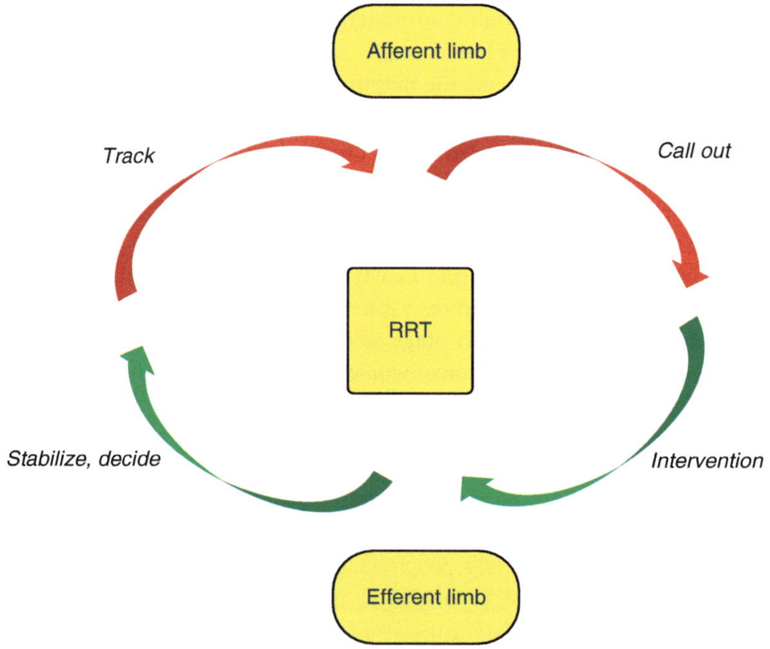

Fig. 48.1 The RRT flow: tracking of patient condition, recognition of early warning signs, and callout constitutes the afferent limb. RRT intervention, stabilization, and decision-making represents the efferent limb

48.2.2 Scoring Systems

Early Warning Systems (EWS) have revealed a high sensitivity in identifying patients who need escalation of care [10]. The National Early Warning Score (NEWS), by the Royal College of Physicians in the UK, is a nursing tool widely used in the identification and escalation of care of patients who may be deteriorating [11]. It consists of six physiological parameters, including the respiratory rate, oxygen saturation, systolic BP, pulse rate, level of consciousness, and temperature. Escalation of care is triggered when the aggregate score is ≥5 or ≥3 for any individual parameter [9]. The Modified Early Warning Score (MEWS), proposed by Stenhouse et al., included urine output as one of the criteria [12]. A retrospective cohort study compared the efficacy of NEWS, MEWS, Systemic Inflammatory Response Syndrome (SIRS), Between the Flags (BTF), and Quick Sequential Sepsis-Related Organ Failure Assessment (qSOFA) as risk assessment tools. The relative performance of these scoring systems was compared through 1.5 million hospitalizations across 28 hospitals in the USA. In this study, NEWS revealed greater discrimination in the identification of patients who were at risk of dying compared to other scoring systems in the overall cohort and in patients suspected to have infection [13].

Most rapid response systems also provide the option for activation based on the clinical judgment of the reporter even if objective criteria based on standard scoring systems are not met. The proviso for judgment-based activation has enabled the identification of patients and situations that may have been missed based on objective callout criteria alone [14].

48.2.3 Reporting: Relay of Information

Abnormal vital signs may be noted by nursing staff, but delays in communication may lead to clinical deterioration before appropriate corrective measures are initiated [14]. Nursing staff may feel reluctant to report worsening of clinical parameters due to fear of criticism or rebuke [15]. A rigid, non-receptive organizational culture may discourage communication, especially among junior-level staff [16]. Furthermore, a fixed, hierarchical escalation process could lead to failure in communication at various levels. Junior-level staff may be dissuaded from reporting due to concerns regarding unfavorable response from senior staff, including fear of intimidation or humiliation [17].

The efficacy of an automated advisory system based on vital parameters was evaluated in a before-after study from the UK [18]. The automated system monitored vital signs and notified ward nurses and RRT members regarding possible clinical deterioration through a paging device. RRT calls increased significantly after the introduction of the automated system. Hospital mortality and the incidence of cardiac arrests reduced significantly during the intervention period. This study suggested that an automated advisory system may lead to improvement in key clinical outcomes including hospital mortality.

48.2.4 Delays in the Activation of Rapid Response Systems

Failure to activate rapid response systems has been associated with adverse clinical outcomes including mortality. In a retrospective observational cohort study, a delay of more than 1 h between the documentation of an abnormal vital parameter and RRT activation led to higher mortality and a longer hospital stay [19]. In another study, the frequency of callouts was lower during night hours and led to a failure to rescue during this vulnerable period [20]. These studies strongly suggest that the timely activation of rapid response systems is crucial in optimizing clinical outcomes.

Although abnormal vital signs are recognized, latency may occur in escalation and initiation of action, leading to adverse outcomes. In up to 84% of patients, physiological deterioration is identified and recorded by caregivers, but timely and appropriate action does not ensue [21, 22]. The ACADEMIA study evaluated the incidence of abnormal physiological parameters that preceded adverse events including ICU admissions, cardiac arrests, and in-hospital deaths across 90 hospitals in the UK, Australia, and New Zealand [23]. Hypotension and altered level of consciousness were the most common antecedents to adverse events. Cardiac arrest occurred in 22.1% of adverse events. Most patients who suffered cardiac arrest (79.4) experienced physiological deterioration before the event; many had abnormal physiological parameters recorded for up to 4 h before the event. A failure to escalate care in the face of worsening physiological parameters was encountered in 14% of cases.

48.2.5 RRT Intervention

Critically ill patients often receive suboptimal care prior to ICU transfer, resulting in adverse clinical outcomes [24]. Rapid response systems aim to act speedily to address a deteriorating clinical situation by providing expertise and healthcare resources at the point of care, to enable a favorable modification of the disease trajectory. Common interventions performed by the RRT include airway management, initiation of ventilator support, fluid resuscitation, and vasopressor support as appropriate.

48.3 Efficacy of Rapid Response Systems: The Evidence

Rapid response systems are expected to intervene early and prevent a downward spiral of the clinical state, thereby improving outcomes. Do they fulfill this objective (Table 48.1)?

The MERIT cluster-randomized controlled trial (RCT) included 125,132 patients from 23 hospitals in Australia [25]. A medical emergency team (MET) was introduced as a rapid response system in 12 hospitals; the existing level of care was maintained in 11 hospitals. The incidence of emergency callouts increased

Table 48.1 Controlled studies that evaluated the impact of introduction of rapid response systems

Study/year	Design	Intervention	Control	Outcomes
Hillman et al. (MERIT, 2005) [25]	Comparative study between hospitals that introduced a MET system with those who continued with usual care	The MET system was introduced in 12 hospitals	11 hospitals continued with usual care	Significant increase in emergency callouts in the MET hospitals during the study period. The composite outcome of cardiac arrest, unexpected mortality, and unplanned ICU admission not different between MET vs. no MET hospitals. Individual components of the primary outcome not different
Priestley et al. (2004) [27]	Pragmatic design; a critical care outreach service was introduced in a phased manner to the acute care wards of an 800-bed hospital	A nurse-led team including critical care physicians offered a 24-h outreach service to acute care wards	Wards that continued with usual care	Hospital mortality reduced significantly in wards where the outreach service was operational
Jung et al. (2016) [28]	Retrospective study. The impact of RRT was compared with hospitals that continued with usual care	Intensivist-led RRT with 24-h coverage was introduced in one hospital	3 hospitals that continued with usual care	RRT establishment was associated with reduction in the unexpected mortality rate compared to control hospitals. Overall hospital mortality was lower after introduction of RRT compared to the pre-RRT period

MET medical emergency team, *RRT* rapid response team

significantly during the study period in hospitals that introduced MET (3·1 vs. 8·7/1000 admissions, $p = 0·0001$). The composite primary outcome including cardiac arrest, unexpected mortality, and unplanned admission to the ICU was not significantly different between hospitals that had MET compared to control hospitals (5·86 vs. 5·31/1000 admissions, $p = 0·640$). The incidence of the individual components of the composite outcome was also similar in both groups of hospitals. However, in the MET group of hospitals, 30% of patients who suffered cardiac arrest had fulfilled the callout criteria for more than 15 min prior to the event. Similarly, no callout was made in half of the instances that resulted in unplanned ICU admission or unexpected mortality. Thus, a substantial number of patients did not actually receive the planned escalation of care through the rapid response system; this could likely explain the lack of benefit observed [26].

Sixteen acute care wards of a UK general hospital were included in a pragmatic, cluster- randomized trial to assess the impact of a critical care outreach service. The outreach unit included nurses and doctors with experience in critical care who offered a 24-h service. The outreach service was introduced in a phased manner across the hospital. This study, including 2903 patients, revealed a significant reduction in hospital mortality in wards where the outreach service was operational compared to those that did not [two-level odds ratio: 0.52 (95% CI 0.32–0.85)]. The hospital length of stay was unexpectedly longer in patients who received outreach service; however, this finding was not supported on confirmatory and sensitivity analysis [27].

A retrospective study from France evaluated the impact of RRT implementation in one hospital and compared outcomes with three hospitals that acted as controls. The establishment of an RRT was associated with a significant reduction in the unexpected mortality rate compared to the three control hospitals (17.4 vs. 21.9/1000 discharges; $p = 0.002$). Besides, the overall hospital mortality also decreased significantly after RRT implementation compared to the pre-RRT period [28].

Tirkonnen et al. evaluated outcomes following RRT intervention. This systematic review of 29 studies that analyzed 157,383 activations revealed that RRT review may enable decision-making regarding limitation of care. Limitation of care occurred in 8.1% of RRT callouts, while 23% led to ICU transfer. The median hospital mortality following RRT intervention was 26% with a 30-day mortality of 29% [29].

Several meta-analyses have evaluated the efficacy of rapid response systems. Maharaj et al. analyzed 29 cluster RCTs or before-after studies. Implementation of rapid response systems was associated with an overall reduction in hospital mortality. A significant reduction in cardiopulmonary arrests was also observed. However, there was no difference in the number of ICU admissions [30]. Solomon et al. included 30 before-after studies, cluster-randomized trials, or cohort studies in their meta-analysis. The introduction of an RRT or MET was associated with significantly lower hospital mortality and cardiac arrests outside the ICU [31].

Key Points

- Hospitalized patients often experience unexpected deterioration in their clinical status, leading to adverse outcomes, including mortality.
- Rapid response systems act as safety nets aimed at the early identification of patients who are at risk of deterioration. They provide clinical expertise and timely intervention at the point of care.
- The key components of rapid response systems include early identification of patients with a declining clinical status and prompt activation of the responder team followed by appropriate intervention by the RRT to enable rescue.

- The large, MERIT cluster randomized controlled trial did not reveal a significant impact on cardiac arrests, unexpected mortality, or unplanned admission to the ICU; however, rapid response activation was not performed in a relatively large number of patients who experienced clinical deterioration.
- Several observational studies and meta-analyses lend support to the establishment of rapid response systems with improved clinical outcomes including a reduction in hospital mortality.
- Rapid response systems may also facilitate decision-making regarding end-of-life care in patients who are terminally ill.

References

1. Schimmel EM. The hazards of hospitalization. Ann Intern Med. 1964;60:100–10.
2. Thomas EJ, Studdert DM, Burstin HR, Orav EJ, Zeena T, Williams EJ, et al. Incidence and types of adverse events and negligent care in Utah and Colorado. Med Care. 2000;38(3):261–71.
3. Brennan TA, Localio AR, Leape LL, Laird NM, Peterson L, Hiatt HH, et al. Identification of adverse events occurring during hospitalization. A cross-sectional study of litigation, quality assurance, and medical records at two teaching hospitals. Ann Intern Med. 1990;112(3):221–6.
4. Silber JH, Williams SV, Krakauer H, Schwartz JS. Hospital and patient characteristics associated with death after surgery. A study of adverse occurrence and failure to rescue. Med Care. 1992;30(7):615–29.
5. Andersen LW, Kim WY, Chase M, Berg KM, Mortensen SJ, Moskowitz A, et al. The prevalence and significance of abnormal vital signs prior to in-hospital cardiac arrest. Resuscitation. 2016;98:112–7.
6. Jones D, Duke G, Green J, Briedis J, Bellomo R, Casamento A, et al. Medical emergency team syndromes and an approach to their management. Crit Care. 2006;10(1):R30.
7. Steel AC, Reynolds SF. The growth of rapid response systems. Jt Comm J Qual Patient Saf. 2008;34(8):489–95.
8. Kronick SL, Kurz MC, Lin S, Edelson DP, Berg RA, Billi JE, et al. Part 4: Systems of care and continuous quality improvement: 2015 American heart association guidelines update for cardiopulmonary resuscitation and emergency cardiovascular care. Circulation. 2015;132(18 Suppl 2):S397–413.
9. Aiken LH, Cimiotti JP, Sloane DM, Smith HL, Flynn L, Neff DF. Effects of nurse staffing and nurse education on patient deaths in hospitals with different nurse work environments. Med Care. 2011;49(12):1047–53.
10. Gardner-Thorpe J, Love N, Wrightson J, Walsh S, Keeling N. The value of modified early warning score (MEWS) in surgical in-patients: a prospective observational study. Ann R Coll Surg Engl. 2006;88(6):571–5.
11. National Early Warning Score (NEWS) 2 [Internet]. RCP London. 2017. https://www.rcplondon.ac.uk/projects/outputs/national-early-warning-score-news-2. Accessed 25 May 2022.
12. Stenhouse C, Coates S, Tivey M, Allsop P, Parker T. Prospective evaluation of a modified early warning score to aid earlier detection of patients developing critical illness on a general surgical ward. Br J Anaesth. 2000;84(5):663P.
13. Liu VX, Lu Y, Carey KA, Gilbert ER, Afshar M, Akel M, et al. Comparison of early warning scoring systems for hospitalized patients with and without infection at risk for in-hospital mortality and transfer to the intensive care unit. JAMA Netw Open. 2020;3(5):e205191.

14. Parr MJ, Hadfield JH, Flabouris A, Bishop G, Hillman K. The medical emergency team: 12 month analysis of reasons for activation, immediate outcome and not-for-resuscitation orders. Resuscitation. 2001;50(1):39–44.
15. Burke JR, Downey C, Almoudaris AM. Failure to rescue deteriorating patients: a systematic review of root causes and improvement strategies. J Patient Saf. 2022;18(1):e140–55.
16. Brinkert R. A literature review of conflict communication causes, costs, benefits and interventions in nursing. J Nurs Manag. 2010;18(2):145–56.
17. Johnston M, Arora S, King D, Stroman L, Darzi A. Escalation of care and failure to rescue: a multicenter, multiprofessional qualitative study. Surgery. 2014;155(6):989–94.
18. Subbe CP, Duller B, Bellomo R. Effect of an automated notification system for deteriorating ward patients on clinical outcomes. Crit Care. 2017;21(1):52.
19. Barwise A, Thongprayoon C, Gajic O, Jensen J, Herasevich V, Pickering BW. Delayed rapid response team activation is associated with increased hospital mortality, morbidity, and length of stay in a tertiary care institution. Crit Care Med. 2016;44(1):54–63.
20. Churpek MM, Edelson DP, Lee JY, Carey K, Snyder A. American heart association's get with the guidelines-resuscitation investigators. Association between survival and time of day for rapid response team calls in a national registry. Crit Care Med. 2017;45(10):1677–82.
21. Franklin C, Mathew J. Developing strategies to prevent inhospital cardiac arrest: analyzing responses of physicians and nurses in the hours before the event. Crit Care Med. 1994;22(2):244–7.
22. Schein RM, Hazday N, Pena M, Ruben BH, Sprung CL. Clinical antecedents to in-hospital cardiopulmonary arrest. Chest. 1990;98(6):1388–92.
23. Kause J, Smith G, Prytherch D, Parr M, Flabouris A, Hillman K. A comparison of antecedents to cardiac arrests, deaths and emergency intensive care admissions in Australia and New Zealand, and the United Kingdom—the ACADEMIA study. Resuscitation. 2004;62(3):275–82.
24. McQuillan P, Pilkington S, Allan A, Taylor B, Short A, Morgan G, et al. Confidential inquiry into quality of care before admission to intensive care. BMJ. 1998;316(7148):1853–8.
25. Hillman K, Chen J, Cretikos M, Bellomo R, Brown D, Doig G, et al. Introduction of the medical emergency team (MET) system: a cluster-randomised controlled trial. Lancet. 2005;365(9477):2091–7.
26. Buist M, Harrison J, Abaloz E, Van Dyke S. Six year audit of cardiac arrests and medical emergency team calls in an Australian outer metropolitan teaching hospital. BMJ. 2007;335(7631):1210–2.
27. Priestley G, Watson W, Rashidian A, Mozley C, Russell D, Wilson J, et al. Introducing critical care outreach: a ward-randomised trial of phased introduction in a general hospital. Intensive Care Med. 2004;30(7):1398–404.
28. Jung B, Daurat A, De Jong A, Chanques G, Mahul M, Monnin M, et al. Rapid response team and hospital mortality in hospitalized patients. Intensive Care Med. 2016;42(4):494–504.
29. Tirkkonen J, Tamminen T, Skrifvars MB. Outcome of adult patients attended by rapid response teams: a systematic review of the literature. Resuscitation. 2017;112:43–52.
30. Maharaj R, Raffaele I, Wendon J. Rapid response systems: a systematic review and meta-analysis. Crit Care. 2015;19:254.
31. Solomon RS, Corwin GS, Barclay DC, Quddusi SF, Dannenberg MD. Effectiveness of rapid response teams on rates of in-hospital cardiopulmonary arrest and mortality: a systematic review and meta-analysis: rapid response team meta-analysis. J Hosp Med. 2016;11(6):438–45.

Part IX

Coagulopathy and Transfusion

Transfusion Thresholds in Non-Bleeding Critically Ill Patients

49

More than two centuries ago, James Blundell, a British obstetrician, performed the first successful human-to-human transfusion in a lady who had developed severe postpartum hemorrhage. Mr. Waller, a surgical colleague, had sought his assistance for the patient who was on the verge of death, "lying on her back, pale as a sheet, with no apparent respiration…" Using a syringe, Blundell drew four ounces of blood from the husband and transfused it to his wife, saving her life [1]. He proceeded with this novel intervention in several patients over the next decade and suggested rational indications for blood transfusion.

Anemia is all too common among critically ill patients, with 30–50% of patients receiving red cell transfusion [2]. The etiology of anemia in the ICU is multifactorial, contributed to by intravenous fluid resuscitation with the resulting hemodilution, repeated blood sampling, low erythropoietin levels induced by inflammatory cytokines, and abnormalities of iron metabolism. A hemoglobin level of 10 g/dL was proposed by Adam and Lundy among surgical patients in 1942 [3]; they averred that "when the concentration of hemoglobin is less than 8 to 10 g per 100 cm^3 of whole blood, it is wise to give a blood transfusion before operation." The 10/30 rule was embraced wholeheartedly by clinicians for decades before evidence emerged supporting lower thresholds in most clinical situations, particularly among critically ill patients.

J. Chacko et al., *Controversies in Critical Care*,
https://doi.org/10.1007/978-981-19-9940-6_49

49.1 Red Cell Transfusion and Oxygen Delivery

Oxygen delivered per minute is the product of the cardiac output and the arterial oxygen content.

$$\text{Oxygen delivery} = \text{cardiac output} \times \left[\left(1.39 \times \text{hemoglobin} \times SaO_2\right) + \left(PaO_2 \times 0.003\right)\right]$$

According to this equation, a rise in hemoglobin concentration increases oxygen delivery. However, the interplay of several other factors impedes oxygen delivery following the transfusion of stored blood. Nitric oxide levels diminish over time with storage, leading to vasoconstriction and reduction in blood flow. The 2,3 diphosphoglycerate levels also decrease during storage, shifting the oxygen-dissociation curve to the left, leading to impaired oxygen delivery at the tissue level. Furthermore, transfused red cells may lead to platelet activation and aggregation that may predispose to the occlusion of blood vessels [4].

In the past two decades, a restrictive transfusion strategy has gained ground, with the Transfusion Requirements in Critical Care (TRICC) trial by the Canadian Critical Care Trials group being the harbinger of change [5]. However, does one size fit all, or do we need to tailor transfusion strategy among specific patient populations (Table 49.1)?

Table 49.1 Important studies that evaluate transfusion thresholds in critically ill patients

Study/year	Population	Restrictive strategy	Liberal strategy	Outcomes
General ICU patients				
Hébert et al. (TRICC, 1999) [5]	General ICU patients	Transfusion if Hb ≤ 7 g/dL; aim for Hb between 7.0 and 9.0 g/dL	Transfusion if Hb ≤ 9.0 g/dL; aim for Hb between 10 and 12 g/dL	Overall trend toward reduced 30- and 60-day mortality with a restrictive strategy; effect most pronounced when APACHE II score ≤20 and age ≤55 years
Sepsis				
Holst et al. (TRISS, 2014) [6]	Septic shock, with Hb ≤9 g/dL	Transfusion if Hb ≤ 7 g/dL	Transfusion if Hb ≤ 9 g/dL	90-day mortality similar. No difference in ischemic events, use of life support between groups
Bergamin et al. (TRICOP, 2017) [7]	Adult cancer patients with septic shock	Transfusion if Hb ≤ 7 g/dL	Transfusion if Hb ≤ 9 g/dL	28-day mortality similar. Requirement for mechanical ventilation, inotropic support, and renal replacement therapy similar. ICU and hospital LOS similar duration. 90-day mortality was lower with a liberal strategy (secondary outcome, not powered)

Table 49.1 (continued)

Study/year	Population	Restrictive strategy	Liberal strategy	Outcomes
Cardiac surgical				
Hajjar et al. (TRACS, 2010) [10]	Adults undergoing cardiac surgery	Transfusion if Hb ≤ 8 g/dL	Transfusion if Hb ≤ 10 g/dL	Composite primary outcome including the 30-day all-cause mortality, cardiogenic shock, ARDS, and AKI requiring RRT similar. Number of red cell units transfused was an independent predictor of death or the development of complications at 30 days
Murphy et al. (TITRe, 2015) [11]	Elective cardiac surgery	Transfusion if Hb ≤ 7.5 g/dL	Transfusion if Hb ≤ 9 g/dL	No difference in the composite primary outcome of serious infection or an ischemic event, including myocardial infarction, bowel ischemia, or AKI, within 3 months of randomization. Higher overall mortality with restrictive strategy
Mazer et al. (TRICS III, 2017) [12]	Cardiac surgery, EUROSCORE 1 ≥ 6	Transfusion if Hb ≤ 7.5 g/dL	Transfusion if Hb ≤ 9 g/dL	No difference in the composite primary outcome of death, MI, stroke, AKI requiring RRT at hospital discharge or by day 28 (whichever was earlier)
Acute coronary syndrome				
Ducrocq et al. (REALITY, 2021) [15]	Acute MI, Hb level 7–10 g/dL	Transfusion if Hb ≤ 8 g/dL	Transfusion if Hb ≤ 10 g/dL	MACE at 30 days similar. All-cause mortality, recurrent MI, requirement for emergency revascularization, acute stroke, similar
Weaning from mechanical ventilation				
Hébert et al. (2001) [17]	Patients who underwent mechanical ventilation in the TRICC trial	Transfusion if Hb ≤ 7 g/dL; aim for Hb between 7.0 and 9.0 g/dL	Transfusion if Hb ≤ 9.0 g/dL; aim for Hb between 10 and 12 g/dL	Mean duration of ventilation, ventilator-free days, extubation success similar. Results similar with prolonged ventilation >7 days

(continued)

Table 49.1 (continued)

Study/year	Population	Restrictive strategy	Liberal strategy	Outcomes
Walsh et al. (2013) [18]	Patients undergoing mechanical ventilation ≥4 days	Transfusion if Hb ≤ 7 g/dL; aim for Hb between 7.1 and 9.0 g/dL	Transfusion if Hb ≤ 9 g/dL; aim for Hb between 9.1 and 11.0 g/dL	Trend toward lower 180-day mortality with the restrictive strategy. Similar trend after adjustment for age, gender, presence of IHD, APACHE II score, non-neurological SOFA score
Acute neurological injury				
McIntyre et al. (2006) [20]	Patients with moderate to severe TBI in the TRICC trial	Transfusion if Hb ≤ 7 g/dL; aim for Hb between 7.0 and 9.0 g/dL	Transfusion if Hb ≤ 9.0 g/dL; aim for Hb between 10 and 12 g/dL	30-day all-cause mortality, multiorgan dysfunction, median ICU and hospital LOS similar
Robertson et al. (2014) [21]	Severe TBI	Transfusion threshold of 7 g/dL	Transfusion threshold of 10 g/dL	Neither IV erythropoietin nor higher transfusion threshold resulted in improved neurological outcomes at 6 months

APACHE acute physiology and chronic health evaluation, *LOS* length of stay, *ARDS* acute respiratory distress syndrome, *AKI* acute kidney injury, *RRT* renal replacement therapy, *MI* myocardial infarction, *MACE* major adverse cardiovascular events, *IHD* ischemic heart disease, *TBI* traumatic brain injury, *SOFA* sequential organ failure assessment

49.2 TRICC: The Landmark Trial

The TRICC trial compared a restrictive to a liberal transfusion strategy in critically ill patients. In this multicenter study conducted by the Canadian Critical Care Trials Group, 838 critically ill patients were randomized to a restrictive or a liberal red cell transfusion strategy [5]. In the restrictive strategy group, red cells were transfused if the Hb level dropped below 7 g/dL and maintained between 7 and 9 g/dL. In the liberal group, red cells were transfused if Hb dropped below 10 g/dL and maintained between 10 and 12 g/dL. The 30-day mortality, the primary outcome, was similar between the two groups. The hospital mortality was significantly lower in the restrictive group. Furthermore, on subgroup analysis, younger patients, less than 55 years old, and patients with an APACHE II score ≤ 20 had significantly lower mortality with restrictive transfusion. This landmark trial suggested that in general critically ill patients, a transfusion trigger of 7 g/dL may be appropriate, except for patients with acute myocardial infarction and unstable angina, who may need a higher transfusion trigger.

49.3 Restrictive Vs. Liberal Transfusion Strategy in Septic Shock

Anemia in critically ill patients may be associated with heart failure, poor physiological reserve, and reduced oxygen-carrying capacity due to low Hb levels. Anemia may worsen sepsis-induced cardiac dysfunction and lower the oxygen carrying-capacity further, leading to worsening of septic shock. Would a lower transfusion threshold be appropriate in patients with septic shock?

The TRISS trial randomized 988 patients with septic shock across 32 ICUs in Norway, Sweden, Denmark, and Finland to a restrictive or liberal transfusion strategy [6]. Leuco-reduced red cells were transfused if the Hb level dropped below 7 g/dL in the restrictive and 9 g/dL in liberal group. The most common source of infection was respiratory, followed by intra-abdominal, urinary, and soft tissue infection. Patients in the restrictive group received a median of one unit (IQR 0–3) of red cells, while the liberal group received four (IQR 2–7). The 90-day mortality was similar between the two groups. Besides, the incidence of ischemic events, defined as acute myocardial, cerebral, intestinal, and limb ischemia, was similar. Severe adverse reactions and the requirement for life support, including mechanical ventilation, vasopressor support, or renal replacement therapy, were not significantly different between groups. Patients with acute coronary syndrome were not included in the study. This study established the safety of a restrictive transfusion strategy in patients with septic shock.

The TRICOP trial was a single-center RCT that randomized 300 oncology patients with septic shock to a restrictive or a liberal transfusion strategy [7]. A transfusion trigger of 7 g/dL was followed in the restrictive and 9 g/dL in the liberal group. The median number of units of red cells transfused was 0 (IQR 0–2) in the restrictive compared with 1 (IQR 0–3) in the liberal group. There was no significant difference in the 28-day mortality between the two groups. Among the secondary outcomes, the requirement for mechanical ventilation, inotropic support, and renal replacement therapy was similar in both groups. The length of ICU and hospital stay were also similar. However, the 90-day mortality was lower with a liberal strategy. The TRICOP study suggested a trend toward possible benefit of a liberal strategy in oncology patients with septic shock. The study was powered based on a mortality difference of 16% on the 28-day mortality, the primary outcome. However, the mortality difference at 90 days was only 11.6%; although the difference was statistically significant, the validity of this finding needs to be corroborated in adequately powered trials.

49.4 Cardiac Surgical Patients and Transfusion Thresholds

The consumption of blood products, including red cells, may often border on profligacy in cardiac surgical patients. Indeed, cardiac surgical patients are among the highest consumers of blood products [8]. Correction of anemia makes physiological sense, and a sense of satisfaction follows among caregivers as the numbers rise. A retrospective study revealed that the transfusion rate following coronary artery bypass grafting was between 43–54% and 54–67% after valve surgery. In combined CABG and valve surgery, the transfusion rate was 80–88% [9]. Would a restrictive approach be safe and effective in patients who undergo cardiac surgery?

The TRACS trial was a single-center RCT from Brazil, including 502 patients who underwent cardiac surgery under cardiopulmonary bypass. Patients were randomized to a restrictive transfusion strategy aiming for a hematocrit ≥24% compared with ≥30% in the liberal group [10]. The composite primary outcome, including the 30-day all-cause mortality, cardiogenic shock, acute respiratory distress syndrome, and acute kidney injury requiring renal replacement therapy, was similar between the two groups. Furthermore, the number of red cell units transfused was an independent predictor of death or the development of clinical complications at 30 days in both groups of patients.

A multicenter RCT evaluated patients undergoing elective cardiac surgery in 17 centers in the UK. Patients with a postoperative Hb level of less than 9 g/dL were randomized to a restrictive transfusion threshold of <7.5 g/dL compared to a liberal threshold of <9 g/dL. In the liberal group, 92.2% of patients received red cell transfusion compared with 53.4% in the restrictive group. The primary outcome was a composite of a serious infection or an ischemic event, including myocardial infarction, bowel ischemia, or acute kidney injury, within 3 months of randomization. There was no significant difference between the two groups in the primary outcome. The overall mortality was low and higher with a restrictive compared to a liberal strategy. However, mortality was only a secondary endpoint and could not be explained on the basis of postoperative complications [11].

Different transfusion thresholds were compared among patients undergoing cardiac surgery in the TRICS III RCT. In the restrictive threshold arm, the red cell transfusion threshold was <7.5 g/dL. The liberal group had two thresholds depending on patient location: <9.5 g/dL in the theater or ICU and <8.5 g/dL in the ward. The transfusion strategy was followed starting from induction of anesthesia. Red cells were transfused in 52.3% of patients in the restrictive compared with 72.6% in the liberal arm. The primary composite outcome included all-cause mortality, acute myocardial infarction, stroke, or acute kidney injury requiring dialysis at hospital discharge or by day 28, whichever occurred earlier. The primary outcome occurred in 11.4% of patients in the restrictive arm, compared with 12.5% in the liberal arm, establishing the non-inferiority of a restrictive strategy. There was no significant difference in mortality between the two groups [12].

49.5 Transfusion Strategy in Acute Coronary Syndrome

Anemia may jeopardize the ischemic myocardium due to impaired oxygen-carrying capacity. Patients with acute myocardial infarction are often anemic, and a higher Hb level is often targeted to optimize oxygen delivery in this population. Previous studies with varying Hb thresholds as transfusion triggers have yielded conflicting results. In the CRIT trial, 45 patients with acute myocardial infarction were randomized to a threshold hematocrit of 30% to maintain a range between 30 and 33% in the liberal group. In the restrictive group, the transfusion threshold was a hematocrit of 24%, and the target ranges between 24 and 27%. In this pilot study of a small sample size, the composite outcome of death in hospital, recurrent myocardial infarction, or new-onset or worsening heart failure occurred more often with a liberal compared to a restrictive transfusion strategy [13]. However, in another underpowered randomized controlled trial, a liberal transfusion strategy (Hb >10 g/dL) revealed a trend toward fewer major cardiac events and mortality compared to a restrictive strategy with red cell transfusion below a threshold of 8 g/dL [14].

Against the background of uncertainty regarding different transfusion thresholds, the REALITY trial randomized 668 patients with acute myocardial infarction and Hb levels between 7 and 10 g/dL in an RCT. The restrictive transfusion strategy used a transfusion trigger of Hb ≤8 g/dL; the liberal strategy followed a trigger of Hb ≤10 g/dL. The primary outcome studied was major adverse cardiovascular events at 30 days (MACE: a composite of all-cause mortality, acute stroke, recurrent myocardial infarction, or ischemia requiring emergency revascularization). In the liberal arm, 99.7% of patients were transfused compared to 35.7% in the restrictive arm. MACE occurred in 11% of patients in the restrictive compared with 14% of patients in the liberal group. All-cause mortality, recurrent myocardial infarction, the requirement for emergency revascularization, and acute ischemic stroke were similar in both groups. This study demonstrated the non-inferiority of a transfusion trigger of Hb ≤8 mg/dL in patients with acute myocardial infarction and anemia, compared to a higher trigger of ≤10 g/dL [15]. Adverse events were uncommon; transfusion-associated acute lung injury occurred in seven patients in the liberal arm compared to one patient in the restrictive arm. Although underpowered to demonstrate superiority, the REALITY trial strongly suggests that MACE events are comparable between a restrictive and a liberal transfusion strategy in patients with acute myocardial infarction.

49.6 Restrictive Versus Liberal Transfusion Practices for Weaning from Mechanical Ventilation

Among mechanically ventilated patients, 7–14% undergo a process of slow, prolonged weaning [16]; nearly all develop anemia, and many undergo red cell transfusion. Anemia may adversely impact the weaning process; transfusion of red cells and improved oxygen delivery may potentially reduce respiratory workload during spontaneous breathing trials and facilitate liberation from mechanical ventilation. Would aiming for a higher target Hb enable more rapid weaning and liberation from mechanical ventilation?

Hébert et al. analyzed 713 patients who required invasive mechanical ventilation from the TRICC trial. The liberal transfusion group used a trigger of 10 g/dL with the maintenance of Hb levels between 10 and 12 g/dL; the restrictive strategy aimed to maintain Hb levels between 7 and 9 g/dL with a transfusion trigger of 7 g/dL. The baseline characteristics were similar between patients who were transfused at the two different transfusion thresholds. The mean duration of mechanical ventilation and ventilator-free days were similar between the two groups. Extubation success was also similar; after adjusting for confounding variables, including age, the APACHE II score, and comorbidities, the relative risk of extubation success with a restrictive strategy was 1.07 (95% CI, 0.96–1.26; $p = 0.43$); the results were similar among patients who received mechanical ventilation for >7 days. This study clearly demonstrated that neither the duration of mechanical ventilation nor successful extubation was related to a liberal compared with a restrictive transfusion strategy [17].

A pilot study evaluated 100 patients aged 55 years or more, on mechanical ventilation for at least 4 days across six ICUs in the UK [18]. The transfusion trigger in the restrictive group was ≤7 g/dL with the maintenance of Hb levels between 7.1 and 9.0 g/dL; in the liberal group, the transfusion trigger was 9 g/dL aimed to maintain the Hb level between 9.1 and 11.0 g/dL. The target Hb level was maintained for the duration of ICU stay, or 14 days, whichever was longer. The restrictive strategy group was associated with a trend toward lower 180-day mortality. A similar trend was observed on post hoc analysis after adjustment for age, gender, presence of ischemic heart disease, the APACHE II score, and non-neurological SOFA scores.

A retrospective, observational study evaluated tracheostomized patients on prolonged mechanical ventilation admitted to a weaning center. Ninety-eight percent of patients were anemic on admission. Red cell transfusion was an independent predictor of prolonged weaning and prolongation of hospital stay. Furthermore, there was a trend toward increased hospital mortality among patients who received red cell transfusion [19].

49.7 Transfusion Strategy in Neuro-Intensive Care

Considering the physiological plausibility of the injured brain being more vulnerable to hypoxic insults, red cell transfusions are often considered important in patients with acute neurological injury.

A subgroup analysis of the TRICC trial included 67 critically ill patients with moderate to severe traumatic brain injury (TBI). The 30-day all-cause mortality, multiorgan dysfunction, and median duration of ICU and hospital stay were similar between the restrictive and liberal transfusion strategies [20]. Robertson et al. compared the efficacy of intravenous erythropoietin and transfusion thresholds of 7 and 10 g/dL in patients with severe TBI in an RCT. Neither intravenous erythropoietin nor maintaining a Hb level of >10 g/dL led to improvement in neurological outcomes at 6 months [21]. A feasibility study of 44 patients compared a transfusion threshold of 7 vs. 9 g/dL in patients with moderate to severe TBI. The incidence of post-TBI vasospasm was less with a liberal strategy, as evidenced by lower flow velocities in the middle cerebral artery. Although not powered for clinical outcomes, hospital mortality was higher in the restrictive arm in this study [22].

Currently, there are three major RCTs underway on this topic including the TRAIN [23], HEMOTION, [24], and the SAHARA [25] trials.

Key Points

- Anemia is common among critically ill patients. Transfusion of red cells is often resorted to with the aim of augmenting oxygen delivery to the tissues. However, a complex interplay of several factors hinders a proportional rise in oxygen delivery. Paradoxically, both anemia and red cell transfusion may be associated with organ dysfunction and adverse outcomes.
- Historically, physicians have often followed tradition-bound transfusion thresholds; the TRICC trial heralded a trigger for change in transfusion thresholds in critically ill patients.
- A higher Hb target has often been targeted in septic patients; however, oxygen delivery is usually well-maintained in sepsis. A transfusion threshold of 7 g/dL has been shown to be as effective compared to a more liberal transfusion strategy.
- Cardiac surgical patients often undergo red cell transfusion to attain higher target Hb levels; however, three RCTs clearly establish that a Hb threshold of 7.5–8 compared to 9–10 does not lead to adverse clinical outcomes.
- Considering the possibility of compromised myocardial oxygen delivery, higher levels of Hb has often been targeted in patients with acute myocardial infarction. However, the large REALITY trial suggested that a restrictive threshold of 8 g/dL is at least equally safe compared with a higher threshold of 10 g/dL.
- The available evidence suggests that higher transfusion thresholds are unnecessary in patients who require prolonged weaning from mechanical ventilation.
- Adequately powered, controlled trials comparing transfusion thresholds are conspicuously absent among patients with neurological injury. In TBI, a transfusion threshold of 7 g/dL seems appropriate under most clinical circumstances.

References

1. Waller C. Case of uterine hemorrhage, in which the operation of transfusion was successfully performed. Lond Med Phys J. 1825;54(320):273–7.
2. Napolitano LM. Anemia and red blood cell transfusion. Crit Care Clin. 2017;33(2):345–64.
3. Adams RC, Lundy JS. Anesthesia in cases of poor surgical risk: some suggestions for decreasing the risk. Anesthesiology. 1942;3(5):603–7.
4. Silvain J, Pena A, Cayla G, Brieger D, Bellemain-Appaix A, Chastre T, et al. Impact of red blood cell transfusion on platelet activation and aggregation in healthy volunteers: results of the TRANSFUSION study. Eur Heart J. 2010;31(22):2816–21.
5. Hébert PC, Wells G, Blajchman MA, Marshall J, Martin C, Pagliarello G, et al. A multicenter, randomized, controlled clinical trial of transfusion requirements in critical care. N Engl J Med. 1999;340(6):409–17.

6. Holst LB, Haase N, Wetterslev J, Wernerman J, Guttormsen AB, Karlsson S, et al. Lower versus higher hemoglobin threshold for transfusion in septic shock. N Engl J Med. 2014;371(15):1381–91.
7. Bergamin FS, Almeida JP, Landoni G, Galas FRBG, Fukushima JT, Fominskiy E, et al. Liberal versus restrictive transfusion strategy in critically ill oncologic patients: the transfusion requirements in critically ill oncologic patients randomized controlled trial. Crit Care Med. 2017;45(5):766–73.
8. Huang D, Chen C, Ming Y, Liu J, Zhou L, Zhang F, et al. Risk of massive blood product requirement in cardiac surgery: a large retrospective study from 2 heart centers. Medicine (Baltimore). 2019;98(5):e14219.
9. Brouwers C, Hooftman B, Vonk S, Vonk A, Stooker W, te Gussinklo WH, et al. Benchmarking the use of blood products in cardiac surgery to stimulate awareness of transfusion behaviour. Neth Heart J. 2017;25(3):207–14.
10. Hajjar LA, Vincent JL, Galas FRBG, Nakamura RE, Silva CMP, Santos MH, et al. Transfusion requirements after cardiac surgery: the TRACS randomized controlled trial. JAMA. 2010;304(14):1559.
11. Murphy GJ, Pike K, Rogers CA, Wordsworth S, Stokes EA, Angelini GD, et al. Liberal or restrictive transfusion after cardiac surgery. N Engl J Med. 2015;372(11):997–1008.
12. Mazer CD, Whitlock RP, Fergusson DA, Hall J, Belley-Cote E, Connolly K, et al. Restrictive or liberal red-cell transfusion for cardiac surgery. N Engl J Med. 2017;377(22):2133–44.
13. Cooper HA, Rao SV, Greenberg MD, Rumsey MP, McKenzie M, Alcorn KW, et al. Conservative versus liberal red cell transfusion in acute myocardial infarction (the CRIT randomized pilot study). Am J Cardiol. 2011;108(8):1108–11.
14. Carson JL, Brooks MM, Abbott JD, Chaitman B, Kelsey SF, Triulzi DJ, et al. Liberal versus restrictive transfusion thresholds for patients with symptomatic coronary artery disease. Am Heart J. 2013;165(6):964–971.e1.
15. Ducrocq G, Gonzalez-Juanatey JR, Puymirat E, Lemesle G, Cachanado M, Durand-Zaleski I, et al. Effect of a restrictive vs liberal blood transfusion strategy on major cardiovascular events among patients with acute myocardial infarction and anemia: the REALITY randomized clinical trial. JAMA. 2021;325(6):552–60.
16. Funk GC, Anders S, Breyer MK, Burghuber OC, Edelmann G, Heindl W, et al. Incidence and outcome of weaning from mechanical ventilation according to new categories. Eur Respir J. 2010;35(1):88–94.
17. Hébert PC, Blajchman MA, Cook DJ, Yetisir E, Wells G, Marshall J, et al. Do blood transfusions improve outcomes related to mechanical ventilation? Chest. 2001;119(6):1850–7.
18. Walsh TS, Boyd JA, Watson D, Hope D, Lewis S, Krishan A, et al. Restrictive versus liberal transfusion strategies for older mechanically ventilated critically ill patients: a randomized pilot trial. Crit Care Med. 2013;41(10):2354–63.
19. Ghiani A, Sainis A, Sainis G, Neurohr C. Anemia and red blood cell transfusion practice in prolonged mechanically ventilated patients admitted to a specialized weaning center: an observational study. BMC Pulm Med. 2019;19:250.
20. McIntyre LA, Fergusson DA, Hutchison JS, Pagliarello G, Marshall JC, Yetisir E, et al. Effect of a liberal versus restrictive transfusion strategy on mortality in patients with moderate to severe head injury. Neurocrit Care. 2006;5(1):4–9.
21. Robertson CS, Hannay HJ, Yamal JM, Gopinath S, Goodman JC, Tilley BC, et al. Effect of erythropoietin and transfusion threshold on neurological recovery after traumatic brain injury: a randomized clinical trial. JAMA. 2014;312(1):36–47.
22. Gobatto ALN, Link MA, Solla DJ, Bassi E, Tierno PF, Paiva W, et al. Transfusion requirements after head trauma: a randomized feasibility controlled trial. Crit Care. 2019;23(1):89.
23. Taccone F. Transfusion strategies in acute brain injured patients. A prospective multicenter randomized study. [Internet]. clinicaltrials.gov; 2021. Report No.: NCT02968654. https://clinicaltrials.gov/ct2/show/NCT02968654. Accessed 1 Sep 2022.

24. Turgeon DA. HEMOglobin transfusion threshold in traumatic brain injury optimization: the HEMOTION trial [Internet]. clinicaltrials.gov; 2022. Report No.: NCT03260478. https://clinicaltrials.gov/ct2/show/NCT03260478. Accessed 1 Sep 2022.
25. Ottawa Hospital Research Institute. Aneurysmal subarachnoid hemorrhage—red blood cell transfusion and outcome (SAHaRA): a randomized controlled trial [Internet]. clinicaltrials.gov; 2021. Report No.: NCT03309579. https://clinicaltrials.gov/ct2/show/NCT03309579. Accessed 1 Sep 2022.

Tranexamic Acid in the Bleeding Patient 50

50.1 Introduction

Tranexamic acid is an antifibrinolytic agent used to prevent or treat life-threatening hemorrhage [1]. In the early 1960s, Utako Okamoto, and her husband Shosuke Okamoto, working from their laboratory in Tokyo, Japan, discovered this novel drug that seemed to be magically effective in reducing bleeding. Initially used to treat heavy menstrual blood loss, tranexamic acid use became more widespread later, especially during elective surgery. Over the years, clinical use has extended to wider subgroups of bleeding patients, including trauma, intracerebral hemorrhage, and postpartum hemorrhage.

50.2 Pharmacology and Mechanism of Action

During the fibrinolytic process, plasminogen, through its lysine binding sites, binds to fibrin. The plasminogen-fibrin complex is cleaved by tissue plasminogen activator (tPA) with the conversion of plasminogen to plasmin. The plasmin thus formed degrades the fibrin to break down the clot. Tranexamic acid competitively binds to the fibrin-binding sites on the plasminogen molecule, with a reduction in the formation of plasminogen-fibrin complexes. Hence, there is less conversion of plasminogen to plasmin by tPA, with inhibition of fibrinolysis. Prevention of fibrin dissolution leads to stabilization of the clot, thus preventing hemorrhage (Fig. 50.1).

The bioavailability of tranexamic acid after oral administration in humans is approximately 30–50% of the ingested dose and unaffected by food intake. It is approximately 3% protein-bound in plasma at therapeutic concentrations. However, it does not bind to serum albumin.

J. Chacko et al., *Controversies in Critical Care*,
https://doi.org/10.1007/978-981-19-9940-6_50

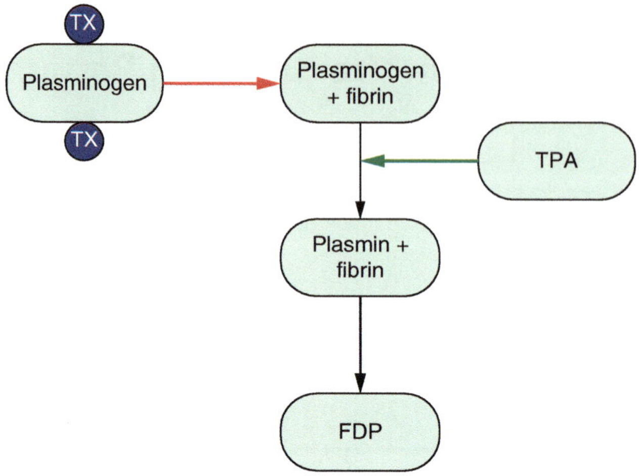

Fig. 50.1 During fibrinolysis, the plasminogen binds to fibrin; the plasminogen-fibrin complex is acted upon by the tissue plasminogen activator (tPA) with conversion of plasminogen to plasmin. The plasmin breaks down the clot through the process of fibrinolysis. Tranexamic acid (TX) competitively binds to the fibrin-binding sites on the plasminogen molecule. Plasminogen-fibrin complexes can no longer be formed (red arrow), and tPA cannot act on these complexes to generate plasmin. The reduction in plasmin generation leads to less clot lysis

Tranexamic acid metabolism is poorly characterized. Urinary excretion is the primary route of elimination, with >95% of an administered dose excreted in the urine as the unchanged drug. The rate of excretion is dependent on the route of administration, with approximately 90% of an intravenously administered dose excreted within 24 h; only 39% of an orally administered dose is excreted within the same time frame [1]. Following intravenous administration, the apparent elimination half-life is approximately 2 h and the mean terminal half-life, 11 h.

50.3 Adverse Effects

High doses of tranexamic acid may cause seizures. It may increase the excitability of neuronal networks by reducing inhibitory neurotransmission, either through the GABA-A or the glycine receptors [2]. Although there is a potential risk of thrombosis, it seems to be unusual in clinical practice. Hypersensitive and anaphylactic reactions may occur. Dose adjustment is required in renal failure.

50.4 The Evidence

Tranexamic acid has been extensively evaluated in different clinical situations leading to severe hemorrhage. Early studies date back to the 1960s; there has been renewed interest in its use, particularly following severe trauma. Table 50.1 summarizes important RCTs that have evaluated the use of tranexamic acid in clinical practice.

Table 50.1 Landmark RCTs that have evaluated the safety and efficacy of tranexamic acid

Study/year	Population	Intervention	Control	Outcomes
Shakur et al. (CRASH-2, 2010) [4]	Trauma with significant bleeding or high risk of bleeding	TXA 1 g over 10 min, followed by 1 g in 8 h	Placebo	Lower all-cause hospital mortality at 28 days and reduced risk of death due to bleeding with TXA. Lower mortality with TXA administration ≤3 h of injury
Spinella et al. (TAMPITI, 2020) [5]	Severe trauma	TXA 2 g or 4 g (2 intervention arms)	Placebo (3-armed study)	No difference in mortality or use of blood products with TXA
Guyette et al. (STAAMP, 2020) [6]	Patients at risk of hemorrhage after trauma. Systolic BP <90 mmHg, HR >110/min	1 g TXA before arrival at hospital. After arrival, either no TXA, 1 g over 8 h, or a bolus of 1 g followed by 1 g over 8 h	Placebo	30-day all-cause mortality similar. 30-day all-cause mortality lower when TXA administered within 1 h of injury. 30-day mortality less in patients with systolic BP <70 mmHg. Improved survival with a total of 3 g TXA. Thrombotic complications similar
CRASH-3 (2019) [9]	TBI within 3 h of injury, GCS 12 or less, or intracranial bleed	TXA 1 g over 10 min, followed by 1 g over 8 h	Placebo	TBI-related death at 28 days similar. Pre-specified subgroup analysis showed no difference in 28-day mortality after excluding patients with GCS 3 or bilateral fixed pupils. TBI-related death lower in mild to moderate, but not in severe TBI. Vaso-occlusive events similar
Sprigg et al. (TICH-2, 2018) [11]	Primary intracerebral hemorrhage	TXA 1 g bolus, 1 g over 8 h	Placebo	Functional status at 90 days by the modified Rankin score similar. 7-day mortality lower with TXA; 90-day mortality similar. Subgroup analysis showed benefit with TXA if systolic BP <170 and baseline hematoma volume 30–60 mL
WOMAN (2017) [13]	Postpartum hemorrhage	TXA 1 g; second dose of 1 g if continued bleed or recurrent bleed within 24 h	Placebo	Death due to continued bleed lower with TXA; effect most prominent with TXA administration within 3 h of delivery. Hysterectomy rates similar. Composite endpoint of all-cause mortality or hysterectomy similar. Thrombotic complications similar

(continued)

Table 50.1 (continued)

Study/year	Population	Intervention	Control	Outcomes
Myles et al. (ATACAS, 2017) [15]	Patients scheduled for CABG	TXA 100 mg/kg 30 min after induction of anesthesia. The dose was halved in the latter part of the study	Placebo	No difference in the composite primary outcome of death and thrombotic complications at 30 day postop. TXA associated with significant reduction in the requirement for postop blood product transfusion. Major bleed, pericardial tamponade requiring re-exploration lower with TXA. Higher incidence of seizures with TXA. Thrombotic complications similar at 30 days
HALT-IT (2020) [18]	Patients with significant upper of lower GI bleeding	TXA 1 g over 10 min, 3 g over 24 h	Placebo	Death due to bleeding at 5 days similar. Venous thromboembolic events higher with TXA. Arterial thromboembolic events similar

RCT randomized controlled trial, *TXA* tranexamic acid, *CABG* coronary artery bypass graft, *GI* gastrointestinal

50.5 Trauma

Coagulopathy associated with trauma is considered to be secondary to hyperfibrinolysis with an estimated incidence of 20% [3]. In trauma patients, endothelial injury and tissue ischemia induce the release of TPA, which, in turn, triggers fibrinolysis. Early administration of tranexamic acid may stop or slow down this process.

50.5.1 CRASH-2 Trial

The CRASH-2 randomized controlled trial (RCT) assessed the effects of early administration of a short course of tranexamic acid on death, vascular occlusive events, and the receipt of blood transfusion in trauma patients. The study patients experienced significant bleeding or were at high risk of bleeding. A total of 20,211 patients were recruited from 274 hospitals across 40 countries, within 8 h of injury. The patients were randomly assigned within 8 h of injury to receive either tranexamic acid at a loading dose of 1 g over 10 min followed by 1 g over 8 h, intravenously, or a matching placebo. The all-cause in-hospital mortality within 4 weeks of injury, the primary outcome, was significantly lower with tranexamic acid compared to placebo (14.5% vs. 16%, $p = 0.003$). Besides, the risk of death due to bleeding was also significantly lower. Thus, tranexamic acid safely reduced the risk of death in bleeding trauma patients [4]. The study was limited by a patient population with relatively low injury severity; besides, the incidence of penetrating trauma was relatively low. The majority of patients were recruited from low-income countries with less developed trauma systems.

50.5.2 TAMPITI Trial

This single-center RCT was primarily aimed at evaluating the effect of tranexamic acid on monocyte activation in bleeding trauma patients with severe injury. The three-armed study compared a 2 g or 4 g dose of intravenous tranexamic acid bolus with placebo in severe trauma. There were 50 patients in each study group. There was no difference in clinical outcomes, including mortality and the use of blood products given following tranexamic administration, compared to the control group. Thromboembolic events were more common with tranexamic acid use [5].

50.5.3 STAAMP Trial

The STAAMP (Study of Tranexamic acid during Air Medical Prehospital Transport) trial assessed the efficacy and safety of pre-hospital administration of tranexamic acid, among patients at risk of hemorrhage following severe trauma. The study was a phase 3, multicenter, double-blind, placebo-controlled RCT. The patients included had pre-hospital hypotension with systolic blood pressure <90 mmHg or tachycardia with a heart rate >110/min; they arrived at the trauma center within 2 h of injury. Tranexamic acid, 1 g intravenously, was administered before arrival to hospital in 447 patients while 456 patients received a placebo. After arrival to the hospital, in the tranexamic acid group, patients received either no additional tranexamic acid, 1 g tranexamic acid over 8 h, or a further bolus dose of 1 g followed by 1 g over 8 h. The 30-day all-cause mortality, the primary outcome, was not significantly different between the two groups (tranexamic acid vs. placebo, 8.1% vs. 9.9%). On post hoc analysis, the 30-day mortality was less in patients who received tranexamic acid within 1 h of injury (4.6% vs. 7.6%, $p < 0.002$). Besides, the 30-day mortality was significantly lower among patients in severe shock with a systolic blood pressure of ≤70 mmHg (18.5% vs. 35.5%, $p < 0.003$). Prespecified dose-response analysis revealed improved survival with tranexamic acid in patients who received a repeat dosing with a total of 3 g of tranexamic acid (two 1 g boluses over 10 min and 1 g in 8 h). Adverse events, including thrombotic complications, were comparable between the two groups [6].

50.6 Traumatic Brain Injury

In TBI, continued intracranial hemorrhage leads to an increase in intracranial pressure (ICP). Increase in fibrinolysis, evidenced by high concentrations of fibrin degradation products, suggests expansion of intracranial hemorrhage. If the ICP remains uncontrolled, brain herniation, and death often ensue. Tranexamic acid may be a beneficial adjunct in this situation by reducing bleeding through the inhibition of fibrin. Two small RCTs, including 510 patients [7, 8], were published prior to the CRASH-3 RCT. A meta-analysis of these two trials had demonstrated significant reduction in mortality with the use of tranexamic acid.

50.6.1 CRASH-3 Trial

The CRASH-3 trial assessed the effect of tranexamic acid in patients with TBI. This RCT was conducted across 175 hospitals in 29 countries. Adult patients with TBI within 3 h of injury, with Glasgow Coma Scale (GCS) score of 12 or less, or any intracranial bleeding on CT scan were included in the study. The study included a total of 12,737 patients, randomly allocated to receive tranexamic acid or a matching placebo. Tranexamic acid was administered as a loading dose of 1 gram over 10 min followed by an infusion of 1 g over 8 h. TBI-related death in hospital within 28 days of injury in patients who were treated within 3 h of injury, the primary outcome, was not significantly different between the two groups (tranexamic acid vs. placebo, 18.5% vs. 19.8%, RR: 0.94; 95% CI 0.86–1.02). On prespecified subgroup analysis, after excluding patients with a GCS 3 or bilateral unreactive pupils, the 28-day mortality was similar between groups. TBI-related death was significantly lower with tranexamic acid in mild-to-moderate TBI, defined as GCS 9–15; however, there was no significant mortality difference with severe TBI, defined as GCS 3–8. In mild-to-moderate TBI, early treatment was more effective compared to later treatment; but time to administration of tranexamic acid did not affect outcomes in severe TBI. The risk of vascular occlusive events was similar between groups [9].

50.7 Primary Intracerebral Hemorrhage: The TICH-2 Trial

Spontaneous intracerebral hemorrhage (ICH) carries a high mortality, with a median case fatality at 1 month of nearly 40% [10]. The mortality related to ICH has remained static over time, with relatively few interventions that alter clinical outcomes. Expansion of the hematoma occurs most often within the first few hours and is the leading cause for poor outcomes.

The TICH-2 trial was an international, multicentric RCT that aimed to evaluate the efficacy of tranexamic acid in reducing hematoma expansion and thereby, improve outcomes in ICH. The study was conducted across 124 hospitals in 12 countries and included a total of 2325 patients. Patients were randomized to receive a bolus of 1 g intravenous tranexamic acid followed by an 8-h infusion of 1 g within 8 h of symptom onset or placebo. The primary outcome was functional status at day 90, based on the modified Rankin scale. The functional status at 90 days did not differ significantly between the two groups. The 7-day mortality was lower in the tranexamic acid group; however, the case fatality at 90 days was similar. On pre-specified subgroup analysis, tranexamic acid was beneficial if systolic BP was <170 and with a baseline hematoma volume of 30–60 mL. Overall, this study revealed no impact on long-term clinical outcomes with the use of tranexamic acid following primary intracerebral hemorrhage although early deaths and adverse events were fewer [11].

50.8 Postpartum Hemorrhage: The WOMAN Trial

Postpartum hemorrhage (PPH) continues to be a leading cause of maternal mortality. Early activation of fibrinolysis occurs after childbirth. The TPA levels increase sharply after delivery, likely due to tissue damage during childbirth; normalization of the fibrinolytic system occurs in 3–4 days [12]. On the basis of results of its favorable effects in trauma, the efficacy of tranexamic acid has been evaluated in primary PPH refractory to uterotonic agents, or if the bleeding is suspected to be due to trauma.

The WOMAN trial aimed to evaluate the effects of early administration of tranexamic acid on death, hysterectomy, and other important clinical outcomes in patients with PPH. This multicentric RCT was conducted across 193 hospitals in 21 countries. Patients with a clinical diagnosis of PPH after vaginal delivery or cesarean section were included. In the intervention arm, patients received 1 g tranexamic acid intravenously. A second dose of 1 g could be administered for continuous bleeding after 30 min, or for recurrent bleed within 24 h of the first dose. Patients in the control group received a matching placebo. A total of 20,060 women were included in the study. Death due to continued bleeding was significantly lower in the tranexamic acid group (1·5% vs. 1·9% $p = 0·045$). The effect on mortality was most profound in patients who received tranexamic acid within 3 h of childbirth. The requirement for hysterectomy was not different between groups. The composite endpoint of all-cause mortality or hysterectomy was also similar. The incidence of adverse events, including thrombotic complications was similar in both groups. The WOMAN trial suggests that tranexamic acid may be beneficial in reducing PPH-related death. The study is limited by a change in the primary endpoint through the course of the trial after the initial observation that the decision to perform hysterectomy was often made at the time of randomization. This led to a change in the statistical methodology and adjustment of the sample size with mortality as the primary endpoint [13].

50.9 Coronary Artery Surgery: The ATACAS-Tranexamic Acid Trial

Major hemorrhage with the requirement for blood transfusions often occurs in patients who undergo cardiac surgery. Surgical re-exploration may be required in some cases, leading to adverse clinical outcomes. Antifibrinolytic therapy has the potential to reduce the risk of bleeding, requirement for transfusion, and re-exploration in patients undergoing cardiac surgery [14]. The putative benefits of tranexamic acid in this setting need to be balanced with possible thrombotic events including perioperative myocardial infarction, stroke, and seizures.

The ATACAS-tranexamic acid trial included patients scheduled to undergo coronary artery surgery who were at risk for perioperative complications. Tranexamic acid was administered in a dose of 100 mg/kg intravenously 30 min after induction of anesthesia and compared with placebo. The dose was halved during the course of the study as seizures were reported with tranexamic acid use and was considered to be dose-related. The primary composite outcome was death and thrombotic complications in the 30-day postoperative period. The thrombotic complications evaluated included myocardial infarction, stroke, pulmonary embolism, or bowel ischemia. The primary outcome was similar between the two groups (tranexamic acid vs. placebo, 16.7% vs. 18.1%). Tranexamic acid administration was associated with a significant reduction in the requirement for blood product transfusion during hospitalization (4331 vs. 7994 units, $p < 0.001$). Major hemorrhage or pericardial tamponade requiring re-exploration was significantly lower with tranexamic acid use. However, there was a significantly higher incidence of seizures with tranexamic acid use. The ATACAS-tranexamic acid trial suggested a lower incidence of bleeding with the use of tranexamic acid in patients who undergo coronary artery surgery, with no increase in the risk of death or thrombotic complications in the 30-day postoperative period [15].

50.10 Gastrointestinal Bleeding: The HALT-IT Trial

Acute gastrointestinal bleeding often leads to adverse clinical outcomes, including mortality. Upper gastrointestinal bleeding carries a mortality of approximately 10%; lower gastrointestinal bleeding may result in a mortality of up to 3% [16]. The HALT-IT RCT was conducted against a background of substantial mortality reduction reported in a meta-analysis of patients who received tranexamic acid for upper gastrointestinal bleeding [17].

The multicentric RCT was conducted across 164 hospitals in 15 countries. The patients included in the study had significant upper or lower gastrointestinal tract bleeding. In the intervention group, tranexamic acid was administered as a loading dose of 1 g over 10 min, followed by an infusion of 3 g over 24 h; the control group received matching placebo. Death due to bleeding within 5 days of randomization, the primary outcome, was similar between the two groups (4% in both groups; RR 0·99, 95% CI 0·82–1·18). Concerningly, the incidence of venous thromboembolic events, including deep vein thrombosis and pulmonary embolism, was higher with tranexamic acid (0.8% vs. 0.4%, RR: 1·85; 95% CI: 1·15–2·98). Arterial thromboembolic events, including myocardial infarction and stroke, were similar in both groups. This large RCT revealed no mortality benefit with tranexamic acid on gastrointestinal bleeding; besides, it suggested an increased rate of venous thromboembolism [18].

Key Points

- Fibrinolysis perpetuates bleeding in many clinical situations. Tranexamic acid competitively binds to the lysine-binding sites on plasminogen and inhibits formation of the plasminogen-fibrin complex. Fibrinolysis is suppressed, leading to stabilization of the clot.
- When administered to medical, elective, and emergency surgical patients, tranexamic acid may reduce bleeding and transfusion requirements.
- Tranexamic acid reduces severe trauma-related bleeding and mortality, especially if administered within the first 3 h of injury.
- In postpartum hemorrhage, tranexamic acid administration within 3 h of delivery has been shown to reduce mortality due to continued bleeding.
- The requirement for transfusion of blood products may be reduced with tranexamic acid administration in patients who undergo coronary artery bypass grafting. Tranexamic acid may also reduce major hemorrhage or pericardial tamponade requiring re-exploration in this patient population.
- Tranexamic acid may reduce TBI-related death in patients with mild to moderate injury if administered within the first 3 h; however, the beneficial effect was observed only on a subgroup analysis of the CRASH-3 trial and needs corroboration in future trials.
- In primary intracerebral hemorrhage, tranexamic acid did not lead to an improved functional status at day 90 in the TICH-2 RCT.
- Tranexamic acid has no beneficial effect on patients with acute gastrointestinal bleeding.
- There is no evidence to suggest an increase in thromboembolic complications associated with tranexamic acid use.

References

1. Relke N, Chornenki NLJ, Sholzberg M. Tranexamic acid evidence and controversies: an illustrated review. Res Pract Thromb Haemost. 2021;5(5):e12546.
2. Lecker I, Wang DS, Whissell PD, Avramescu S, Mazer CD, Orser BA. Tranexamic acid-associated seizures: causes and treatment. Ann Neurol. 2016;79(1):18–26.
3. Banerjee A, Silliman CC, Moore EE, Dzieciatskowa M, Kelher M, Sauaia A, et al. Systemic hyperfibrinolysis after trauma: a pilot study of targeted proteomic analysis of superposed mechanisms in patient plasma. J Trauma Acute Care Surg. 2018;84(6):929–38.

4. Shakur H, Roberts I, Bautista R, Caballero J, Coats T, et al. The CRASH-2 collaborators. Effects of tranexamic acid on death, vascular occlusive events, and blood transfusion in trauma patients with significant haemorrhage (CRASH-2): a randomised, placebo-controlled trial. Lancet. 2010;376(9734):23–32.
5. Spinella PC, Thomas KA, Turnbull IR, Fuchs A, Bochicchio K, Schuerer D, et al. The immunologic effect of early intravenous two and four gram bolus dosing of tranexamic acid compared to placebo in patients with severe traumatic bleeding (TAMPITI): a randomized, double-blind, placebo-controlled, single-center trial. Front Immunol. 2020;11:2085.
6. Guyette FX, Brown JB, Zenati MS, Early-Young BJ, Adams PW, Eastridge BJ, et al. Tranexamic acid during prehospital transport in patients at risk for hemorrhage after injury: a double-blind, placebo-controlled, randomized clinical trial. JAMA Surg. 2020;156:11.
7. Perel P, Al-Shahi Salman R, Kawahara T, Morris Z, Prieto-Merino D, Roberts I, et al. CRASH-2 (Clinical randomisation of an antifibrinolytic in significant haemorrhage) intracranial bleeding study: the effect of tranexamic acid in traumatic brain injury--a nested randomised, placebo-controlled trial. Health Technol Assess. 2012;16(13):iii–xii, 1–54.
8. Yutthakasemsunt S, Kittiwatanagul W, Piyavechvirat P, Thinkamrop B, Phuenpathom N, Lumbiganon P. Tranexamic acid for patients with traumatic brain injury: a randomized, double-blinded, placebo-controlled trial. BMC Emerg Med. 2013;13:20.
9. CRASH-3 trial collaborators. Effects of tranexamic acid on death, disability, vascular occlusive events and other morbidities in patients with acute traumatic brain injury (CRASH-3): a randomised, placebo-controlled trial. Lancet. 2019;394(10210):1713–23.
10. van Asch CJ, Luitse MJ, Rinkel GJ, van der Tweel I, Algra A, Klijn CJ. Incidence, case fatality, and functional outcome of intracerebral haemorrhage over time, according to age, sex, and ethnic origin: a systematic review and meta-analysis. Lancet Neurol. 2010;9(2):167–76.
11. Sprigg N, Flaherty K, Appleton JP, Al-Shahi Salman R, Bereczki D, Beridze M, et al. Tranexamic acid for hyperacute primary IntraCerebral Haemorrhage (TICH-2): an international randomised, placebo-controlled, phase 3 superiority trial. Lancet. 2018;391(10135):2107–15.
12. Kruithof EK, Tran-Thang C, Gudinchet A, Hauert J, Nicoloso G, Genton C, et al. Fibrinolysis in pregnancy: a study of plasminogen activator inhibitors. Blood. 1987;69(2):460–6.
13. WOMAN Trial Collaborators. Effect of early tranexamic acid administration on mortality, hysterectomy, and other morbidities in women with postpartum haemorrhage (WOMAN): an international, randomised, double-blind, placebo-controlled trial. Lancet. 2017;389(10084):2105–16.
14. Ker K, Edwards P, Perel P, Shakur H, Roberts I. Effect of tranexamic acid on surgical bleeding: systematic review and cumulative meta-analysis. BMJ. 2012;344:e3054.
15. Myles PS, Smith JA, Forbes A, Silbert B, Jayarajah M, Painter T, et al. Tranexamic acid in patients undergoing coronary-artery surgery. N Engl J Med. 2017;376(2):136–48.
16. Oakland K, Guy R, Uberoi R, Hogg R, Mortensen N, Murphy MF, et al. Acute lower GI bleeding in the UK: patient characteristics, interventions and outcomes in the first nationwide audit. Gut. 2018;67(4):654–62.
17. Bennett C, Klingenberg SL, Langholz E, Gluud LL. Tranexamic acid for upper gastrointestinal bleeding. Cochrane Database Syst Rev. 2014;11:CD006640.
18. HALT-IT Trial Collaborators. Effects of a high-dose 24-h infusion of tranexamic acid on death and thromboembolic events in patients with acute gastrointestinal bleeding (HALT-IT): an international randomised, double-blind, placebo-controlled trial. Lancet. 2020;395(10241):1927–36.

Dengue-Related Thrombocytopenia and Platelet Transfusion

51

Dengue is an arboviral disease transmitted by *Aedes aegypti* and *Aedes albopictus* mosquitoes. The clinical features are highly variable, ranging from mild disease to severe dengue, leading to capillary leak, hemorrhage, and impaired organ function. Low platelet counts are commonly observed in dengue fever; several reports reveal that 79–100% of patients develop significant thrombocytopenia [1, 2]. Platelet transfusions are regularly administered by clinicians, often as prophylaxis, using varying thresholds of platelet counts. In a survey of 306 physicians from 20 countries, 38% of respondents supported prophylactic platelet transfusions at cutoff levels ranging from less than 5000–50,000/mm^3 [3]. In a single-center retrospective study during the dengue epidemic of 2013 in Delhi, the authors concluded that up to 23.2% of platelet transfusions may have been unnecessary [4].

51.1 Why Does Thrombocytopenia Occur in Dengue?

The platelet counts begin to drop during the febrile stage of dengue; defervescence heralds the onset of the toxic stage when the counts drop to a nadir. Bone marrow depression with impaired production of platelets is one of the key mechanisms of thrombocytopenia (Fig. 51.1). Platelet destruction occurs, as evidenced by reduced platelet survival times [5]. Dengue virus-infected platelets release cytokines and chemokines and adhere to activated vascular endothelium. Adherence to infected endothelial cells leads to the lysis of platelets [6]. Platelets also aggregate with leukocytes, triggering the release of inflammatory mediators by neutrophils and monocytes. Furthermore, the dengue virus infects stromal cells and hematopoietic precursors, thereby inhibiting the generation of megakaryocytes, the precursors of platelets [7].

J. Chacko et al., *Controversies in Critical Care*,
https://doi.org/10.1007/978-981-19-9940-6_51

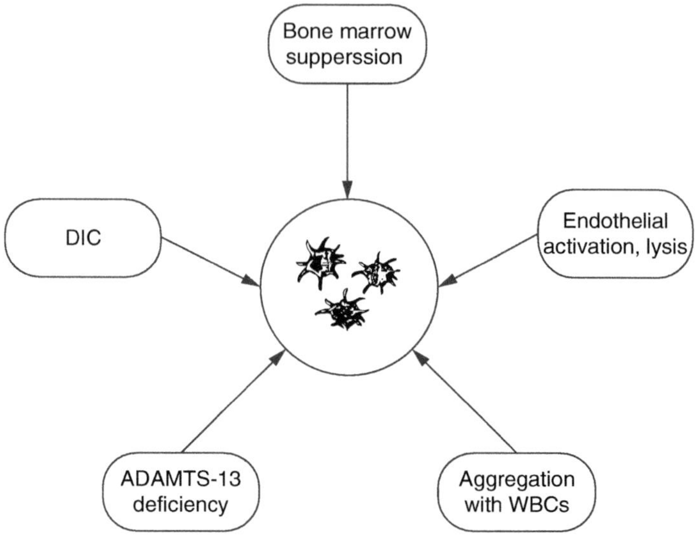

Fig. 51.1 Mechanisms of thrombocytopenia in dengue

Another possible mechanism for thrombocytopenia in dengue is through the release of von Willebrand factor (vWF) from the Weibel Palade bodies of endothelial cells. Platelets adhere to vWF to form plugs, as part of the normal hemostatic mechanism. The ultra-large vWf multimers are cleaved by ADAMTS 13, a metalloprotease enzyme, to keep the hemostatic mechanism in balance and prevent excessive platelet adhesion. However, deficiency of ADAMTS 13 has been shown to occur in acute infective processes, including dengue fever that results in thrombocytopenia [8]. Failure to cleave vWF multimers leads to extensive platelet adhesion to vWf, leading to microthrombi formation and organ failure. Similar to hemolytic uremic syndrome and thrombotic thrombocytopenic purpura, this mechanism may play an important role in dengue-associated thrombocytopenia [9]. Considering this putative mechanism of thrombocytopenia in dengue, prior transfusion with fresh frozen plasma to replenish the ADAMTS 13 levels before platelet administration may be beneficial [10].

51.2 Possible Harmful Effects of Prophylactic Platelet Transfusion

Injudicious transfusion of blood products can lead to potential harm. Prophylactic platelet transfusions in dengue may lead to fluid overload, especially in children [11], and transfusion-associated lung injury (TRALI) [12]. Recovery of platelet count in dengue fever is stimulated by the generation of thrombopoietin, the physiological response to thrombocytopenia. However, transfusion of platelets may inhibit thrombopoietin generation and delay the recovery of platelet counts [13, 14]. The efficacy of prophylactic platelet transfusion in reducing clinically significant bleeding in dengue fever is shrouded in controversy.

51.3 Prophylactic Platelet Transfusions and Outcomes in Dengue

Apart from a transient increase in counts, do platelet transfusions in dengue improve platelet function and clot strength? Thromboelastography (TEG) is commonly used during major surgery involving significant hemorrhage and involves the assessment of the tensile force that develops during the process of clotting, arising from the interaction between glycoprotein IIb/IIIa receptors and fibrin. Sundar et al. evaluated dengue patients who developed bleeding complications and underwent transfusion with random or single donor platelets [15]. In this study of 74 patients, platelet transfusion increased the mean platelet count by 10,210/mm^3 at 24 h compared to pre-transfusion levels. However, there was no significant increase in clot strength evident on TEG. Besides, platelet transfusion did not have any impact on the incidence of clinical bleeding.

Lee et al. conducted a single-center, retrospective observational study of 7500 dengue patients over a 4-year period [16]. Among these patients, 788 (10.5%) developed thrombocytopenia of <20,000/mm^3. Four hundred and eighty-six (61.7%) of these patients received platelet transfusion, with a median volume of 240 mL (range: 100–618 mL). Clinically significant bleeding occurred in 18.2% of patients who received platelet transfusion compared to 23.5% among those who did not, the difference being non-significant ($p = 0.08$). Increase in platelet counts to 50,000/mm^3 was delayed by a median of 1 day in the transfused compared to the control group (3 vs. 2 days, $p < 0.0001$). Platelet transfusion was also associated with a longer median duration of hospital stay (6 vs. 5 days, $p < 0.0001$ days). The incidence of severe disease requiring intensive care was similar between the two groups of patients. On propensity-matched analysis adjusting for possible confounders, prophylactic platelet transfusion was not associated with a lower incidence of clinically significant bleeding.

A single-center randomized controlled trial (RCT) from Pakistan studied patients with platelet counts of less than 30,000/mm^3 with either no bleeding or mild (WHO grade 1 or 2) bleeding [17]. The treatment group (43 patients) was administered single-donor platelets; the control group (44 patients) received standard care alone. The mean increase in platelet count at 24 and 72 h was significantly higher in the treatment group compared to the control group. There was no new incidence of bleeding in patients without bleeding at baseline in either group. Among patients with WHO grade 1 or 2 bleeding, progression to more severe, grade 3 bleeding was observed in one patient in the treatment group. The mean time to cessation of bleeding was also not different in patients with WHO grade 1 or 2 bleeding at baseline.

Adverse events were noted in the treatment group; three patients (7%) developed severe anaphylaxis with hypotension. Two deaths occurred in the treatment group, one due to TRALI, while the cause of death in the other patient was multifactorial. This study revealed no potential benefit from prophylactic platelet transfusions, with a relatively higher likelihood of severe adverse events.

The efficacy of prophylactic platelet transfusion in the prevention of bleeding was evaluated in a retrospective cohort study of dengue patients [18]. The study included patients with a platelet count of less than 20,000/mm^3 without clinical bleeding. Prophylactic platelet transfusions were administered at the discretion of the clinician. Outcomes were compared between 188 patients who received prophylactic platelet transfusion with 68 who did not. The incidence of clinical bleeding was low; one patient (0.5%) developed clinical bleeding in the group that received prophylactic transfusion compared to two patients (2.9%) who did not. The bleeding was mild in both cases and did not require any further intervention. The platelet count 24 h after it dropped below 20,000/mm^3 was higher in those who were not transfused compared with those who received a transfusion. The median duration for the platelet count to reach 50,000/mm^3 was similar between the two groups of patients. The length of hospital stay was also similar between the two groups of patients. This study also demonstrated that prophylactic platelet transfusion was ineffective in preventing bleeding in dengue fever.

Lye et al. performed an RCT in adult patients with dengue admitted to five hospitals in Singapore and Malaysia [19]. Patients had confirmed or probable dengue and thrombocytopenia of <20,000/mm^3; those with persistent mild bleeding or severe bleeding were excluded. Of the 372 patients enrolled, 188 patients were randomized to receive prophylactic platelet transfusion and 184 to supportive care alone. In the prophylactic transfusion arm, 4 units of pooled platelets were administered each day if the platelet count was less than 20,000/mm^3. Patients in the transfusion arm received a mean of 4·71 ± 2·17 units of platelets. Clinical bleeding by day 7 or until hospital discharge, the primary outcome, occurred in 40/188 (21%) patients in the transfusion arm compared to 48/181 (26%) patients in the control group; the difference was not statistically significant. Clinically important bleeding by day 21 was also not different between the two groups (transfused vs. control: 22% vs. 27%; $p = 0{\cdot}34$). Severe bleeding was rare; three (2%) patients in the transfusion group and seven (4%) patients in the control group experienced severe bleeding by day 21. In subgroups of patients with platelet counts of <10,000/mm^3 and < 5000/mm^3, the incidence of clinical bleeding was not significantly different between patients who received prophylactic transfusion compared with controls. Plasma leakage, defined as an increase of at least 20% in serum hematocrit, was also similar between groups. Adverse events were significantly more common in the transfusion group and included anaphylaxis, TRALI, and transfusion-associated fluid overload. This RCT clearly demonstrated that prophylactic platelet transfusion for platelet counts <20,000/mm^3 was not superior to supportive care alone in the prevention of clinical bleeding in dengue fever; besides, adverse effects are more likely to occur in patients who undergo transfusion. Important studies that evaluated the impact of platelet transfusion in dengue are summarized in Table 51.1.

Table 51.1 Main studies evaluating the impact of platelet transfusion in patients with dengue

Study/ year	Design	Population	Intervention	Control	Outcomes
Lee et al. (2016) [16]	Retrospective observational	Dengue patients with thrombocytopenia <20,000/mm^3 without bleeding	Platelet transfusion	No platelet transfusion	Increase in platelet counts to 50,000/mm^3 delayed by 1 day (median) with platelet transfusion. Longer duration of hospital stay in the transfused group. No reduction in the incidence of bleeding with platelet transfusion
Assir et al. (2013) [17]	RCT	Dengue patients with thrombocytopenia <30,000/mm^3 with mild bleeding or no bleeding	Single donor platelets	Standard care	Platelet count increased at 24–72 h with transfusion. No new bleeding in either group. Adverse events in the transfused group—severe anaphylaxis in 3 patients, two deaths, including one death due to TRALI
Lye et al. (2009) [18]	Retrospective cohort study	Dengue patients with thrombocytopenia <20,000/mm^3 with no bleeding	Prophylactic platelet transfusions at clinician discretion	Control group that did not receive transfusion	Platelet count at 24 h after dropping below <20,000/mm^3 was higher in patients who did not receive transfusion. Median time to a count of <50,000/mm^3 similar whether transfused or not. Duration of hospital stay similar

(continued)

Table 51.1 (continued)

Study/ year	Design	Population	Intervention	Control	Outcomes
Lye et al. (2017) [19]	RCT	Confirmed or probable dengue with thrombocytopenia <20,000/mm^3. Excluded patients with persistent mild or severe bleeding	4 units of pooled platelets daily if count <20,000/ mm^3	Standard care	Similar incidence of clinical bleeding by day 7, day 21, or discharge. Severe bleeding was rare and not significantly different. In patients with platelet counts <10,000 and < 5000/mm^3, no significant difference in the incidence of clinical bleeding. Plasma leakage similar between groups. Adverse events including anaphylaxis, TRALI, and TACO more common with platelet transfusion

RCT randomized controlled trial, *TRALI* transfusion-associated lung injury, *TACO* transfusion-associated circulatory overload

Key Points

- Thrombocytopenia is typically present in most patients with dengue fever and occurs due to reduced generation of platelets in the bone marrow and increased peripheral destruction.
- Conventionally, prophylactic platelet transfusions are administered based on arbitrary cutoff levels.
- Although platelet transfusions lead to a transient rise, they may delay recovery of platelet counts in the long term.
- Prophylactic platelet transfusions have not been shown to reduce the incidence of clinical bleeding; furthermore, adverse events may occur, including volume overload, TRALI, and anaphylaxis. Besides the likelihood of adverse events, injudicious transfusions lead to pressure on blood banks during epidemics and increase the cost of care.

- In dengue fever, the incidence of severe bleeding appears to be unrelated to the extent of decrease in platelet counts even to levels below 10,000/mm^3.
- Robust evidence suggests that platelet transfusions be confined to patients who experience severe bleeding, thereby conserving a scarce blood product for those who really need it.

References

1. Chaudhary R, Khetan D, Sinha S, Sinha P, Sonker A, Pandey P, et al. Transfusion support to dengue patients in a hospital based blood transfusion service in North India. Transfus Apher Sci. 2006;35(3):239–44.
2. Lee MS, Hwang KP, Chen TC, Lu PL, Chen TP. Clinical characteristics of dengue and dengue hemorrhagic fever in a medical center of southern Taiwan during the 2002 epidemic. J Microbiol Immunol Infect. 2006;39(2):121–9.
3. Whitehorn J, Roche RR, Guzman MG, Martinez E, Gomez WV, Nainggolan L, et al. Prophylactic platelets in dengue: survey responses highlight lack of an evidence base. PLoS Negl Trop Dis. 2012;6(6):e1716.
4. Chaurasia R, Zaman S, Chatterjee K, Das B. Retrospective review of platelet transfusion practices during 2013 dengue epidemic of Delhi, India. Transfus Med Hemother. 2015;42(4):227–31.
5. Isarangkura P, Tuchinda S. The behavior of transfused platelets in dengue hemorrhagic fever. Southeast Asian J Trop Med Public Health. 1993;24(Suppl 1):222–4.
6. Funahara Y, Ogawa K, Fujita N, Okuno Y. Three possible triggers to induce thrombocytopenia in dengue virus infection. Southeast Asian J Trop Med Public Health. 1987;18(3):351–5.
7. Quirino-Teixeira AC, Andrade FB, Pinheiro MBM, Rozini SV, Hottz ED. Platelets in dengue infection: more than a numbers game. Platelets. 2022;33(2):176–83.
8. Sosothikul D, Seksarn P, Pongsewalak S, Thisyakorn U, Lusher J. Activation of endothelial cells, coagulation and fibrinolysis in children with dengue virus infection. Thromb Haemost. 2007;97(4):627–34.
9. Djamiatun K, van der Ven AJAM, de Groot PG, Faradz SMH, Hapsari D, Dolmans WMV, et al. Severe dengue is associated with consumption of von Willebrand factor and its cleaving enzyme ADAMTS-13. PLoS Negl Trop Dis. 2012;6(5):e1628.
10. Sellahewa K, Samaraweera N, Thusita K, Fernando J. Is fresh frozen plasma effective for thrombocytopenia in adults with dengue fever? A prospective randomised double blind controlled study. Ceylon Med J. 2008;53(2):36.
11. Lum LCS, Abdel-Latif MEA, Goh AYT, Chan PWK, Lam SK. Preventive transfusion in dengue shock syndrome-is it necessary? J Pediatr. 2003;143(5):682–4.
12. Karoli R, Bhat S, Fatima J, Verma P. Acute lung injury after platelet transfusion in a patient with dengue fever. Asian J Transfus Sci. 2014;8(2):131–4.
13. Cardier JE, Balogh V, Perez-Silva C, Romano E, Rivas B, Bosch N, et al. Relationship of thrombopoietin and interleukin-11 levels to thrombocytopenia associated with dengue disease. Cytokine. 2006;34(3–4):155–60.
14. Shinjo K, Takeshita A, Nakamura S, Naitoh K, Yanagi M, Tobita T, et al. Serum thrombopoietin levels in patients correlate inversely with platelet counts during chemotherapy-induced thrombocytopenia. Leukemia. 1998;12(3):295–300.
15. Sundar V, Bhaskar E. Effect of platelet transfusion on clot strength in dengue fever with thrombocytopenia related bleeding: a thromboelastography-based study. Transfus Med Hemother. 2019;46(6):457–60.

16. Lee TH, Wong JGX, Leo YS, Thein TL, Ng EL, Lee LK, et al. Potential harm of prophylactic platelet transfusion in adult dengue patients. PLoS Negl Trop Dis. 2016;10(3):e0004576.
17. Assir MZK, Kamran U, Ahmad HI, Bashir S, Mansoor H, Anees SB, et al. Effectiveness of platelet transfusion in dengue fever: a randomized controlled trial. Transfus Med Hemother. 2013;40(5):362–8.
18. Lye DC, Lee VJ, Sun Y, Leo YS. Lack of efficacy of prophylactic platelet transfusion for severe thrombocytopenia in adults with acute uncomplicated dengue infection. Clin Infect Dis. 2009;48(9):1262–5.
19. Lye DC, Archuleta S, Syed-Omar SF, Low JG, Oh HM, Wei Y, et al. Prophylactic platelet transfusion plus supportive care versus supportive care alone in adults with dengue and thrombocytopenia: a multicentre, open-label, randomised, superiority trial. Lancet. 2017;389(10079):1611–8.

Part X

Burns

Thermal Injury Resuscitation 52

52.1 Introduction

Each year in Australia, approximately 1% of the population sustains a thermal injury [1]. The great majority of these burns are minor; however patients with severe burns (defined as area of burn > 20% of total body surface area or those necessitating intensive care admission) experience considerable morbidity and mortality [2]. Burn injury resuscitation is complex and has been the subject of significant controversy for the last seven decades. There is very little high-quality evidence to guide clinical practice in the critical care management of the severely burnt patient [3, 4]. Appropriate fluid resuscitation is a critical component of the initial management of major burn injury and has resulted in significant improvement in morbidity and mortality [5].

52.2 Burn Pathophysiology

A unique feature of a severe thermal injury is the subsequent response to the insult. Immediately post injury, both systemic and local stress responses ensue.

The "Jackson Burn Wound Model" assists in understanding the pathophysiology of a burn wound at a local level. In 1947 Jackson described three zones of a burn wound. The primary injury is the *zone of coagulation* nearest the heat source [6]. This zone has irreversible tissue necrosis at the center of the burn due to exposure to heat, chemicals, or electricity. The extent of this injury depends on duration of exposure and the maximal temperature (or concentration). Immediately adjacent to the central zone of necrosis is the *zone of stasis* in which there is a reduced dermal perfusion; this tissue is damaged but potentially viable.

J. Chacko et al., *Controversies in Critical Care*,
https://doi.org/10.1007/978-981-19-9940-6_52

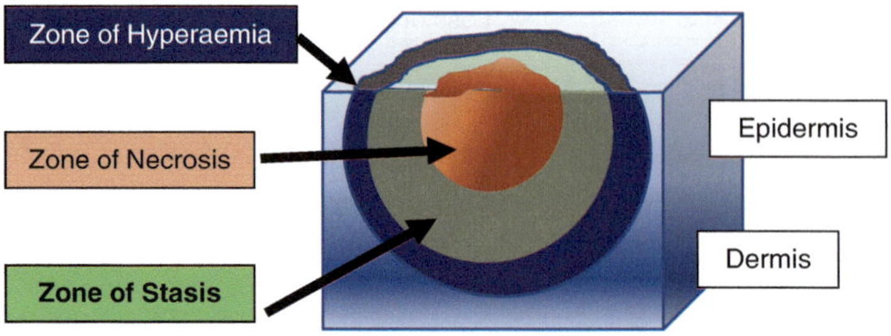

Fig. 52.1 Schematic representation of local burn zones

The principle goal of burn resuscitation is to increase tissue perfusion to this area and prevent the damage becoming irreversible [7]. This ischemic zone may progress to full necrosis unless perfusion is re-established. At the periphery of the burn is the third zone, the *zone of hyperemia* characterized by a reversible increase in blood flow and inflammation. It is important to recognize these three zones of a burn are three dimensional (see Fig. 52.1) and further loss of viable tissue results in both wound deepening as well as surface extension [8].

The pathophysiology of large surface area burns (>20%) is extremely complex and requires a detailed understanding to facilitate appropriate resuscitation. Patients are at risk of developing "burn shock" is if they have greater than 20% of their total body surface area (TBSA) involved with deep or partial thickness burns [9]. The extent of the shock not only depends on the depth and extent of the burn, but also on pre-existing illness, the presence of inhalational injury, age of the patient, and timing of resuscitation.

52.3 Factors Influencing "Burn Shock"

1. Patient age
2. Depth of burn
3. Surface extent of burn
4. Presence of inhalation injury
5. Need for escharotomies/fasciotomies
6. Time delay to resuscitation
7. Associated injuries

Burn pathophysiology is characterized by a series of predictable phases. The principal insult is the loss of the integument and hence body fluid and temperature homeostasis. The initial phase of injury is characterized by markedly increased capillary permeability and transmembrane cellular changes. The increased capillary permeability results from a massive and sustained cytokine release into the systemic circulation following injury and includes vasoactive substances, interleukins, histamine, and prostaglandins. This results in a distributive type pattern of shock, which is further exacerbated by fluid loss into the interstitium. Increased capillary

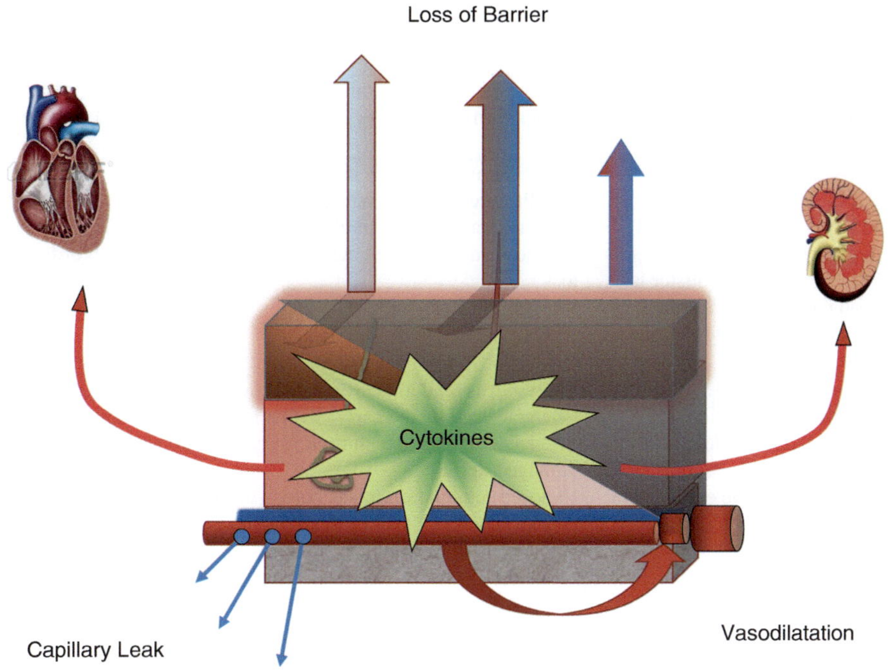

Fig. 52.2 Burn shock. Local and systemic effects of severe burns leading to multifactorial shock

permeability, mediated by these cytokines, results in a loss of intravascular proteins and intravascular oncotic pressure [10]. Concomitantly the interstitial oncotic pressure may rise, further encouraging volume loss from the intravascular compartment. It is highly likely that this initial "cytokine storm" may have directly negative effects on both myocardial and renal function [11]. The cytokine-mediated decrease in myocardial contractility leads to a depressed cardiac output which is further exacerbated by impaired intracellular calcium homeostasis. It is now accepted that burns with 20% of total body surface area or more will result in systemic inflammatory response. The outpouring of cytokines and inflammatory mediators into the circulation results in decreased microvasculature integrity, vasodilation, and compromised myocardial function (Fig. 52.2).

52.4 Clinical Assessment of the Burns Patient

The assessment of a burns patient is complex and requires a disciplined and methodical approach. The approach should be no different to that for any other patient with severe multi trauma but is then followed up by a detailed evaluation of the depth and extent of the burn (Table 52.1). To make an accurate assessment of the burn severity, the clinician requires experience, but more importantly diligence. The evolving nature of a burn makes it essential to reassess these burn wounds at least within 48 h, when exudate and edema have started to resolve.

Table 52.1 Burn depth

Burn depth	Clinical features
Superficial epidermal burns: Involves the epidermis	Hyperemic, erythematous, and painful Blister formation and skin desquamation are delayed for few days
Superficial dermal partial thickness burns: Involves the epidermis and papillary dermis Skin overlying the blister is dead and separated from the base by inflammatory edema fluid	Very painful secondary to sensory nerve exposure Capillary return brisk with preserved vasculature Blisters characteristic on the pink papillary dermis is exposed. Desiccation of exposed dermis can increase the depth of tissue loss
Deep dermal burns: Extensive destruction of dermal vascular plexus Exposed reticular dermis The dermal nerve endings are also damaged	These burns tend to be dry, with diminished fluid exudates Characterized by the early (within hours) development of extensive blisters, which rupture early to expose deep damaged dermis Exposed reticular dermis is pale in color due to damage to dermal blood vessels or red secondary to extravasation of red blood cells from damaged vessels Markedly decreased capillary return, with no or sluggish blanching Sensation is reduced
Full thickness burns: Epidermis and dermis destroyed May penetrate more deeply into underlying structures—fat, muscle, and bone	Dense white, waxy, or even charred appearance. The sensory nerves in the dermis are destroyed in a full thickness burn, and so sensation is lost. The coagulated dead skin, which has a leathery appearance is referred to as an eschar

52.5 Burn Depth

Establishing the depth of a burn is critical to developing a formal resuscitation plan [12]; it is also important in determining the potential for subsequent wound healing and the prognosis. The history and injury pattern often afford the clinician a good idea as to the likely severity of injury. On examination of the burn, the extent and speed of capillary refill is useful in helping establish burn depth. The clinician needs to be cognizant that burn wound evolution frequently results in increased depth of burn injury when subsequently reviewed. Depending on the depth of tissue damage, burns are classified as either epidermal, superficial dermal partial thickness, deep dermal partial thickness, or full thickness (Table 52.2).

Superficial burns and severe deep burns are readily diagnosed; it is those of intermediate or mixed thickness that are more problematic. It is also important to recognize that most burn wounds, especially those involving larger surface areas, are not homogenous in depth. They are usually a mixture of areas of different depths, and only diligent clinical examination will establish the true extent of injury [9].

Table 52.2 Examples of available burn resuscitation formulae

Name of the formula	Strategy
Brooke formula	First 24 h Lactated Ringer's at 1.5 mL/kg/% TBSA burn and colloid at 0.5 mL/kg/% TBSA burn
Modified Brooke	First 24 h: LR at 2 mL/kg/% TBSA burn, one half in the first 8 h and half in the remaining 16 h
Parkland formula	First 24 h Lactated Ringer's at 4 mL/kg/% TBSA Half in first 8 h and the remaining fluid over next 16 h
Rule of tens	% TBSA × 10 = initial fluid rate mL/h For every 10 kg > 80 kg increase rate by 100 mL/h

52.6 Total Body Surface Area

The establishment of burn surface area is an important component of the initial assessment and is critical to determining resuscitation requirements and the need for transfer to a specialist burns center. The extent of injury is documented using the percentage of the total body surface area that affected by the burn. It is important that erythematous areas (superficial burn) are not be included when calculating burn area.

Several studies have compared a range of methods of estimating burn surface area. The surface area of a patient's palm (including fingers) is about 1% total body surface area (Fig. 52.3). Palmar surface can be used to estimate the size of a burn. The accuracy of this method, however, tends to decline when used to estimate larger surface areas. It remains a useful strategy in difficult or austere environments.

The Lund-Browder charts (Fig. 52.4) appear more accurate than either the Wallace rule of nines (Fig. 52.5) or palm size in determining the percentage of body surface area involved in a burn. The rule of nines is however convenient and easily applied in burn patients with the caveat. That it is potentially inaccurate in children or obese people.

While conducting the primary survey, reliable intravenous access must be established. Intravenous cannulas may be placed through the burned area; if there is no other viable option, it is then necessary to suture the cannula in place to prevent dislodgement. Intraosseous access is an excellent short-term alternative while more reliable access is achieved.

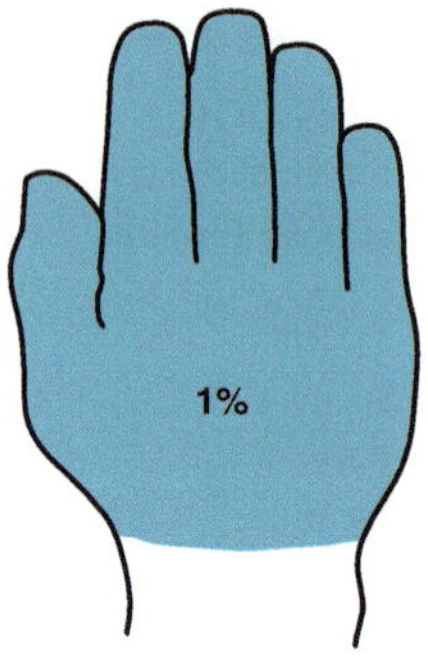

Fig. 52.3 Palmer surface for estimating burn size

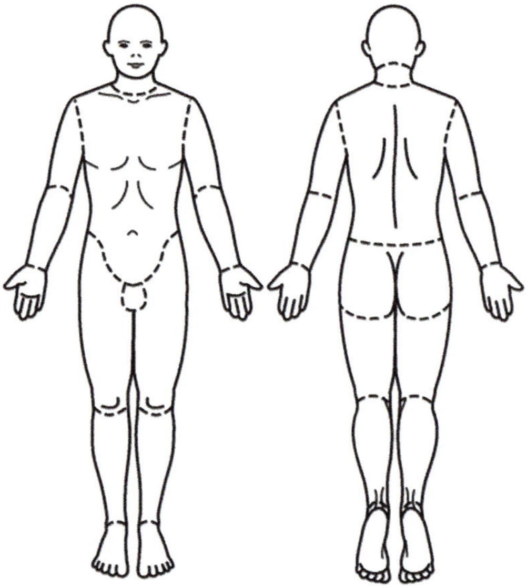

	Birth 1 yr.	1–4 yrs.	5–9 yrs.	10–14 yrs.	15 yrs.	Adult	Burn size estimate
Head	19	17	13	11	9	7	
Neck	2	2	2	2	2	2	
Anterior trunk	13	13	13	13	13	13	
Posterior trunk	13	13	13	13	13	13	
Right buttock	2.5	2.5	2.5	2.5	2.5	2.5	
Left buttock	2.5	2.5	2.5	2.5	2.5	2.5	
Genitalia	1	1	1	1	1	1	
Right upper arm	4	4	4	4	4	4	
Left upper arm	4	4	4	4	4	4	
Right lower arm	3	3	3	3	3	3	
Left lower arm	3	3	3	3	3	3	
Right hand	2.5	2.5	2.5	2.5	2.5	2.5	
Left hand	2.5	2.5	2.5	2.5	2.5	2.5	
Right thigh	5.5	6.5	8	8.5	9	9.5	
Left thigh	5.5	6.5	8	8.5	9	9.5	
Right leg	5	5	5.5	6	6.5	7	
Left leg	5	5	5.5	6	6.5	7	
Right foot	3.5	3.5	3.5	3.5	3.5	3.5	
Left foot	3.5	3.5	3.5	3.5	3.5	3.5	

Total BSAB ____________

Fig. 52.4 The Lund-Browder chart

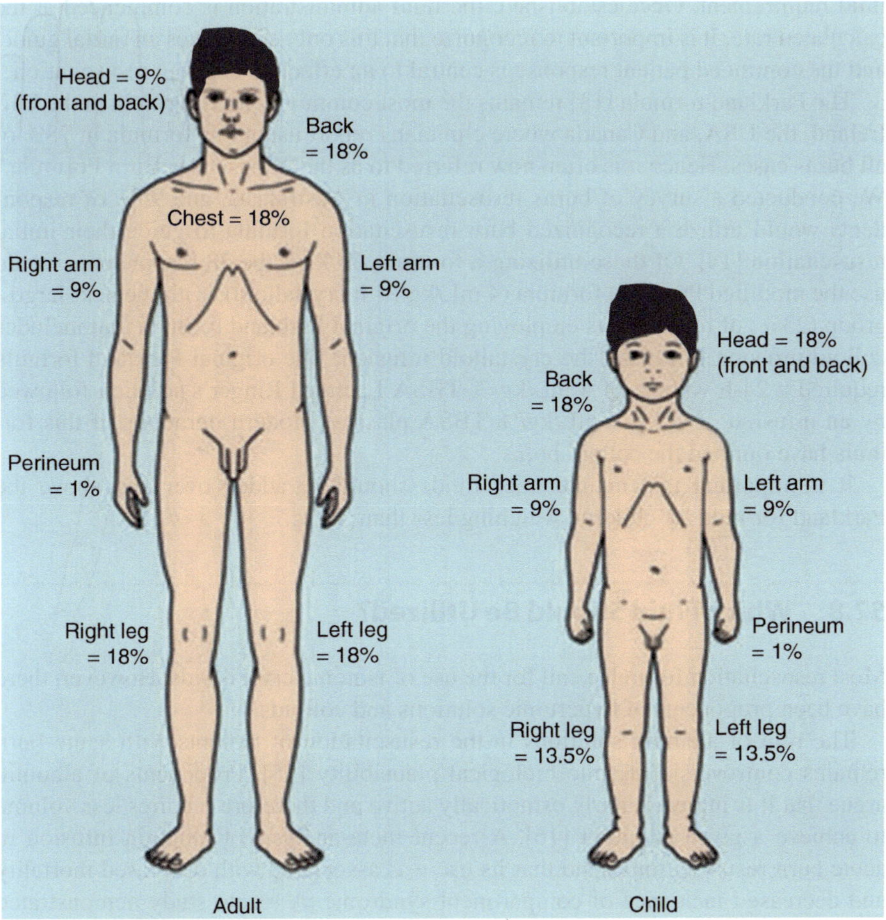

Fig. 52.5 Wallace rule of nines

52.7 Which Burn Formula Should Be Utilized?

The principal aims of fluid resuscitation following a severe burn is to ensure appropriate end-organ tissue perfusion and minimize extension of the injury in the zone of stasis (Fig. 52.1). This task can be extremely difficult to efficiently achieve because of the complex pathophysiology involved in a burn injury.

Our understanding of burn resuscitation has progressed significantly over the last five decades. The optimal formula, most appropriate fluid, and the best resuscitation endpoints remain contentious. Any burn resuscitation strategy requires a reliable estimate of both depth of the burn and percentage body surface area involved. In addition to this information, the patient's weight is critical to compute the initial fluid requirement. Once established, the fluid administration is commenced at the calculated rate. It is important to recognize that this only constitutes an initial guide, and the continued patient response is central to an effective ongoing resuscitation.

The Parkland formula [13] remains the most commonly used formula in the UK, Ireland, the USA, and Canada where clinicians report using this formula in 78% of all burns cases. Hence it is often now referred to as the "Consensus Burn Formula." We conducted a survey of burns resuscitation in Australasia, and 95% of respondents would utilize a recognized burn resuscitation formula to guide their initial resuscitation [14]. Of those utilizing a formula, 74% of the 78 respondents would use the modified Parkland formula (4 mL/kg/24 h crystalloid), with the next largest group (23%) of respondents employing the original Parkland formula that includes colloid infusion following the crystalloid infusion. The original Parkland formula required a 24-h volume of 4 mL/kg/% TBSA Lactated Ringer's solution followed by an infusion of 0.3–0.5 mL/kg/% TBSA plasma. Modern iterations of this formula have omitted the colloid bolus.

It is important that maintenance fluids should be added over and above the Parkland formula for children weighing less than 30 kg.

52.8 Which Fluid Should Be Utilized?

Most resuscitation formulae call for the use of isotonic crystalloids. However, there have been proponents of hypertonic solutions and colloids.

The role of albumin solutions in the resuscitation of patients with acute burn remains controversial despite biological plausibility [15]. Proponents of albumin argue that it is intravascularly osmotically active and therefore requires less volume to achieve a given endpoint [16]. A recent meta-analysis of albumin infusion in acute burn resuscitation found that its use was associated with decreased mortality and decreased incidence of compartment syndrome. A recent study demonstrated that 20% albumin infusions in burn patients and healthy volunteers increased the rate of urine flow by 35% and 97%, respectively, presumably on the basis of plasma volume expansion by the albumin. The Cochrane analysis of the use of albumin in critical illness has highlighted the need for more well-conducted studies on colloid use in burns [17]. The analysis provides no evidence that albumin is unsafe for the initial resuscitation of uncomplicated burns. Thus, there are not only many inconsistencies, but also a striking absence of any high-quality evidence regarding the effect of albumin resuscitation on clinical outcomes. The ABRUPT-2 study (ClinTrials.gov NCT0435659) randomizing patients to Lactated Ringer's or Lactated Ringers +5% albumin between 8 and 12 h postburn may provide guidance [18]. The primary outcomes are the volume of resuscitation fluids at 24 and 48 h, and secondary outcomes include survival and various measures of morbidity.

A randomized controlled trial demonstrated that plasma resuscitation reduced 24-h fluid volumes and reduced subsequent development of abdominal compartment syndrome compared with crystalloid use. Plasma may also have the advantage of preserving the microvascular endothelium by protecting the cell wall glycocalyx

[19]. However, there is sufficient evidence to provide a recommendation on plasma resuscitation [20].

The use of hypertonic saline has been considered as a possible strategy to minimize volume for burn injury resuscitation. There is limited evidence to support hypertonic saline use and more concerning are the reports that its use has been associated with hypernatremia and higher risk of acute kidney injury [21]. At the current time, the use of hypertonic saline resuscitation cannot be recommended.

The term "fluid creep" has been coined [22], suggesting that many patients are over-resuscitated with resultant complications. Over-resuscitation can result in "resuscitation morbidity," a term used to describe complications of secondary to excess fluid delivery including pulmonary edema and orbital/extremity/abdominal compartment syndromes [23]. All of these are associated with increased morbidity and mortality.

52.9 Burn Resuscitation Endpoints?

The initial fluid rate selected is not as important as the resuscitation itself, which must be closely monitored and adjusted by a diligent clinician [12]. For burns > 20% TBSA, we would recommend the following:

1. Insert a central venous catheter.
2. Insert a urinary (Foley) catheter.
3. Consider hemodynamic monitoring/echocardiography to guide resuscitation.
4. Monitor intra-abdominal (bladder) pressure every 4 h during the initial resuscitation.

Resuscitation should be targeted to a compilation of various endpoints which are continually reviewed by the attending clinician [24, 25]. There is a paucity of level I evidence to direct resuscitation; however, by thoughtfully selecting targets and achieving them without detriment to the patient is a reasonable approach (Table 52.3 Burn resuscitation endpoints).

The American Burn Association Practice Guidelines for Burn Shock Resuscitation continue to recommend a urine output of 0.5 mL/kg/h in adults and 0.5–1.0 mL/kg/h in children (<30 kg) [26]. Urine output dropping below these standards within the first 48 h postburn often is indicative of inadequate resuscitation.

Table 52.3 Burn resuscitation endpoints

Parameter	Value in the acute phase
Urine output	0.5 mL/kg/h
Blood pressure	Mean arterial pressure (MAP) > 65 mmHg
Heart rate	<120 beats/min
Hemoglobin/Hct	100–150 g/L
Lactate	<2.5 mmol/L

There has been substantial interest in the value of invasive monitoring endpoints. Hemodynamic markers including central venous oxygen saturation ($ScvO_2$), CVP, and arterial pulse waveform analysis and echocardiography have been evaluated [27]. Hemodynamic resuscitation endpoints are highly controversial, and there is neither sufficient evidence nor consensus on the best monitoring approach during burn shock resuscitation to currently provide a strong recommendation. Markers of cellular perfusion have demonstrated utility in some studies. Arterial base deficit is a nonspecific, global marker of acidosis [28]. An elevated base deficit after a significant thermal injury burn has been associated with increased organ dysfunction and higher mortality. Similarly lactate levels have may be confounded by hypothermia, alcohol intoxication, hypercarbia, and carbon monoxide poisoning. There is some evidence to suggest blood lactate levels and lactate clearance in the first 24 h of burn injury correlate with mortality.

The aim of resuscitation is to ensure effective organ perfusion while avoiding over-resuscitation and the consequences of excess fluid. Excess fluid resuscitation often referred to as "fluid creep" has been associated with increased incidence of pulmonary edema, compartment syndromes, and the requirement for escharotomies or even fasciotomies [29, 30]. Fluid creep is reported in 30%–90% of patients with major burns and the incidence increases with increasing burn extent. Recent reports suggest progressive edema formation in unburned areas, which is recognized to occur 8 h beyond burn injury, in patients receiving excess fluid. Furthermore, excessive resuscitation has been associated with the occurrence of abdominal compartment syndrome and other serious complications. The risk complications of over-resuscitation increase when resuscitation is greater than a predicted total resuscitation volume of 6 mL/kg/% TBSA. Strategies to reduce fluid creep may therefore include the avoidance of early over-resuscitation, potentially substitution of colloid in crystalloid non-responders, and the use and adherence to well-considered burn resuscitation protocols.

Key Points

- Burn pathophysiology is complex and makes resuscitation challenging.
- It is imperative to accurately assess the depth and extent of the burn.
- The use of resuscitation formulae simply serves as a guide and conventional clinical endpoints need to be meticulously and continuously evaluated to effectively titrate the resuscitation.
- In the first instance, a balanced crystalloid is the favored fluid, with the potential use of albumin when fluid requirements exceed calculated predicted volume.
- There is little compelling evidence for invasive cardiac monitoring to guide resuscitation.
- "Fluid creep" is now recognized as a potentially very significant complication of burns resuscitation and is to be avoided.

References

1. Holley AD, Reade MC, Lipman J, Delaney A, Udy A, Lee R, Litton E, Cheung W, Turner A, Garside T, Macken L, Reddi B, Kol M, Kazemi A, Phillips M, Shah A, Townsend S, Cohen J. Survey of critical care practice in Australian and New Zealand burn referral centres. Crit Care Resusc. 2019;21(4):303–4.
2. Moore EC, Pilcher DV, Bailey MJ, Stephens H, Cleland H. The Burns Evaluation and Mortality Study (BEAMS): predicting deaths in Australian and New Zealand burn patients admitted to intensive care with burns. J Trauma Acute Care Surg. 2013;75(2):298–303.
3. Henschke A, Lee R, Delaney A. Burns management in ICU: quality of the evidence: a systematic review. Burns. 2016;42(6):1173–82.
4. Campbell JM, Kavanagh S, Kurmis R, Munn Z. Systematic reviews in burns care: poor quality and getting worse. J Burn Care Res. 2017;38(2):e552–e67.
5. Aikawa N, Ishibiki K, Naito C, Abe O, Yamamoto S, Motegi M, et al. Individualized fluid resuscitation based on haemodynamic monitoring in the management of extensive burns. Burns Incl Therm Inj. 1982;8(4):249–55.
6. Hettiaratchy S, Dziewulski P. ABC of burns: pathophysiology and types of burns. BMJ. 2004;328(7453):1427–9.
7. Middelkoop E, Vloemans AF. Response to burns in the elderly: what is pathophysiology and what is physiology? EBioMedicine. 2015;2(10):1314–5.
8. Ganapathy M. Body's response to heat—pathophysiology of burns. Nurs J India. 2012;103(6):279–81.
9. Murphy P, Colwell C, Pineda G, Bryan T. Burning issues. By understanding the pathophysiology of burns, providers can give patients their best chance at good outcomes. EMS Mag. 2009;38(10):83–90.
10. Keck M, Herndon DH, Kamolz LP, Frey M, Jeschke MG. Pathophysiology of burns. Wien Med Wochenschr. 2009;159(13–14):327–36.
11. Abu-Sittah GS, Sarhane KA, Dibo SA, Ibrahim A. Cardiovascular dysfunction in burns: review of the literature. Ann Burns Fire Disasters. 2012;25(1):26–37.
12. Tricklebank S. Modern trends in fluid therapy for burns. Burns. 2009;35(6):757–67.
13. Sjoberg F. The 'Parkland protocol' for early fluid resuscitation of burns: too little, too much, or … even … too late …? Acta Anaesthesiol Scand. 2008;52(6):725–6.
14. Holley AD, Reade MC, Lipman J, Delaney A, Udy A, Lee R, et al. Survey of critical care practice in Australian and New Zealand burn referral centres. Crit Care Resusc. 2019;21(4):303–4.
15. Blanco-Schweizer P, Sánchez-Ballesteros J, Bendito B, Martín AI, Fernández L, Piqueras JM, et al. Resuscitation with albumin using BET formula keeps at bay fluid administration in burned patients. An observational study. Burns. 2020;46(4):860–7.
16. Comish P, Walsh M, Castillo-Angeles M, Kuhlenschmidt K, Carlson D, Arnoldo B, et al. Adoption of rescue colloid during burn resuscitation decreases fluid administered and restores end-organ perfusion. Burns. 2021;47(8):1844–50.
17. Lewis SR, Pritchard MW, Evans DJ, Butler AR, Alderson P, Smith AF, et al. Colloids versus crystalloids for fluid resuscitation in critically ill people. Cochrane Database Syst Rev. 2018;8(8):Cd000567.
18. Greenhalgh DG. Burn resuscitation: the results of the ISBI/ABA survey. Burns. 2010;36(2):176–82.
19. Gurney JM, Kozar RA, Cancio LC. Plasma for burn shock resuscitation: is it time to go back to the future? Transfusion. 2019;59(S2):1578–86.
20. Cartotto R, Callum J. A review on the use of plasma during acute burn resuscitation. J Burn Care Res. 2020;41(2):433–40.
21. Huang PP, Stucky FS, Dimick AR, Treat RC, Bessey PQ, Rue LW. Hypertonic sodium resuscitation is associated with renal failure and death. Ann Surg. 1995;221(5):543–54; discussion 54–7.

22. Rogers AD, Karpelowsky J, Millar AJ, Argent A, Rode H. Fluid creep in major pediatric burns. Eur J Pediatr Surg. 2010;20(2):133–8.
23. Oda J, Yamashita K, Inoue T, Harunari N, Ode Y, Mega K, et al. Resuscitation fluid volume and abdominal compartment syndrome in patients with major burns. Burns. 2006;32(2):151–4.
24. Peeters Y, Lebeer M, Wise R, Malbrain ML. An overview on fluid resuscitation and resuscitation endpoints in burns: past, present and future. Part 2- avoiding complications by using the right endpoints with a new personalized protocolized approach. Anaesthesiol Intensive Ther. 2015;47:15.
25. Peeters Y, Vandervelden S, Wise R, Malbrain ML. An overview on fluid resuscitation and resuscitation endpoints in burns: past, present and future. Part 1- historical background, resuscitation fluid and adjunctive treatment. Anaesthesiol Intensive Ther. 2015;47:6.
26. Pham TN, Cancio LC, Gibran NS, American BA. American burn association practice guidelines burn shock resuscitation. J Burn Care Res. 2008;29(1):257–66.
27. Holley A, Lukin W, Paratz J, Hawkins T, Boots R, Lipman J. Review article: part one: goal-directed resuscitation—which goals? Haemodynamic targets. Emerg Med Australas. 2012;24(1):14–22.
28. Holley A, Lukin W, Paratz J, Hawkins T, Boots R, Lipman J. Review article: part two: goal-directed resuscitation—which goals? Perfusion targets. Emerg Med Australas. 2012;24(2):127–35.
29. Shah A, Pedraza I, Mitchell C, Kramer GC. Fluid volumes infused during burn resuscitation 1980-2015: a quantitative review. Burns. 2020;46(1):52–7.
30. Dulhunty JM, Boots RJ, Rudd MJ, Muller MJ, Lipman J. Increased fluid resuscitation can lead to adverse outcomes in major-burn injured patients, but low mortality is achievable. Burns. 2008;34(8):1090–7.

Index

J. Chacko et al., *Controversies in Critical Care*,
https://doi.org/10.1007/978-981-19-9940-6

GPSR Compliance

The European Union's (EU) General Product Safety Regulation (GPSR) is a set of rules that requires consumer products to be safe and our obligations to ensure this.

If you have any concerns about our products, you can contact us on ProductSafety@springernature.com

In case Publisher is established outside the EU, the EU authorized representative is:

Springer Nature Customer Service Center GmbH
Europaplatz 3
69115 Heidelberg, Germany

Batch number: 10726058

Printed by Printforce, the Netherlands